OTHER BOOKS BY EUGENE A. SLOANE

SLOANE'S NEW BICYCLE MAINTENANCE MANUAL
SLOANE'S COMPLETE BOOK OF ALL-TERRAIN BICYCLES
SLOANE'S HANDY POCKET GUIDE TO BICYCLE REPAIR

SLOANE'S

COMPLETE BOOK OF BICYCLING

25TH ANNIVERSARY EDITION

EUGENE A. SLOANE

A FIRESIDE BOOK
Published by Simon & Schuster

NEW YORK ■ LONDON ■ TORONTO ■ SYDNEY ■ TOKYO ■ SINGAPORE

F

FIRESIDE
Rockefeller Center
1230 Avenue of the Americas
New York, New York 10020

First Fireside 25th Anniversary Edition 1995

FIRESIDE and colophon are registered trademarks
of Simon & Schuster Inc.

Designed by Irving Perkins Associates
Manufactured in the United States of America

10   9   8   7   6   5   4   3   2   1

Library of Congress Cataloging-in-Publication Data

Sloane, Eugene A.
    Sloane's complete book of bicycling / Eugene A. Sloane.—25th
anniversary ed., 1st Fireside 25th anniversary ed.
        p.   cm.
    Rev. ed. of: The complete book of bicycling. ©1988.
    "A Fireside book."
    Includes bibliographical references and index.
    1. Cycling.   2. Bicycles.   I. Sloane, Eugene A.   Complete book of
bicycling.   II. Title.   III. Title: Complete book of bicycling.
GV1041.S55   1995   94-46788
796.6—dc20   CIP

ISBN: 0-671-87075-0

CONTENTS

INTRODUCTION

Since the last edition of this book was published some seven years ago the bicycle scene has changed almost beyond recognition. You will find all of these changes in this book, together with new approaches to bicycle safety for you and your family. For example, today's two-wheelers are a techno-biker's dream. Suspension forks, seat posts, stems, and even fully articulated frames with shocks front and rear now let you glide and soar over the roughest of off-road trails. Even your favorite lightweight touring road bike can be equipped with the latest in bump-absorbing suspension technology to ease the slings and arrows of long-distance bike trips, even over the cobblestone streets of old European cities.

If shifting gears has always been a pain, take heart. You can now even shift gears electronically, with derailleur movement precisely controlled by microcomputers. Tired of heavy, cumbersome bikes? Try today's bikes. You will find stronger and lighter frames, thanks to new ways of joining exotic materials such as carbon fiber, alloys of aluminum, titanium, and thinner high-quality steel tubing.

Want more safety on the road? At night, high-powered quartz bike lights, front and rear, rival the lumens from cars, and make night riding much safer. Improved reflective vests and stick-on reflective strips for your helmet make you more visible to drivers. A selection of new, lighter, and better-ventilated helmets for kids as well as for grown-ups offer better head protection. Helmet fit is more exact, with at least two helmets that can be pumped up for a snugger cover on your head. With an assist from federal, state, and local governments, safer, better-marked, and better-policed urban bike routes from home to work are now becoming commonplace in cities.

Management has come to recognize that a healthy employee is a more productive one. Bike lockers and shower and clothing change facilities are being provided by enlightened employers. Some 3.5 million Americans pedal to work, according to the Bicycle Institute of America. It takes far less energy and material to make a bike than it does a car, bike pedalers do not pollute, so the quality of air you breathe will improve, while nonrenewable fossil fuels will be saved for future generations. Between 1983 and 1991, 97.6 million bicycles were sold in this country, according to the Bicycle Manufacturers Association of America.

More of us are bicycle touring throughout the United States and foreign countries, as witnessed by the sales of bike touring gear and the proliferation of experienced tour providers. There are tours for singles, tours that cross China, Europe, and the United States, and tours that go to most commonly visited and even third-world countries, in safety and with all amenities provided. See Chapter 10 for a list of tour organizations.

Most important, many state governments are finally requiring that, at least, cyclists under age sixteen must wear a helmet.

I wish to thank the many manufacturers of bicycles and bicycle components that provided products for me to test and discuss in this book. Above all, my most grateful thanks to Theo Patterson of Portland, Oregon, who was a source of inspiration and a fountain of knowledge for this book. Theo publishes *P.U.M.P.* (*Portland United Mountain Pedalers*), an excellent newsletter for local off-road cyclists. Theo and Frank Branzuela of Anchorage, Alaska, read preliminary drafts of this book and offered much excellent and useful advice.

Finally, I wish to thank Sean Devlin for his superb job of copyediting my manuscript. He was bold in his queries as to fact, intelligent and caring in his treatment of the text, unswerving in his dedication to accuracy and clarity. I am most grateful to him.

Thanks to all of you.
Eugene A. Sloane,
Vancouver, Washington

SLOANE'S COMPLETE BOOK OF BICYCLING

CHAPTER ONE

HOW TO BUY AND FIT THE BIKE THAT'S RIGHT FOR YOU (AND YOUR WALLET)

There's a bicycle out there that's just right for you. A bicycle that fits your body well, transports you in comfort, stops safely at your command, lets you shift gears accurately to traverse hill and dale, and does all that and more within the limits of your budget. I'll tell you where to find it and how to fit it to your body, but let's start with where *not* to look for your ideal bicycle, and why.

I think cut-rate and chain-store outlets are great. They do provide good value for most products. If you want a really inexpensive bike, that's where to buy one. The problem with these bicycles, however, is twofold. First, they may be assembled by people who are not skilled at this work, so they may neglect to safely adjust brakes, for example. I have found that these assemblers are also on piecework, so they may spend as little as 15 minutes to 30 minutes putting the bike together and wheeling it out to the sales floor. By comparison, a good bike shop has skilled mechanics who spend at least one hour and sometimes three hours assembling a bike that comes to them in a carton. Second, chain-store bikes, at least the less expensive ones that sell for less than $150, are quite heavy, have unresponsive frames, and are harder to pedal. They are OK for around-the-block casual riding, but are really most unsuitable for any longer trips. I urge you to shop around for a higher-quality bike in a shop that sells only bicycles.

TYPES OF BICYCLES

Before we discuss what kind of bicycle will best suit your cycling needs, please become familiar with the names of bicycle frame members and component parts. To this end, please study Figs. 1-1 and 1-2, the anatomy of a

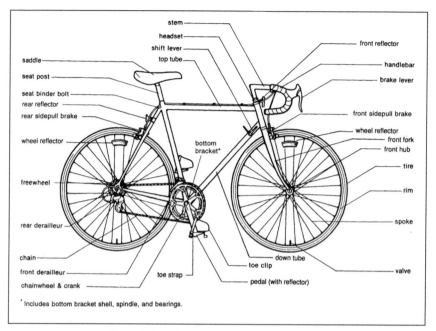

* Includes bottom bracket shell, spindle, and bearings.

F<small>IG</small>. 1-1: Anatomy of a road bicycle.

F<small>IG</small>. 1-2: Anatomy of a mountain bicycle.

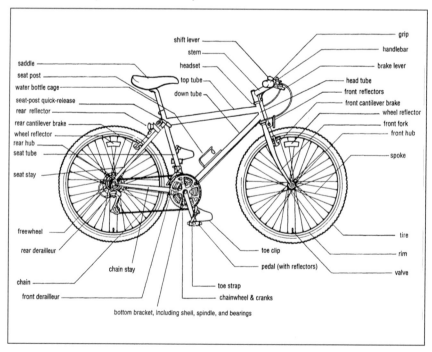

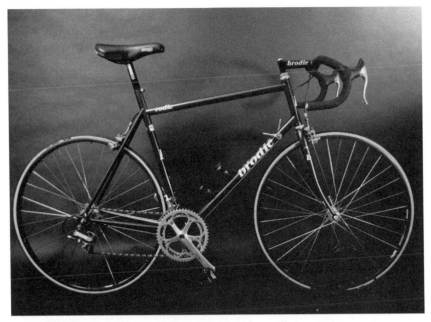

FIG. 1-3: Here is a truly top-grade road bike with excellent components on a strong handbuilt frame of high-carbon steel. Use this type of bicycle for both touring and road and criterium racing. It's made by Brodie Research in Canada.

road and a mountain bicycle, so you can understand references to the parts of a bicycle that follow. First, you need to decide just what kind of riding you will do. For example, if most of your planned riding will be on paved roads, a road bike is what you need.

Road Bicycles

If you commute to work and use the same bike on weekends for longer rides and during vacation for cycle touring and camping, you need a high-quality bike such as the one in Fig. 1-3 that can be, or is, equipped with carriers front and rear to carry panniers (the bicyclist's name for saddlebags). A road bike should have frame-mounted and threaded fittings to which you can fasten carrier and fender struts at the dropouts, carrier mounting fittings on the seat stays and preferably also on the fork blades, and threaded fittings for at least one, and preferably two, water bottle cages.

The more expensive road bikes have powerful sidepull brakes and other top-line components, such as freehub rear hubs with stronger axles, sealed bearing hubs and bottom bracket bearings that go farther with less maintenance, and index shifters with smoother, more accurate gear shifting. As the price of a road bike climbs over $500 and goes as high as $4,500 or even more, look for exotic frame tubes of titanium and carbon fiber composites that combine strength with light weight. I will discuss frame tubing metallurgy in more detail later in this chapter. To sum up, you basically get the quality you pay for. A $350 road bike will have a heavier and less responsive frame, and less costly components, but it will get you there and be reasonably reliable as it does so. The $500 road bike will be a bit lighter, with better components. If you can spend $800 or so you should be able to buy a road bike that is a positive delight to ride. It will have a light yet strong and responsive frame that efficiently translates your muscle power into go power. You will get better components that are easier to maintain and are more reliable.

Among the 111 bicycle manufacturers I counted recently, I can recommend specific manufacturers, even though I cannot give you individual model selections because designs change frequently. Excellent road bikes are made by Brodie, Klein, Bianchi, Fuji, Miyata, Romic, and Terry, to name a few. Terry, by the way, makes bicycles specifically designed for women. (There's more about Terry bicycles in the section on fit in this chapter.)

Before you buy any bicycle, contact the U.S. Consumer Products Safety Commission (CPSC) at their toll free number, 1-800-638-2772, to find out if the model you have in mind has been recalled for safety problems. The CPSC has issued recalls on thousands of bicycles and bicycle components in recent years, for such accident-producing items as defective forks, water bot-

FIG. 1-4: An excellent mountain bike with a handbuilt frame by Brodie Research. The suspension fork smooths out the bumps of trail riding, makes handling safer and easier.

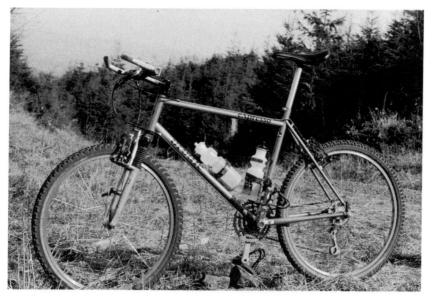

tles, frames, and other parts. When you call the CPSC for this information, please be patient with the voice mail system, which will ask you to dial extensions for specific problems.

Road and Track Racing Bicycles

Bicycles built for criterium and track races are a breed apart. For criterium races (a massed-start race over many laps of a course about a mile long), the bicycle should have a short wheelbase, highly sensitive steering geometry, and an ability to take corners at high speed. I am not going to cover these bikes, or the fixed gear design for track events, because they are specialized, have a limited use, and are very expensive. If you do want to get into racing, I recommend you write the United States Cycling Federation (see Chapter 12) for the USCF representative closest to you.

Mountain Bicycles

First a few words of clarification. Mountain bicycles, until a few years ago, were also called "all-terrain" bicycles. The bicycle industry has decided to use the word "mountain" for this type of bicycle, designed for off-road cycling on rough trails. Some mountain bikes, such as the Brodie in Fig. 1-4, come with suspension forks. Or you can install such a fork on your old mountain bike (see Chapter 8).

Mountain bicycles have shock-absorbing fat tires with knobs that grip the trail for steering control and good traction on slippery surfaces (see Chapter 7 for specific tire tread designs for specific surfaces). These bikes have flat handlebars that help you keep steering under control as the front wheel contacts myriad odd-shaped bumps, rocks, roots, even tree limbs on the trail. These handlebars also let you sit more upright so you can see what's ahead.

Mountain bikes provide a more comfortable ride than road bikes. In fact, more mountain bikes are bought at this writing than any other type of bicycle because they can be used for both trail and road riding. They come with a much wider range of gears than road bikes, gears that make hill climbing a lot easier, especially when the bike is laden with camping gear or when you're towing a trailer. (See Chapter 2 for more on trailers and Chapter 5 for a full discussion of gears and gear tables.)

On the negative side, mountain bikes are generally a bit heavier than comparably priced road bikes, they aren't as responsive to quick turns because of their longer wheelbase, and their fatter tires have about 10 percent greater rolling resistance than high-pressure, skinny road bike tires. But even without a suspension system (see below), mountain bikes are still a lot more comfortable than road bikes, and can go where road bikes cannot, on rough, rock-strewn trails, for example. Their lower-pressure, knobby tires help maintain traction if you have to veer off the pavement onto gravel or grass to escape a maniac in a pickup truck. The skinnier tires of a road bike could in this case slide on the gravel and cause you or your bike to fall.

However, if you never, in your wildest dreams, would consider riding along a remote mountain trail, even with a posse of armed guards along for protection, I'd still suggest a mountain bike just for paved roads, if comfort is important to you. And who knows, you might someday succumb to the lure of a ride in the wilderness, where you can gaze at deer grazing in the distance, view vistas you have only seen in *National Geographic* magazine, see eagles majestically soaring among the clouds, or thrill to speed runs down dusty logging roads curving along a mountainside.

If you use a mountain bike for paved-road cycling, switch to tires with smoother tread and less rolling resistance. You can always change back to knobbies if you go off-road. If you are an apartment dweller, and storage space is tight, think about a high-quality folding mountain bike, such as the one made by Montague. This bike is also ideal for carrying on a boat or even a small private airplane. Write Montague Corp. at 432 Columbia St., Ste. 29, Cambridge, MA 02140, or phone 1-617-491-7200 for a dealer near you.

"Ladies" Frames

In my opinion, bikes without a top tube but with a steeply sloping, longer down tube to accommodate a dress, so-called ladies bikes, are bad news, for two reasons. First, the longer rear brake and both derailleur shift cables have to be routed down along the down tube. The longer cables have more friction, thus can stretch more and make braking and shifting more difficult. Second, without a top tube, the frame is more flexible than a conventional frame, which means that pedaling energy is lost to frame whip. This design is a throwback to the days when women had to wear skirts on a bike.

Suspension Systems for Mountain Bikes

Suspension-equipped bikes are incredibly comfortable. Suspension equipment absorbs jolts and bangs as you ride. You will be able to ride farther with less fatigue because shock absorbers, not the muscles and bones of your body, take up most of the road shock. Pain-sensitive parts of your body will be forever grateful. One rider reports that his suspension fork made it possible to cycle while recovering from a broken arm, but he suffered pain when riding his mountain bike without suspension equipment. The suspension system also prolongs the life of parts subject to damage and undue wear from shock, such as tires and rims, hub and headset bearings. Riders, including myself, have found that a suspension system makes cycling on rough trails much safer because impact jolts that could tear the handlebars right out of your hands are instead usually absorbed by the suspension equipment.

I remember riding a mountain bike without a suspension system a few years ago on a Wisconsin off-road trail. I hit a rock. The impact tore the handlebars from my grasp, permitting the front wheel to turn at a right angle to the bike. The bike came to a sudden stop. I was tossed right over the bars. As I became airborne I felt like an airplane coming in for a landing, except that I landed nose first. I just lost a little skin off my nose, with no harm done except to my ego. I feel certain that had my bike been equipped with a suspension front fork I could have stayed upright and kept going.

Suspension mountain bikes can cost from $800 up to $3,000 or more. The more exotic models have both front and rear suspension (with front and rear shocks). At this writing the bike industry has not figured out how to mount a front fender or a carrier (to hold your panniers) on a suspension fork, so you can have a fender and a carrier only over the rear wheel. If the bike has front and rear suspension, you will have to carry your gear in your backpack, or tow a bike trailer. Suspension forks must be "tuned" to your weight and to the trail itself, either by adjusting the tension if it's an elastomer design, or by changing the air pressure of an air-oil suspension system. For even greater rough-terrain comfort you can add a suspension stem and a suspension saddle to most stock mountain bicycles (see Chapter 8). *Warning!* You will see inexpensive mountain bikes in department stores with what appears to be a suspension fork. These heavy bikes, which sell for around $150, use a steel coil spring in the fork, a design that is virtually useless as a shock absorber.

Hybrids

You can buy a so-called hybrid or city bike that attempts to combine the lighter weight and responsiveness of a road bike with the comfort and upright stance of a mountain bike. Typically such bikes have flat handlebars, have tires that are skinnier than mountain bike tires but wider than road bike tires, use 26-inch or 700C rims, have wide-range gearing, and are moderately priced. They are an excellent compromise bike if you are not really serious about off-road dirt riding but want a bike that will handle well on the occasional trail ride. The Trek Hybrid bicycle, for example, is a good choice, and retails for approximately $340.

A variation is a bike that shifts by itself. The AutoBike is designed for casual riding and costs around $400. If you want a bike that shifts by itself, so you never have to shift up or down for a particular grade, this bike will do it. The shift mechanism is actuated by a counterbalanced sliding weight on the rear wheel. If you go slow or stop and start again, the bike shifts into the low gear. As the rear wheel turns faster the bike shifts into a higher gear, something like an automatic transmission on a car. It's a bit unnerving to hear the chain move up or down by itself, but you get used to it and it is convenient, particularly for city riding. After a stop, the chain starts out again in low gear. AutoBike is at 1076 Black Brook Rd., South Easton, MA 02375.

Tandems

There's nothing like the social togetherness of you and a loved one on a bicycle built for two (Fig. 1-5). There you are, the captain, with the stoker breathing down the back of your neck (backseat biking?). There you are, the stoker, sheltered from the wind, unconcerned about steering, free to muse with the gods of the open road. Tandems come in a variety of price ranges, but a decent model will cost around $950 and can go up to $2,500 or more. You can buy a tandem for the road or in a mountain bike design you can ride on road or trail.

Another major advantage of a tandem is that it is a lot lighter than two comparable road bikes. With the stoker snuggled behind the captain, wind

FIG. 1-5: A bicycle built for two is the way to go when you want your significant other to stay close to you on a bike ride. Besides, with two pedaling, cycling is easier, downhill rides a lot faster.

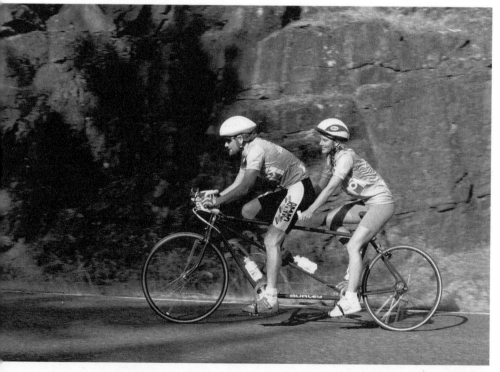

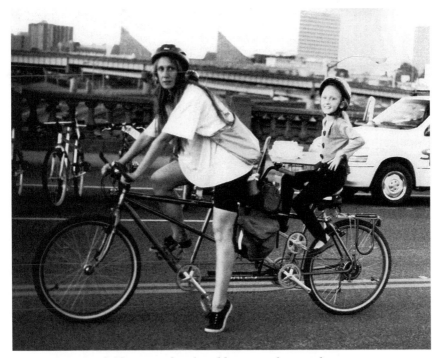

FIG. 1-6: Carry a child on a tandem by adding a crankset on the rear.

resistance for both is a lot less than with two single bikes. You can go faster longer. But a warning. You can also barrel downhill a lot faster, so you have to have good brakes, keep them well adjusted, and use them to keep speed under control.

One final caveat. For happy tandeming the riders should be in synch. The captain has to tell the stoker behind when they will be stopping, making turns, or shifting gears. The stoker must never, and I repeat, never, suddenly stop pedaling, or lean the wrong way on a turn. There's more about safe tandem riding in Chapter 2. For now, though, if you are thinking you want a tandem, I suggest you borrow one and see how it goes. Be patient, remember that even the most inept rider can learn. The rewards are great. You can talk back and forth, comment on the scenery, and pass the time more enjoyably on a tandem. A weaker person can ride behind a stronger captain. You can even add a crankset mounted on the tandem rear seat tube so a child, or a very short person, can pedal along behind you (Fig. 1-6).

Most tandems, like single bikes, can carry two carriers and their panniers. However, this carrying capacity may not be enough for two to travel on a long trip. For example, a single bike can carry about as much as you can carry on a tandem. So for tandem touring over a long distance, I recommend a trailer.

Another tandem disadvantage is really quite minor. Because of its longer wheelbase, a tandem is bit less maneuverable on city streets. However this is merely my observation. I've never heard any complaints from tandem enthusiasts on this point.

Excellent tandems, quite reasonably priced, are made by Burley (check your bike shop for more information).

Recumbents

If you're into a laid-back lifestyle, a recumbent bike may be for you. Today I see recumbents in the bicycle scene about where mountain bikes were in 1980. I remember my own attitude toward mountain bikes back then. I felt that they were just an adult version of kids' BMX bikes, heavy, awkward, and cumbersome. Well, my first mountain bike ride changed my mind just as my first recumbent ride opened my eyes, and my total body, to their comfort.

FIG. 1-7: Recumbent bicycles like this aluminum Linear model are becoming popular because they are comfortable, provide excellent back support, and make cycling easier. This model has an adjustable-length frame, adjustable saddle position, and adjustable steering control.

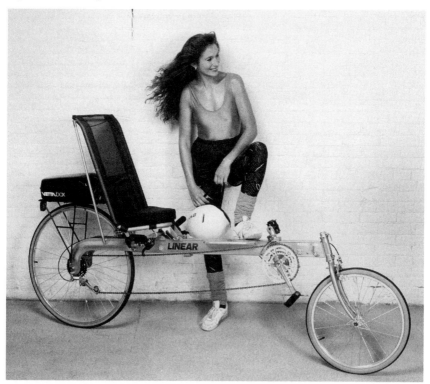

Recumbists (to coin a word) claim their steeds are a lot more comfortable than any other bike, and that they can ride longer and faster than they could on their conventional bike. Recumbents are lower, more streamlined, and have lower wind resistance and are thus less affected by headwinds. Because they are lower, recumbents may be also less visible to car and truck drivers. For safety visibility, install a plastic fishing-rod-type pole with a red flag attached to its top. I've ridden recumbents and can report that the reclining position is indeed comfortable. Depending on the manufacturer, frames may be made of aluminum, carbon fiber, chrome moly steel, high-tensile steel, or the excellent U.S.-made True-Temper steel.

Recumbents also come in a wide variety of frame configurations, such as the Linear (Fig. 1-7). The Linear costs $1,200, has an aluminum frame, weighs 32 pounds, and comes in five sizes to fit inseams of 22 to over 34 inches. The two smaller sizes have 24-inch rear and 16-inch front wheels. Larger sizes have 27-inch rear and 24-inch front wheels. If they are not available at your bike shop, check with Linear for a bike shop near you that does carry their line (P.O. Box 173, Guttenberg, IA 52052, phone 1-319-252-1637 or FAX 1-319-252-3305). Another recumbent is made by Ryan, has a True-Temper high-quality steel frame, weighs 30.5 pounds, and costs $1,295. Ryan also makes a recumbent tandem, price not available at this writing, though I estimate it to be around $1,800. (See your bike shop or contact Ryan directly at One Chestnut St., 4th floor, Nashua, NH 03060). Rans, another recumbent maker, also produces high-quality models, which cost around $1,500. (Rans can be reached directly at 4600 Highway 183 Alternate, Hays, KS 67601, by phone at 1-913-625-6346, by FAX at 1-913-625-2795.) ReBike has a seven-speed model, which retails for $399. For a more upright position with some of the comfort of a recumbent, the ReBike will sit you up straighter. I call this a hybrid recumbent. (Find ReBike at 103 NW 43rd St., Boca Raton, FL 33431.) My suggestion is to ride all the makes and types you can find and buy the one that fits you best and feels most comfortable. For the disabled athlete, Brike, Inc., makes an excellent hand-powered 21-speed recumbent. It has a two-piece frame, which articulates to make a safe turn even at high speed, even while you're cranking away. The frame telescopes for arm length adjustment and breaks down with a ball detent pin for compact stowage or carrying. At $1,995 it's worth the price. (Brike is at 20589 S.W. Elkhorn Ct., Tualitan, OR 97062 and can be reached at 1-800-800-5828.)

A unique recumbent, the three-wheel Pedalcraft Quadraped, lets you use your hands and arms as well as your legs for propulsion and good upper- and lower-body muscle conditioning. You can also stop and remain upright, which makes getting on and off this machine a snap. The many options include a rear cargo panel, head- and taillights, and water bottle mounts. At 43 to 46

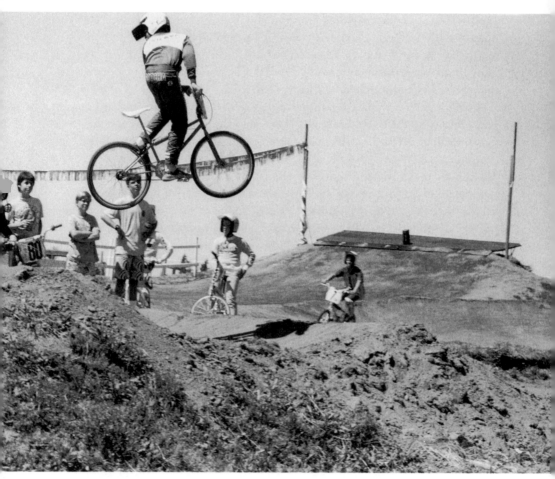

FIG. 1-8: BMX bikes are for kids like this one, who is jumping over hills about three feet high in a track race. Note that the rider is carefully balanced with both pedals parallel to the ground.

pounds, the Quadraped is a tad on the heavy side, but then you wanted a workout, didn't you? The standard model goes for $2,180. (Reach Pedalcraft at 5460 SW Philomath Highway, Corvallis, OR 97333, phone 1-503-752-5035, FAX 1-503-8004.)

BMX Bicycles

BMX means "Bicycle Motocross." These are the little 20-inch-wheel machines you see kids riding around on, pulling wheelies up curbs and over obstacles real or imaginary, becoming airborne briefly down small hills. There are three levels of BMX bikes. Most common is the $85 special available from discount stores. These are the kind kids destroy fairly rapidly, sometimes banging themselves up in the process. Then there are the better bikes, which can cost up to $250. They are still street bikes, unsuitable for much other than play. Most of these bikes are single-speed. Some have caliper brakes on both wheels, others only on the rear wheel. And they are heavy! Kids think they can go like the wind on them, and for a block or two they can actually keep up with me. It gives me great joy to leave them behind. Heft a BMX sometime and compare its weight with that of a road bike in the same price range. The better, more costly BMX bikes have gusseted reinforced frames that can take a lot of abuse. A more costly BMX is made for track racing. These bikes have highest-quality frame tubing (see discussion on frame tubing later in this chapter) and first-class components and can cost as much as $850 or even more. The bikes must be strong enough to stand the impact of airborne jumps over small hills as far apart as 13 feet (Fig. 1-8), slamming around curbs (berms), and banging into bumps and into each other. Unless your child is serious about BMX racing, a competition model at great cost would be a waste of money, in my opinion. The midrange bikes costing between $150 and $250 are very sturdy little machines. They will serve your child well until he or she is old enough to appreciate the advantages of a good mountain or road bike.

Here is a special warning about BMX bicycle pedals. Some BMX bicycles have cranks that are about a half inch longer than the pedals on adult road bikes. This long a crank is not a problem in itself. But some BMX bikes come with pedals that have sawtooth serrated edges. As an expert witness I have been involved in accident case lawsuits in which children have had a foot fall forward off these pedals and get jammed between the pedal and the frame or the ground. With the bike still going forward, there was sufficient momentum in the bike to cause the sawtooth edge of the pedal to sever the Achilles tendon of the child. The reason the child's foot slipped forward off the pedal was that the bike hit a bump hard. You might consider either filing off these teeth and replacing them with road pedals, which do not have these teeth, or installing toe clips (but be sure the toe clip does not contact the tire on a sharp turn).

Do not buy the BMX bike that has a special brake cable fitting that permits the rider to rotate the front wheel 360 degrees without tangling in the brake cables. This design permits the rider to turn the wheel so it's at a right angle to the bike frame, which could bring the bike to a sudden stop. If the front wheel of this type of BMX is reversed, the frame geometry is changed to the point that the bike becomes very unstable and is easily dumped on a turn.

THE BASICS OF BIKE FRAME FIT

Select a bike with a frame that fits you. That may seem obvious, but I have seen too many people riding bikes way too big or too small for them. Ride too big a bike and you could be hurt if your crotch came down hard on the top tube (please see Figs. 1-1 and 1-2 to find the top tube) on an emergency dismount. Ride too small a bike and you risk knee injury from too low a saddle, arm pain from too short a frame lengthwise, and other bodily aches and problems (see Chapter 11 on the health aspects of cycling). In addition to my own experience in 35 years of serious adult cycling, I have relied on Gary Klein of Klein Bicycle Company and other friends in the bike scene for much of the fit data that follow.

Bicycles come in a wide variety of frame sizes. To start, match your height to the bicycle size in Tables 1-1 and 1-2. For example, if you are 6'1" to 6'6" tall, a 56-cm (22") bike should fit you. Measure bicycle frame sizes by the distance from the top of the seat tube to the centerline of the bottom bracket spindle (axle) (see Figs. 1-1 and 1-2).

Use Tables 1-1 and 1-2 as a beginning guide to bike fit. Then straddle the top tube, with both feet on the ground, as shown in Fig. 1-9. Think seriously about pain if you should come off the saddle and your crotch should come down hard on the top tube. There will be times, particularly when riding off-road on a mountain bicycle, when to stay upright you have to move your body

TABLE 1-1: MOUNTAIN BIKES

BIKE SIZE	YOUR HEIGHT
46 cm (18")	5' to 5'4"
48 cm (19")	5'4" to 5'7"
51 cm (20")	5'7" to 5'10"
53 cm (21")	5'10" to 6'
56 cm (22")	6' to 6'6"

TABLE 1-2: ROAD BIKES AND HYBRID BIKES

BIKE SIZE	YOUR HEIGHT
47 cm (18.5")	4'10" to 5'
50 cm (19.7")	5' to 5'2"
51 cm (20.1")	5'2" to 5'4"
54 cm (21.3")	5'4" to 5'6"
56 cm (22.0")	5'6" to 5'8"
58 cm (22.8")	5'8" to 5'11"
60 cm (23.6")	5'11" to 6'1"
62 cm (24.4")	6'1" to 6'3"

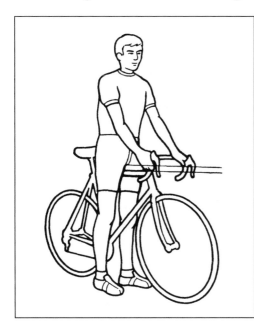

FIG. 1-9: Check bike size fit by straddling the bicycle as shown here. You should have at least two inches between your crotch and the top tube to avoid injury should you have to come down hard on the top tube in an emergency to avoid a spill.

off the saddle, down toward the top tube, and extend a foot out to the ground. Sometimes a situation can crop up in which you simply bounce off the saddle and come down toward the top tube. If you have the correct crotch to top tube clearance you can avoid injury by holding your body up by the pedals and pulling upward on the handlebars. Make sure there is at least one to one and a half inches of clearance between your crotch and the top tube of a road bike (Fig. 1-1), and two to three inches between your crotch and a mountain bike top tube (Fig. 1-2). There are times when you may have to dismount on uneven terrain. The mountain bike bottom bracket shell (see Figs. 1-1 and 1-2) is about one and a half to two inches higher from the ground than that of the road bike, so be aware that mountain bike sizes differ from road bike sizes for the same body length. Mountain bikes need this extra ground clearance for going over obstacles such as rocks and stumps. Adult bicycle sizes are measured by the length of the seat tube from the top of the seat tube to the centerline of the bottom bracket spindle. For example, look at Tables 1-1 and 1-2. The same 5´2˝ to 5´4˝ person should fit a 19.7˝ or 20.1˝ road bike or an 18˝ or 19˝ mountain bike. Remember, bike frame size is not variable, unlike height-adjustable saddles and handlebars. The bike frame has to fit your human frame. Remember too that leg length (inseam measurement) differs between people, so the measurements in Tables 1-1 and 1-2 are only a beginning to selecting the bike that fits you. Later in this chapter I will discuss the variables of frame fit, such as saddle height and tilt and handlebar height, to fine-tune your new bicycle to your torso dimensions.

Tailor-Made Custom Bicycles

There are a number of excellent frame builders who can create a custom frame just to fit you. But custom frames are pricey, because the cost advantage of mass production is lost. A top frame builder, Julian Edwins, has this to say about the advantages of a custom-fitted bicycle:

"An accurate measurement of the human body, as shown in Fig. 1-10, is essential to the custom frame builder. To start with, the builder needs the length of the foot, the distance from floor to knee (flat-footed) and length from knee to femur (greater trochanter). These dimensions determine the seat-tube angle. They are also important because they cover the 12 muscles and muscle groups involved in turning the crank. For all these muscles to perform at peak efficiency (assuming they are in top condition), they must be correctly positioned in relation to the bottom bracket and the pedal axle.

"When you are seated on the bike, your *knee* should be directly above the pedal axle when the crank is parallel to the ground (one crank should be at the three o'clock position). If you try to obtain this position by moving the

FIG. 1-10: Give these body dimensions to a custom frame builder if you are having a bike frame tailor-made to fit you.

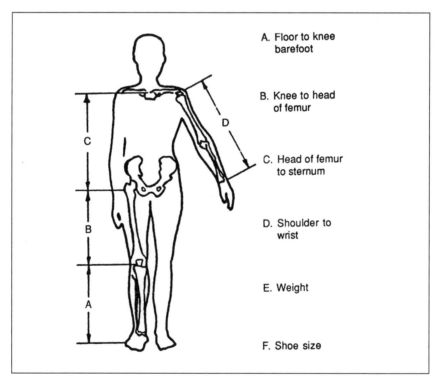

A. Floor to knee
   barefoot

B. Knee to head
   of femur

C. Head of femur
   to sternum

D. Shoulder to
   wrist

E. Weight

F. Shoe size

saddle rearward or forward, you will change the distance of reach to the handlebars, in which case you may be asking for neck and back pain as you strain to see ahead, or have to bend over to reach the handlebars. If the bike is too short and you try to compensate with a very long stem, you'll have more body weight over the front wheel. This is bad for three reasons. First, excess weight over the front wheel makes for poor steering control. Second, the longer stem changes steering response by the rider, because a longer stem gives greater leverage. Third, more weight on the front wheel reduces rear brake effectiveness. This could lead to an end-over if the front brake is grabbed hard, pitching the rider headfirst forward off the bike as the rear wheel comes up off the ground.

"The correct position is best achieved by the seat-tube angle that's compatible with your body dimensions. Such a fit not only helps you get more efficient use of your muscles, but also gives you a good balance between back and stomach muscles. This balance also prevents pelvic tilt, which in turn provides the femur with a fixed pivot point, rather than an unstable one that would reduce efficiency.

"Sending the builder accurate measurements also means that top-tube and handlebar-stem lengths are right for you. Measurements from the head of the femur to the top of the sternum (breast bone) and of the length of the arm from shoulder to wrist combine to determine top-tube and handlebar-stem lengths.

"A final word on behalf of frame builders. If your build and bodily dimensions are unusual (and that includes your weight), be sure to mention them to your builder, who needs all the data he can get. Remember, a custom frame, built to your accurate bodily dimensions, will give you comfort and efficiency. You'll have a frame that makes the best possible use of your own athletic ability. Be sure, too, to let the builder know what you intend to use the bicycle for. For example, do you want a touring bicycle, a mountain bike, or a special racing model?"

Julian Edwins was himself a racing cyclist and has a background in metallurgical engineering and machine design. Julian will be happy to answer your specific questions on frame design. He can be reached at Edwins Cycle Co., P.O. Box 81, Owen Sound, Ontario, Canada N4K 5P1, or 519-376-2852.

Bicycles for Women

There is a line of off-the-shelf bikes made just for women, designed by a woman. These bicycles include road, mountain, hybrid, racing and triathlete designs. They are designed and marketed by Georgena Terry. Terry's designs take into consideration the differences in body dimensions between men and women. She is an engineer with an MBA from the Wharton School of Finance and a science degree from Carnegie Mellon University. Her firm makes a full line of mountain and road bikes for touring, road racing, and tri-athlete events, and makes custom-tailored bikes in all styles. These bikes come in as small a frame size as 16 inches, to fit a woman 4 feet, 11 inches tall. Table I-3 gives the full range of her frame sizes. If your bicycle shop does not carry her line, she can be reached at Terry Precision Bicycles for Women, Inc., 1704 Wayneport Rd., Macedon, NY 14502, 1-800-289-8379, 1-315-986-2103.

Terry notes: "Women have shorter torsos, shorter arms, and smaller hands than a man with the same leg length. Therefore, the top tube must be shorter on a woman's bike. Since diamond frames can't be built under 20 inches with-out compromising frame dimensions, most small women have had to ride a traditional ladies bicycle. This bicycle does not solve the problem of the dis-tance from the saddle to the handlebars." From Table 1-3 you can see that Terry builds a small frame with a 16- or 17-inch seat tube. She does this by using a 24-inch front wheel and a 27-inch rear wheel. For very short women she uses two 24-inch wheels and smaller rear cogs so the gear ratios are the same as they are with bikes having 26- and 27-inch wheels (see Chapter 5 for data on gears and gearing and gear tables).

TABLE I-3: BIKE SIZES FOR WOMEN

Height	Seat Tube	Straddle Height*	Top Tube
Less than 4′11″	16″	26.1″	18.9″
4′11″ to 5′1″	17″	27.3″	19″
5′1″ to 5′2″	18.5″	28.7″	19.3″
5′2″ to 5′4″	20″	30.3″	19.5″ to 21″
5′4″ to 5′7″	21.5″	31.8″	21″
Over 5′7″	23″	33.2″	21.5″

*A function of inseam measurement and bottom bracket height above the ground.

FRAME MATERIALS

Bicycle frames are now available with tubing of steel, aluminum, magnesium, titanium, and carbon fiber composites, and, most lately, even beryllium. Here's a brief review of the pros and cons of each of these materials and the ways in which they are joined. Since I am not a metallurgical engineer, I asked one to write this portion of this chapter. He is Douglas Hayduk, of Boulder, Colorado. He is the author of Bicycle Metallurgy for the Cyclist. He will be happy to send you a copy for $3.95. Write him at 604 Marine St., Boulder, CO 80302.

Doug says: Up to around 1974, choice of material for bicycle frames was simple. It was either steel or nothing. Today, however, you can find bikes made of a wide variety of materials. Some of the more exotic, low production frames alone can cost upward of $800. That's just for the frame. By the time you stick on wheels, cranksets, handlebars, and all the other components, the cost can be in the thousands, and that's for an off-the-shelf bike.

There is a lot of misunderstanding about the pros and cons of various frame materials. Here are a few popular misconceptions: Aluminum is too soft and brittle. It's light but not strong. If an aluminum frame is welded, it's weak at the weld. If it's glued together, it's weak at the glued joints. If it's screwed and glued, it's stronger but may still break at the joints. Magnesium is too brittle. Titanium is too flexible. Titanium frames will waste energy in frame whip that should go into forward movement of the entire bike. Carbon fiber composites may decompose, come apart, crack. All of these statements are false! Steel, aluminum, titanium, magnesium, and carbon fiber composites all have similar strength-to-weight ratios.

Other misconceptions relate to how steel frames are fastened together. Lugged frames are thought to be stronger than unlugged frames. That's totally wrong. Cheap lugged mass-produced frames, however, are usually weaker than a carefully brazed up lugless frame. Any well-made frame has tubing ends accurately mitered so they butt tightly up against the tube they are to be welded, brazed, or lugged to. Inaccurately mitered tubing makes for a weak joint whether it's lugged or not. Electrically welded steel frames of cheap bikes are at least as susceptible to fatigue and impact breakage as any other type of frame. Thermal inert gas welded frames, known as T.I.G. welded, can be as strong as the best hand brazed frame. T.I.G. welded frames are also less expensive than hand-brazed frames because the joining is done by machinery, eliminating a lot of hand labor.

Three Grades of Steel

There are three types of steel used in bicycle frames today. Plain-carbon steel is used for tubing of bicycles that sell for around $100. Low-alloy steel is used for more expensive bicycles. Very-high-strength steel is used for specialty racing bikes and a few super-expensive high-end bikes. Let's start with low-carbon steel.

Low-Carbon Steel

Low- or plain-carbon steel is also called "1020" steel, or "high-tension" steel. You'll see decals on inexpensive bikes bearing one or the other of these names. This seam-welded tubing, unless further treated, can have a weakened section in the vicinity of the seam. Plain-carbon steel is inexpensive, at least compared with better steels, because it contains only iron alloyed with small amounts of carbon (usually 0.2 percent) and manganese. This steel is not as strong as the steel used in better bikes. To make up for its weakness, manufacturers use tubing with heavier walls that are quite thick compared with more costly tubing. The result is a heavier and "deader" feeling, but low-cost, bicycle. The ride of bicycles made with this tubing is sluggish, without the spirited liveliness associated with a truly lightweight frame. The ride will be harsh, so these bicycles are not suited to long-distance touring. The plain-carbon steel tubing in these bikes is also straight gauge, which means that the tubing is the same thickness for its entire length.

Low-Alloy Steel

The steel used to make the tubing of higher-priced bicycles is generically called "low-alloy steel," or just "alloy steel." This steel is an alloy of iron and carbon plus small amounts (5 percent or so) of manganese, molybdenum, vanadium, or nickel. Most of this tubing is seamless, which eliminates the weakened zone where seamed tubing is welded. However, seamed tubing of low-alloy steel can be just as strong as seamless tubing if it is heat-treated after welding. Such tubing is made by True Temper Sports, the only bicycle-tubing manufacturer in the United States.

Low-alloy tubing is made even stronger by a process called "butting" in which tubing walls are thin in the middle and thickened at the ends. You'll see decals on bikes made with tubing that say "double-butted" (such as Reynolds). Better frames have double-butted main tubing as well as double-butted forks and stays. The double-butted ends provide added strength where tubes are brazed or welded together, where the heat of such joining may weaken the tubing. Another type of tubing that has thicker ends is called "tapered gauge." It has a tapered wall thickness throughout most of its length.

All you need know about alloy tubing is that it combines strength with lightness. You get a frame that will absorb road shock well, that feels lively and responsive. It only comes on better, more expensive bikes, usually those that cost from $800 to $1,200 or more.

Very-High-Strength Steel

Examples of the highest-strength bicycle tubing are Reynolds 753, Vitus 983, and Tange Prestige. This tubing is processed to higher strengths than

Reynolds 531, Columbus SL, and SP tubing. Very-high-strength steel tubing is carefully heat-treated and worked to combine lightness (thin walls) with strength. However, Reynolds 753 takes a very skilled and specially trained person to braze it. It's costly, and it has virtually paper-thin walls that are not generally recommended for most bicycles. It is best used for specialty bikes, such as racing machines, where cost is not a factor and where the weight saved, even if only a few ounces, can make the difference between winning and losing a race or establishing a new time trial record.

Tange Prestige and Vitus 983 tubing is not quite as strong as Reynolds 753. Wall thickness of this tubing approaches that of other conventional steel tubes. You will find this tubing used in the most expensive bicycles where a lighter, yet strong frame is desired.

Nonferrous Frame Materials

Here's a quick review of bicycle frames made of materials other than steel. Let's start with aluminum.

Aluminum Frames

Aluminum bicycle frames are not new. They've been made since the late 1890s. What is new is that aluminum frames made today compare very favorably with all steel frames in strength, durability, and ride. Most bike makers include at least one aluminum bicycle in their line.

Aluminum tubing used today is an alloy of other metals as well as aluminum. Some of these alloys are heat-treatable for higher-yield strengths. Other alloys rely on mechanical hardening (cold working) for strength.

For example, Alan and Vitus bicycles use aluminum alloy tubing that has the same diameter of steel tubing, 1 1/8 inches. For strength, these alloys use very thick wall tubes.

Other aluminum-alloy bicycles obtain strength by using larger-diameter tubing, up to 1 1/3 inches. Bicycles with this tubing include Cannondale, Trek, and Klein. In my opinion, this fatter tubing permits a bicycle design of greater strength and lighter weight than are offered by the smaller-diameter, thicker tubing.

It's been claimed that aluminum bikes in general absorb road shock better than steel bikes. The Alan and Vitus bikes do offer a more comfortable ride than some good steel frames. The stiffer frame design of Klein and Cannondale frames, however, provides about the same comfort in terms of road-shock absorption as comparably priced steel frames. Aluminum bicycle frames are also generally lighter than steel bicycle frames, although this weight advantage is marginal in the highest-priced lines, especially compared with very-high-strength steel frames.

One advantage of aluminum alloy frames is that they can be anodized. Anodizing is a hard, thick protective finish layer of oxide formed by chemically treating the tubing in an acid bath. Nearly any color can be added to the anodized layer for an attractive finish that is much more durable and scratch-resistant than any paint finish. Not that you're going to leave your good bike out in the rain, but it may be some comfort to know that aluminum frames won't rust.

Titanium

Titanium has been used successfully in the aerospace and marine vessel industries. The metal is lighter than steel, but heavier than aluminum. Its strength and rigidity are about midway between those of steel and aluminum. Titanium's corrosion resistance is very high, so it doesn't need to be painted or anodized. Its major drawback is still cost. Premium frame builders have apparently solved frame design problems that plagued Speedwell and Teledyne. Titanium bicycles are very competitive as to strength, rigidity, durability, and shock absorption with the best frames of any material.

Composites

The use of composites is one of the most exciting developments in bicycle technology today. Composite material is simply a combination of high-strength reinforcement fibers surrounded and held together in a matrix of epoxy or polymer resin. If you're familiar with tennis racquets, golf clubs, fishing rods, ski poles, or Corvette auto bodies made of composites, you have an idea of the composites used for bicycle-frame tubing. However, instead of glass fibers in an epoxy matrix, composites used for bicycle-frame tubing are graphite fibers embedded in an epoxy or polyester matrix and formed into bicycle tubes.

Let's stop here for a moment of history. The first composite bicycles were made in the late 1800s, of wood or bamboo, materials that are nature's composites. Then carbon-fiber bicycles appeared in the early 1970s with the Exxon Graftek bicycle. This bike was quite popular among racing cyclists. However, it had a number of construction and design problems, so it suffered a fairly early demise.

Today, however, carbon-fiber bicycle-frame development appears to have eliminated the Exxon frame deficiencies. Composite frames made today are very strong and rigid, resistant to impact and fatigue damage. The most attractive feature of these frames is that they are as much as two pounds lighter than their lightest steel-frame counterpart. The only drawback is their price, several hundred dollars more than other top-of-the-line stock frames. For example, the frame alone is around $950. The complete bike will cost around $1,800 minimum. Complete composite frame bicycles are currently being produced (at this writing) by Trek, Peugeot, Eclipse, Guerciotti, Nishiki, Alan, Look, and Vitus.

Combinations

Some frame designers feel that a combination of materials will give desirable characteristics to a frame. For example, Raleigh's Technium line of bicycles uses a combination of aluminum and alloy-steel tubing. The three main tubes (top, down, and seat tubes) are adhesive-bonded into the lugs. Seat stays and chain stays are of chrome-moly tubing, brazed into the lugs and dropouts. Raleigh claims that the bicycle has the best characteristics of both metals, strength and lightness. Prices range from around $250 to around $600, depending on the quality of the steel in the stays and the quality of the components. The $600 model is a good compromise between the stiffness of a road-racing bike and the shock absorbency of a touring bike, and for that reason it should be ideal for triathlon events.

Still another new and at this time unique combination of materials is the Excell CSK tubing, made by Excell of France. This tubing consists of a very thin-walled, high-strength steel tube with a carbon and Kevlar fiber-reinforced epoxy composite tube inside the steel tube for added strength. This tubing is lightweight and very rigid and can be brazed together like a conventional steel frame. The CSK tubing is only available, at this writing, in custom-built frames. It is also *very* expensive.

Chrome-Plating Problems

Chrome-plated bicycle tubing makes for a shiny, attractive bicycle. The finish is highly scratch-resistant. There are, however, several drawbacks to a chrome-plate finish. If the chrome gets scratched, rust can develop that can work its way between the chrome plating and the bicycle tube. The bicycle then has to be polished with chrome rust remover. Doug Hayduk discusses another, more serious problem with chrome plating:

"During the plating, hydrogen atoms may enter the steel and make it more brittle and liable to severe cracking. However, such hydrogen embrittlement is fairly rare and is easily prevented by baking the chromed tubing right after plating at 350 degrees.

"A more serious problem may arise when frame tubes are immersed in an acid bath to clean the steel before plating. If any acid is left in the tubing and is not rinsed out, small amounts of acid left in the tube will eat away the tubing wall from the inside. Later, the frame tubing may fracture or break at the acid-thinned spot. Rinsing the frame in an alkaline bath would neutralize any trapped acid and prevent such tubing failure.

Frame Failure

"Bicycles built today are usually well designed so as to avoid stress risers, places where stress can concentrate and eventually weaken and cause the tubing to break. This is not to say that failure due to improper design or to quality control failures in heat-treating, welding, or brazing do not occur. Such failure does happen, but as I noted, it is rare compared with other types of frame failure.

"These other types of frame failure are caused by impact, running into curbs, hopping off small hills, or stunting with a bike not designed for that great an impact. Other types of frame failure can result, as noted above, from inadequate joint design, improper assembly, such as welding, brazing, adhesive bonding, and so forth. Metallurgists are quite good about coming up with a reason for a frame failure. Their detective work in finding the cause of frame failure has been well established. Metallurgists can tell, usually just by looking at a metal fracture surface, just how the metal failed. They can determine if the failure was due to fatigue, overload, impact, or hydrogen embrittlement."

Julian Edwins, a metallurgical engineer and author of *Metallurgical Considerations in Welding* and a custom bicycle builder, has this to say about various tubing materials:

"Aluminum frames generally give a superior ride, without excessive flexibility. Stress risers are sharp corners, scratches, or score marks, which are an important consideration in aluminum frames. After a fall the frame should be carefully examined. If any damage is found refer the frame to a good frame builder.

"Advanced composites are made of polymeric, metallic carbon, or ceramic materials reinforced with glass, carbon, Kevlar, or ceramic fibers. Frames built without Kevlar would be susceptible to catastrophic failure upon impact or in a fall. Also, the resin holding the fibers together could splinter internally, without any visible external damage. So riders of composite frame bicycles should examine the frame carefully after any impact or fall. Composite frames also have a very hard covering, usually of epoxy. If this covering is damaged the frame fibers will absorb moisture that will delaminate the tubing and lead to frame failure. Think of composite frames as being like plywood, which is strong until the glue fails.

"New metal matrix composites are a recent addition to the bicycle-frame-tubing market. They are a matrix of light alloy, aluminum, magnesium, or titanium, with fibers of some type of ceramic material such as alumina or alumina silica.

Steel Frames Examined

"The exotic composites and expensive metals such as titanium have yet to replace steel for most bicycle frames. A case in point is the fact that 65 percent of all frames used in the 1992 Tour de France race were steel, including that of the winner. The chromium/molybdenum alloy (Cro-Mo) was used for aircraft as long ago as World War I. Another popular alloy of manganese/molybdenum was marketed in 1935. These are the two most popular steels used in bicycle tubing. These steels, and another popular high tensile steel called Hi-Ten, approximate the tensile strength of aluminum, about 115 ksi (one ksi equals 1,000 pounds per square inch). If you are looking for a very strong, very fatigue-resistant steel bike frame, I recommend a modern steel with a tensile strength of at least 130 ksi. If you want your custom builder to make the very strongest frame, ask him to use Aer-Met 100, which has a tensile strength of 280 ksi, and a yield strength of 250 ksi. Air-Met was developed for the F/A 18 jet plane, to withstand a drop rate of 24 feet per second and operate in corrosive sea air. This steel has a strength-to-weight ratio superior to titanium. Titanium has a tensile strength of 145 ksi and a yield strength of 137 ksi and is highly corrosion-resistant but far more expensive than steel. Other excellent steel tubing is made by True-Temper, Columbus, Reynolds, and Excell."

Now, once you have selected the bicycle that fits you and that promises the ride you like, check the bike for assembly and final adjustments.

PROTECT YOURSELF . . . MAKE THESE BICYCLE SAFETY CHECKS

Before you wheel your new bicycle out of the store, I strongly advise that *you* make the following basic safety checks. You can make these tests in a half hour or less, but do them, because your safety depends on them. Later on, as you use the bike, make these same checks every two or three months, or more often if you ride a lot (see the periodic maintenance list in Chapter 2). Needed adjustments can then be done by the shop mechanic. Remember, it is your body and your life that are on the line if a bad adjustment causes an accident. Sure, you can sue the dealer and the manufacturer if you get hurt because of a defectively assembled or designed bicycle, but money is no substitute for a whole, healthy body. Your new bike will have passed this exam by 100 percent if the dealer and the manufacturer have done their jobs correctly. One caveat, however. Unless you are knowledgeable about bicycle mechanics, even these checks may not detect every possible point of poor assembly by the dealer or the manufacturer. The ultimate responsibility for safe assembly and component adjustment rests on both the dealer and the manufacturer. Have the shop mechanic make these tests (and any needed corrections) if you feel safer not making the checks yourself. If possible, watch closely so you can make similar safety inspections from time to time. Again, do not assume that because the bike is new it is in safe working condition.

Look for Toe Overlap

The U.S. Consumer Product Safety Commission (CPSC) has specific regulations about bicycle design and assembly as they relate to the safety of the bicycle user. One of the mandates is that the pedal should have "at least 89 mm (3.5 inches) clearance between the front tire or the fender when [the wheel] is turned in any direction." The purpose of this requirement is that the bicycle shall be so designed that the foot won't hit the wheel or the fender, as shown in Fig. 1-11. This mandate does not apply, says the CPSC, if the pedals have toe clips. The only reason I can think of for eliminating toe-clip-equipped pedals is that some desk jockey decided that toe clips will keep the foot safely back away from the wheel or fender. Yet toe clips, especially if they are the largest of their three sizes, extend even farther than a person's foot. Accidents have happened when pedals both without and with toe clips came too close to the front wheel on a sharp turn. When the rider's foot, or his toe clip, contacts the wheel, loss of control and injury can occur. Check toe overlap this way. Hold the pedal crank arm parallel to the ground. If the pedal has a toe clip, also turn and hold the toe clip parallel to the ground. Then turn the front wheel until it comes as close as possible to the toe clip. If the wheel and toe clip come in contact (Fig. 1-11) that bike is an accident waiting to happen. Look for another bike. Check a bike without toe-clip pedals the same way, but this time have someone measure the distance between the centerline of the pedal axle and the front wheel. If the clearance is less than 3.5 inches, do not buy this bike and also tell the shop people that the bike is in violation of CPSC regulations. If you add fenders to such a bike you are in effect reducing the pedal or toe-clip clearance by a half to one full

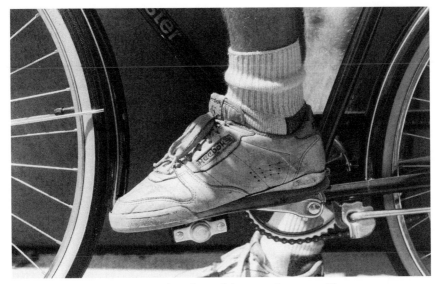

Fig. 1-11: Check any bike you buy for pedal-to-toe clearance. If your toe contacts a fender or the front wheel on a sharp turn you could lose control of the bicycle.

inch. If you plan to bike when it rains I do recommend fenders, though, because they will keep greasy road water from leaving a track up both sides of you.

Brakes

Make these brake tests, and the other safety inspections in this chapter, before you wheel a new bike out of the store. For starters, look at the brake shoes. They should be about ⅟₁₆ to ⅛ inch from the rim (see Chapter 3). Hold the bike up off the ground, or have it in a bike stand. Spin each wheel. Make sure the brake shoes do not rub on the rim when the brake levers are *not* depressed (see Chapter 3).

Now squeeze each brake lever as hard as you can and hold it for a few seconds. Let go of the brake lever. Check brake shoe clearance again. If the shop has removed cable stretch (yes, cables do eventually stretch), brake shoe clearances will not have changed. But if the brake shoes now appear farther from the rim, have the shop readjust these clearances and remove cable stretch as needed. (See Chapter 3 for more data on brake maintenance.)

I recommend you check the brakes on an actual ride in a safe place such as a vacant school playground. Make the following final brake and gear-shift tests outside, in a safe place.

On a safe, flat place, speed up to about 15 miles per hour. Apply first the rear brake, then a second later, the front one. You should be able to come to a complete stop within about 15 feet of where you first applied both brakes. You can stop a bit more quickly if you weigh much less than 150 pounds, a bit more slowly if you weigh much over 150 pounds. The CPSC requires that a rider weighing 150 pounds be able to stop the bike at 15 miles per hour within 15 feet, when riding on a flat paved surface, into a wind velocity no greater than seven miles per hour, without front brake lock-up. If after several tries the bike won't pass this test, I suggest you look for a bike that will.

Some less expensive road bicycles come with so-called safety or extension brake levers in addition to the main brake levers (Fig. 1-12). These levers are supposed to let you apply the brakes without having to move your hands off the handlebars, and without having to move your hands to the main brake levers. Extension levers are in my experience and judgment a major safety hazard. Over time brake cables stretch so gradually you may not be aware that the extension levers, so easy to reach and so habitually used, now must be squeezed all the way down to the handlebars before you can slow or stop. In this case the extension levers will very likely not stop you in time to avoid an accident.

Look at a bike with these levers. Squeeze them and see how close they come to the handlebars. Squeeze the main levers. You will see that the extension levers come closer to the handlebars than the main levers. If you still

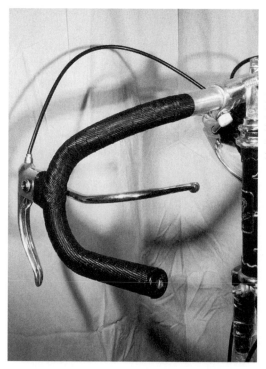

Fig. 1-12:
Remove or have your bike shop remove brake extension levers. (See text for why they can make braking hazardous.)

want this bike, have the shop remove the extension levers and replace the main brake lever axle bolt with a shorter one that won't protrude once the extension levers have been removed. (See Chapter 3 for data on removing these levers on a bike you already own.)

Gear Shifting

The bike of your choice may have passed a gear shift demonstration in the shop. But the reality of shifting under the stress of pedaling is not the same as no-load shifting when the bike is on a stand. After the brake check above, while you are still out on the school playground or other safe place, shift the front and rear derailleurs through all gear combinations. As you shift, ease off on pedal pressure but keep pedaling. Start shifting with the chain on the big front chainwheel and on the small rear freewheel cog. Shift the chain to the next-smallest chainwheel and if the bike has a triple chainwheel then shift the chain to the smallest chainwheel. Repeat this shift test through all the gears. In other words, with the chain on each rear cog shift through each of the chainwheels and vice versa.

If the chain falls off the big chainwheel down onto the crank arm, or off the small chainwheel down onto the bottom bracket shell, the shop should readjust the front derailleur. If the chain jumps between the smallest rear cog and the dropouts, or off the biggest rear cog and onto the spokes, have the shop adjust the rear derailleur. Pedal slowly, being aware that during this shift test the chain might jam between the small cog and the chainstay, or fall off the biggest cog, or any of the chainwheels up front. Then the cranks will suddenly jam, or skip forward, so you may lose control and fall. Now, when you get back to the store make these other quick and simple tests for safe bike part adjustments.

Headset Bearings

Locate the head tube in Fig. 1-2. The headset bearings are inside that tube, where they help make steering smoother. These little bearings take a tremendous beating from road shock. If these bearings are too loose you can get into a horrendous front-wheel shimmy that can cause loss of control, a spill, and injury to you (see Chapter 2 for more data on this and other causes of front-wheel shimmy). Also, if they are too loose or too tight, these little bearings will wear out a lot faster.

Check headset bearing adjustment this way. Straddle the top tube while keeping both feet on the ground (Fig. 1-13). Squeeze the left (front-wheel) brake lever tightly and keep your other hand on the handlebars. Now energetically rock the bike back and forth while you watch the fork crown (the

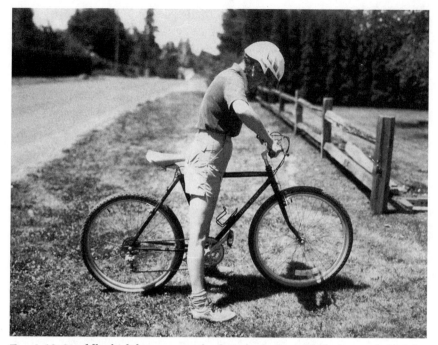

FIG. 1-13: Straddle the bike, squeeze the front brake lever hard, then rock the bike back and forth. If you see movement of the fork where it meets the steerer tube or hear clicks, have the headset bearings readjusted.

top of the fork where it enters the head tube) for movement. At the same time be alert for looseness and clicking sounds from the head tube area. If you detect any looseness from fork movement or hear or feel clicking, have the headset bearings readjusted.

Make this check for headset-bearing overtightness. Let go of the brake lever and lift the front wheel off the ground while still straddling the top tube. Lean the bike to the left and then to the right so the handlebar can move in both directions. If this movement is not smooth, if the handlebar seems to bind, the headset bearings are too tight and should be readjusted by the shop.

Wheel and Hub Bearing Check

Wheels that wobble from side to side, either because they are misaligned or because hub bearings are too loose, can also cause wheel shimmy. Check wheels this way:

1. Check wheel trueness: Place the bike in a bike stand or upside-down on the floor. Spin each wheel. Watch where the rim passes by the brake shoes.

If the rim flat comes closer to, then moves farther away from a brake shoe, the rim is misaligned and should be trued up (see Chapter 7).

2. *Check spoke tension:* Squeeze spokes together in sets of two, on each side of the wheel. If some spokes seem loose and others very tight, spoke tension is uneven. Unevenly tensioned spokes can also cause front-wheel shimmy. Have the shop adjust spoke tension.

3. *Look for loose or tight wheel hub bearings:* Grasp each wheel at the valve stem and move or shake the wheel from side to side. If the wheel moves left or right the hub bearings are too loose. Turn the wheel so the tire valve stem or wheel reflector is at the two o'clock position. Let go of the wheel. The wheel should rotate slowly as the weight of the valve stem or reflector responds to the pull of gravity. If the wheel won't move, or comes to a quick stop as you spin it, hub bearings are too tight.

4. *Make sure that there is a wheel safety retainer clip in place (Fig. 1-14):* These clips are required by the CPSC on front-wheel axles if the front-wheel

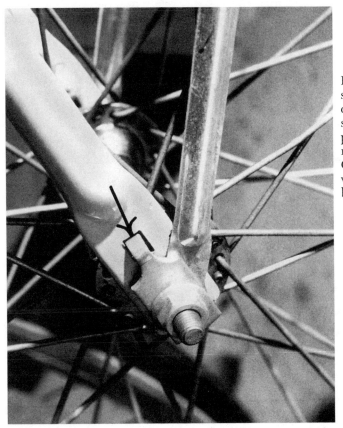

FIG. 1-14: Be sure retention devices are securely in place. They are required by the CPSC on front wheels with bolt-on hubs.

axle is tightened down by an axle nut on each side of the fork. These little clips keep the wheel from falling out of the fork if the hub axle bolt is not safely tight.

5. *Check bolt-on front-wheel tightness:* Lift the front wheel off the ground with one hand and pound down hard on the top of the tire with your other hand. If the wheel moves downward in the fork dropouts, or actually does fall out of the fork, you're in a careless bike shop that has not tightened these bolts to the correct torque (see Chapters 2 and 3). I would probably call a halt to the sale and go elsewhere. However, you may be more forbearing and forgiving than I am. If so, make sure the shop tightens these nuts to 300 to 320 in./lbs. of torque. Bike shops have been known to remove these safety clips because they feel they detract from the bike's appearance. Be sure the shop puts them back. They could save your life. In these litigious days, smart manufacturers also have front-wheel dropout safety clips installed on quick-release front wheels, where they are equally needed.

6. *Check quick-release-equipped front wheels this way:* Again, check tightness by pounding down hard on the tire with the front wheel off the ground. The wheel should not fall out of the fork dropouts. If the wheel does fall out, have the shop tighten the quick-release (*Important!* See Chapter 2 for instructions on use and operation of the quick-release mechanism.) Remove the wheel altogether and take a close look at the fork dropouts. You should see indentations in the dropout where the sawtooth ridges of the quick-release "bit" into the steel of the dropout (see Chapter 2). If the dropout looks smooth, with no "teeth" marks on either side of the dropout, the front-wheel quick-release was never safely tightened. Have the shop explain to you how a quick-release should be adjusted and tightened.

Bottom Bracket and Pedal Bearings

Locate the bottom bracket in Fig. 1-1 or 1-2. The spindle (axle) to which the cranks are attached is inside the bottom bracket, along with spindle ball bearings and the cups in which they rotate as you pedal along. If the adjustable cup (on the left side of the bottom bracket shell) is not accurately adjusted, spindle bearings can be too loose or too tight. Loose or tight bottom bracket bearings (see Fig. 1-1 or 1-2) will cause premature wear of these bearings and an expensive repair, even if you replace the bearings and cups yourself. Check bottom bracket bearings this way: Grasp each crank arm at the pedal and with quick left and right movements move a crank from side to side. If the crank moves or feels loose, bottom bracket bearings are loose. Shift the chain to the small chainwheel, then lift the chain off that chainwheel and let it fall onto the bottom bracket shell. With the chain free, spin the cranks. The cranks and chainwheel should rotate smoothly and come to a gradual stop. If not, bottom bracket bearings are too tight. In either case, have the shop readjust them.

Check pedal bearings by moving each pedal up and down and toward and away from the bike frame. If the pedal feels loose or too tight, their bearings need readjustment. Spin each pedal to check for bearing adjustment.

Handlebars

Twist the handlebar grips. If they move, have the shop replace them with grips that stay tight. Loose grips can cause loss of control and an accident.

Stand in front of the bicycle and hold the front wheel tightly between your legs while you try to turn the handlebars to the left and to the right. If the handlebars move but the wheel does not, the stem expander bolt is not safely tight. The expander bolt may be tight enough to let you steer accurately on the flats, but not on a rough road or trail. If it is loose, have the shop tighten it to a torque of 174 to 260 in./lbs. Now twist the handlebars around in a circular direction. If the handlebars move, the stem handlebar clamp binder bolt (see Chapter 8) is too loose. Have the shop tighten this bolt to 174 to 260 in./lbs.

Saddle and Seat Post

Twist the saddle left and right. If it moves, the seat-post clamp binder bolt, or the quick-release clamp (see Chapter 8) is too loose. Road bike seat-post binder bolts are usually a nut-and-bolt affair, but most mountain bike seat posts are locked in place by a quick-release mechanism. Have the shop do what is necessary to keep the saddle from twisting, or from moving down as you pedal, a rather disconcerting experience, to say the least. I will cover saddle height, tilt, and fore and aft fit adjustments later in this chapter.

Owner's Manual

The CPSC requires that an owner's manual come with every new bike sold. Make sure you receive a copy and that you read it before your first ride. If you do not feel up to making any of the adjustments described in the manual, take your bike to the shop and have them do this work. Again, remember that your safety as you ride depends, at least in part, on the mechanical condition of your bicycle.

FINE-TUNING BIKE FIT

When you have narrowed your search for a new bike down to one that fits your overall height, the type of riding you will do, and your budget, the next step is to fine-tune the variables of bike fit. You can of course make all these changes yourself, or you can have the bike shop do them for you. These variables include saddle height, tilt, distance from the handlebars, and stem height, length, and "rise" in degrees. Other fit options include size of toe clips or fit adjustment of clipless pedals and the location of brake and shift levers. Keep in mind, however, that adjustment of these variables is not engraved in steel. New riders often feel that the bike is too big for them, or that the saddle is too high or too low. Make these basic adjustments as you spend time on the bike, but be flexible and open-minded about them. You can always make further adjustments as comfort dictates. Now here is how to make fit adjustments to tailor your new bike to your body dimensions.

Brake "Reach" Fit Adjustment

Make sure your fingers can reach and grasp the brake levers without strain. Sit on the saddle while leaning against a wall or have someone hold you upright. Now grip the brake levers. If your fingers cannot easily reach and grip the brake levers, adjust the brake lever reach if these levers have such an adjustment on them. See Chapter 3 for instructions.

Saddle Height and Frame Size

Before making any of the fit adjustments below, make sure the bike fits you. I have already mentioned this at the beginning of the chapter, but I want to repeat the safety importance of bike frame size and fit. If the bike is too small, there will be more than an inch and half of air between you and the top tube. Too small a bike means too short a top tube and too high a saddle for the bike frame size. If you have to raise the saddle up high to prevent knee injury (see below) you may be too far away from the handlebars and have to strain to reach them, which means an unbalanced position on the saddle, with more of your weight over the front wheel. Ideally, your weight should be closely balanced between both wheels. If your saddle is too high you have to strain to reach the pedals, which promotes knee, back, and ankle injuries. You also will have difficulty in handling road shock by putting a pedal down and taking up bumps through your leg while you lift yourself up off the saddle. If the saddle is too high you may also have balance problems that can affect steering and control. If your saddle is too low, you cannot get full leg extension as you pedal. Partial leg extension means you cannot exert full leg muscle power to the pedals. If you try to do so while your knee is not bent far enough, you could strain or tear a knee ligament, particularly on hill climbs.

Find the correct saddle height for your leg length this way. Have a friend hold your bike or balance yourself against a wall. With one pedal at the 12 o'clock position and the other pedal at the 6 o'clock position, your knee should be slightly bent, at about a five-degree angle (Fig. 1-15).

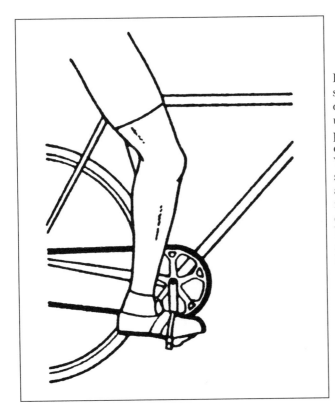

FIG. 1-15: Sit on the saddle while someone holds the bike upright. Move a pedal to the six o'clock position. Your knee should show a slight bend, as shown. If not, move the saddle up or down as needed by loosening the seat-post quick-release clamp bolt.

Mounting and Taking Off

Put one foot on the pedal and move that pedal to the two-o'clock position. Take off by pushing the pedal hard while at the same time hoisting your bottom onto the saddle. Practice this maneuver until it becomes automatic. Get off the saddle by leaning the bicycle slightly sideways and at the same time extending a leg to reach the ground. Hold the front brake lever closed to keep the bicycle from moving as you get off the bicycle.

To move the saddle up or down on a mountain bike, turn the quick-release lever to the open position, adjust saddle height, then turn the quick-release lever to its closed position (please review the quick-release adjustment and tightening procedure in Chapter 2). To move the saddle up or down on a road bike, loosen the seat-post binder bolt, adjust saddle height, then tighten the binder bolt to 147 to 347 in./lbs. (See Chapter 3 for a discussion of torque as it applies to the safe tightening of nuts and bolts on your bicycle.) I suggest you move the saddle up or down about one-quarter inch at a time. Then ride the bike for a couple of hours to check your comfort level. Make further saddle height adjustments in quarter-inch increments until you find the saddle height that produces the most comfort. Make sure that you have *at least* three inches of the seat post *inside* the seat tube (Fig. 1-16). Most seat posts

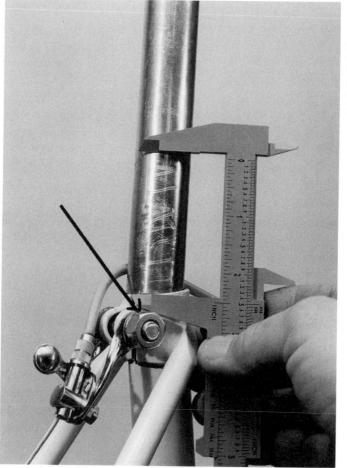

FIG. 1-16: Keep at least three inches of the seat post inside the seat tube.

have a safe height line scribed on them with a warning that this line must not show above the seat tube. That's an important warning, because less than three inches of the seat post inside the seat tube can damage the frame, even snap off the top of the seat tube. Remember Archimedes and the lever. Think of the seat tube as such a lever. The force exerted by this lever can, as I said, damage the bike frame unless there's enough of that lever inside the seat tube. A snapped-off seat tube or seat tube cluster can cause loss of control and an accident as you ride.

Saddle to Handlebar Distance

Adjust the saddle fore and aft position to suit your leg, torso, and arm length. If the saddle is too far forward, you put undue stress on your arms, wrists, and hands because too much of your body weight is too far forward. If the saddle is too far away from the handlebars you will find yourself pulling up on the handlebars on hard pedaling when your legs should be doing most of the work. Ideally, your lower body should be supported mostly by the saddle, with your upper torso supported at least in part by your hands when placed on the handlebars.

First try adjusting the saddle horizontal movement about in the middle of its range—that is, about in the middle of the saddle rail. Just loosen the clamp bolt(s), move the saddle and tighten the clamp bolt(s) (see Chapter 8) to a torque of 140 to 160 in./lbs. If you have a long torso but shorter legs, try moving the saddle back one-quarter inch. If your legs are long but your torso is comparatively shorter, move the saddle forward one-quarter inch. Ride the bike for at least one hour before making additional fore or aft adjustments. Remember that the best position for you is the one that is the most comfortable.

Saddle Tilt

Most riders seem to prefer the nose of the saddle tilted slightly upward from a position horizontal to the ground. For example, I prefer just a slight upward tilt, about 10 degrees from horizontal. This position more evenly distributes body weight between the handlebars and the saddle. If your saddle chafes your skin, try tilting it down a bit. If your arms or the palms of your hands are sore because too much of your weight is pushed forward onto the handlebars, tilt the saddle up slightly. Ride for about an hour after each tilt adjustment before changing it. To change saddle tilt, loosen the saddle clamp bolt or bolts, tilt the saddle up or down and retighten the clamp bolt(s) to 140 to 160 in./lbs. of torque.

Handlebar Height Adjustments

If your handlebars are too low, you have to lean too far forward to reach them. This degree of lean can cause some discomfort. If you have to lean far forward you also have to strain your neck muscles to hold your head up at an angle at which you can see the road ahead. This strain on a long ride can create a lot of pain in your neck and shoulder muscles, believe me. To relieve this pain you will tend to look too often down at the road immediately before you and not up at the traffic ahead, which I am sure you don't need me to tell you is dangerous to life and limb. You will also not be able to absorb road shock with your arms as well you could with the handlebars at the correct height, because your arms will be straight out, without the benefit of a slight bend in your elbows.

If the handlebars are too high, you can't bend into an aerodynamic position on a road bike to lessen wind resistance. On all bikes your arm reach to

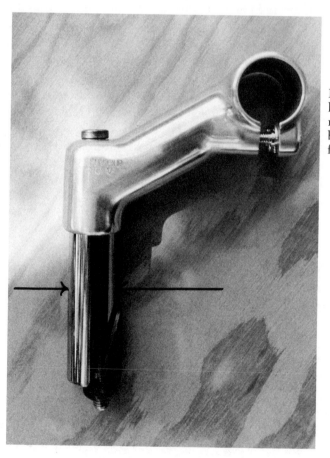

FIG. 1-17: Keep at least 2½ inches, arrow, of the handlebar stem inside the fork steerer tube.

the handlebars will be too short to permit pulling up on the bars on a stiff road climb.

Before you make any handlebar height adjustments, keep these two warnings in mind. *First,* if you raise the bars on any bicycle you must keep at least 2½ inches of the stem inside the fork steerer tube (Fig. 1-17). Look for a scribe mark on the stem, which must not show. Otherwise the stem could snap off and you would lose all steering control. *Second,* if you raise or lower the handlebars on a mountain bike and your brake cable is routed through the stem, you will have to readjust brake shoe rim clearance. If you raise the handlebars, the brake shoes will rub and bind on the rim. If you lower the handlebars, the brake shoes will be too far from the rim, so braking efficiency will be reduced to where you may have little or no braking power left. See Chapter 3 for brake shoe adjustments.

Raise or lower the handlebars about a half inch at a time. Test ride for 10 or 15 minutes to check your comfort level. Do not raise the handlebars more than one inch, ever. If your body configuration, such as short arms, requires handlebars to be repositioned more than one inch, the bike shop can do this in two ways. First, they can install a Delta Stem Raiser (available from your bike shop), which can raise your stem up to four inches. The Stem Raiser comes in 22-mm or 25.4-mm diameters, so install the one that fits your steerer tube. Second, they can install a mountain bike stem with a greater degree rise or greater length (extension). For example, Control Tech makes mountain bike stems with rises of 0°, 10°, and 25°. The 0° and 10° stems come in 90-, 105-, 120-, 135-, and 150-mm extensions. The 25° rise comes in 80-, 100-, and 120-mm extensions. Fig. 1-18 shows some of these stems. Stems for road bikes are available from Control Tech in 0° and 15° rises in extensions from 80 to 140 mm in 10-mm increments. Remember, stems also come in widths of 1 inch, 1⅛ inches, and 1¼ inches to fit your particular steerer tube. Stems come to fit the two most popular diameters of handlebars, 25.4 mm and 26 mm. Be sure you get the right size.

To raise or lower your handlebars, loosen the stem expander bolt with the appropriate wrench five or six turns, then tap it down with a plastic mallet, or put a block of wood over the bolt and tap on that with a hammer. Adjust the handlebar height, then tighten the expander bolt to 174 to 260 in./lbs. (See Chapter 3 for information on torque and the use of a torque wrench.) The expander bolt has a wedge-shaped nut, which when tightened is forced against the inside wall of the steerer tube to hold the stem in place.

Road Bike Handlebar Tilt

The drops on road bicycle handlebars can be adjusted for upward or downward tilt. A slight downtilt with respect to the top tube is one I find com-

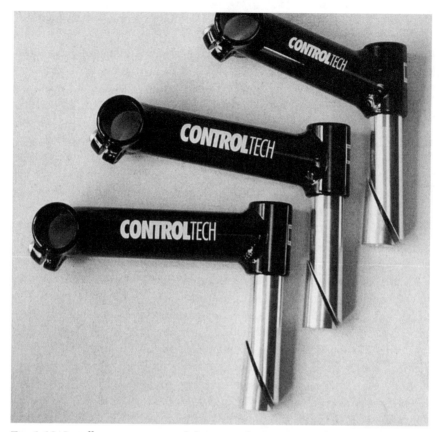

Fig. 1-18: Install a new mountain bike stem, if necessary, to fit your reach. Use a longer or shorter stem or one with the rise to fit your torso height. A stock bike may not come with the stem that's right for you. Shown are stems of various lengths and degrees of rise.

fortable and is also recommended by Klein Bicycle Corporation. You can change the tilt by loosening the stem handlebar binder bolt, tilting the handlebar as you wish, then tightening this bolt to 180 in./lbs.

The fit data above do not necessarily apply to recumbents. The recumbent bike industry is really in its infancy. There are many producers, all with different frame configurations and relatively low-volume production, which explains why their prices are relatively high. However, most recumbent frames or their saddles (seats, really) can be moved to fit your torso.

Now that you know how to buy the bike that fits you, let's get into how to ride it safely.

Chapter Two

SAFETY TIPS THAT PRESERVE LIFE AND LIMB

Most bicycle accidents are avoidable. In this chapter you will learn how to keep yourself safe at all times, how to ride with the peace of mind that comes from an awareness of road and trail hazards and how to avoid them. Before we get into the specifics of accident prevention, here is a summary of what causes most bicycle accidents, in my experience of over 25 years as an expert witness involved in related litigation:

1. Rider error (I think this is a conservative percentage): 75 percent.
2. Vehicle driver error (bicyclist could not escape): 5 percent.
3. Poor bicycle maintenance (see maintenance and adjustment chapters in this book): 5 percent.
4. Defective bicycle assembly at retail level (see Chapter 1): 5 percent.
5. Defective bicycle trail design or dangerous road condition: 4 percent.
6. Defective bicycle owner's manual (inadequate instructions): 3 percent.
7. Defective bicycle (manufacturer assembly, design of frame or component—see Chapter 1 for details): 3 percent.

Safety awareness is what brings you back from a bike trip all in one piece, unscathed and happy. Sometimes, as I ride down a city street, the thought goes through my mind, like an old refrain, over and over again: "The alert cyclist is the safe cyclist." In this chapter, I'll try to explain what I mean by the word "alert," because in that word lie a host of survival skills. After hundreds of thousands of miles of bicycling in city and country, in the United

States and abroad, on city streets, rural roads, and off-road trails, I exercise most of these skills almost subconsciously. I know, for example, that if I don't make eye contact with a car driver at an intersection, I can't be sure I have been seen. I also know, without thinking about it, even if I am sure the driver has seen me, that he or she won't run into me. There are literally hundreds of safety-related decisions you *must* make every time you take a bike trip. These decisions must be based on accurate information. What will that driver do now? Can I escape into a ditch? Jump a curb to get away from a car or even a pedestrian? How should I cross this intersection? Will that driver coming out of the shopping mall driveway wait until I pass? Is this a safe road for me? How can I tell by the driver's actions if the car coming from behind will pass me safely on this narrow two-lane road? What am I doing on this narrow two-lane road in the first place? Will the car coming from behind me and the car coming toward me pass right where I am? (It's amazing how many drivers do this.) Will the prevailing winds and the big semi truck rig coming toward or passing me combine to suck me into the rig or blow me off the road, and which way should I lean the bike to counteract these winds? These are just a few examples of the myriad decisions you must make every mile of a bike ride. You simply have to learn to recognize these road and trail safety signals almost without conscious effort on your part. Because if you have to stop to think about what you must do in a particular situation, it may be too late. Remember, even at the slow speed of 10 miles per hour, you are traveling 14.66 feet per second. A car moving at only 25 miles per hour is covering almost 37 feet per second (See Table 2-1).

TABLE 2-1: SECONDS TO TRAVEL A STANDARD CITY BLOCK OF 280 FEET
(to Convert mph to fps Multiply mph by 1.4667)

MILES PER HOUR	FEET PER SECOND	SECONDS PER BLOCK
5	7.33	38.99
10	14.66	19.04
15	22.00	12.72
20	29.33	9.66
25	36.66	7.66
30	44.00	6.36
35	51.33	5.45
40	58.67	4.94
45	66.00	4.24
50	73.34	3.80
55	80.66	3.47
60	88.00	3.18
65	95.34	2.94
70	102.67	2.73
75	110.00	2.55

Correct action in a split second is often the only way to avoid an accident on a bicycle. It doesn't help much to reflect that the skills you learned as a car driver cannot save you on a bicycle.

TABLE 2-2: CHANGE IN PERCENT OF DEATHS BY AGE BETWEEN 1982 AND 1992 IN BICYCLE-RELATED ACCIDENTS*

YEAR	BYCYCLES IN USE (MILLIONS)	DEATHS	DEATH RATE†	PERCENT AGE 0–14	PERCENT AGE 15–24	PERCENT AGE 25 AND OVER
1982	84.1	1,100	1.31	35	27	38
1992	110.0	700	0.64	39	11	50

* *Accident Facts*, 1993 edition: The National Safety Council.
† Per 100,000 bicycles in use.

As you can see in Table 2-2, between 1982 and 1992, total fatalities due to bicycle accidents shrank from 1,100 to 700 while at the same time during this period the number of bicycles in use jumped from 84.1 million to 110.0 million. In other words, over this 10-year period, the number of bicycles in use grew by 31 percent while total fatalities in bicycle-related accidents shrank 57 percent. We may think of teenagers as the most accident-prone of all bicyclists, yet during this 10-year period the percent of bicycle-accident-related deaths dropped from 27 to only 11 in the age group 15 to 24 years of age. What is most significant, at least to me, is that adults aged 25 and over accounted for 38 percent of bike-accident-related fatalities in 1982 but in 1992 that figure jumped to 50 percent of all bicycle-accident-related deaths. This says to me that more people over 25 are riding bikes, and that this group needs to hone the safety skills needed to survive on the road on a bike. This is what this chapter is all about, getting you out there and back, safely, on your bicycle. Let's start with your noggin.

Wear a Helmet at All Times!

I would not go two feet on my bicycle without a helmet on my head. Studies have clearly shown that fatal head injuries of bicyclists involved in an accident are at least 60 percent more likely to occur to the rider who is *not* wearing a helmet. Your brain is the most complex and impact-vulnerable part of your body. An impact that would only bruise an arm or a leg could kill you if it involved your helmetless head.

One of the most frustrating aspects of helmet safety training is getting youngsters to wear a helmet. Kids up to the late teens think wearing a helmet is "dorky" and simply won't cooperate. Peer pressure prevails. So you as a parent must insist that your child wear a helmet or lose the privilege of riding the bicycle. I have lectured kids in grade and high school about all the aspects of safety in this chapter and discovered one ear- and eye-catching way to focus their attention on helmets. Try this demo. Take a wok or other large pot. Place it on the floor. Hand your child an egg. Have him or her hold the egg about three feet above the pot. Say: "Now, this egg is your head. When I say *drop*, let go of the egg, let it fall into the pot." The egg will hit the pot with an audible smashing, squishing sound and you will hear a gasp from the child. I tried this in elementary-school classrooms, and it did impress the kids, as if it were their first ever dropped-egg sound. If you are in a group of kids, immediately pass the pot, with the shell fragments and the yellow yolk and white stuck to the side, around to each of the kids. I guarantee they will look into that pot with intensity. Tell them that their brains could be splattered just like that egg, and that a helmet will keep their brains from splashing like the egg if they themselves should fall off their bicycle. Excellent helmets, for adults and children, are available from Bell, Giro, Protec, Headway, and other manufacturers.

Helmets are cheap compared to brain surgery or to the lifetime medical costs of a paraplegic or even a quadriplegic. Good helmets can be had for as little as $45. Pricier helmets (more stylish, colorful, and attention getting) are available in bike stores for up to $150 or so. At whatever price, a helmet is very cost effective, considering the consequences of not wearing one. I know of accidents in which the rider, just waiting at a stop light, lost balance, fell, struck his helmetless head on a curb, and died from the impact.

I was astounded and shocked when I learned of the Oregon bicycle industry's opposition to a proposed law requiring bicycle helmets. I'd like to share a letter I wrote about this to *The Oregonian,* Portland, Oregon's, leading daily newspaper.

As an expert witness on bicycle accidents, I am involved in such lawsuits throughout the United States and Canada. Had the bicyclist been wearing a helmet, many of the fatalities and serious head injuries in these accidents would not have occurred.

I am in total disagreement with Tom Wolbert of the Bicycle Federation of Oregon when he says that a law requiring every bicyclist to wear a helmet would be "practically impossible to enforce." Oregon and now Washington both require motorcyclists to wear a helmet, and enforcement is simple. A quick look at the head is all that's needed. The same holds true for bicyclists.

No, the real reason that Wolbert and other people involved in bicycling discourage a mandatory bicycle helmet law is much more cold-blooded. As Wolbert himself told the Oregon Senate Judiciary Committee, a mandatory helmet law would "discourage" potential riders. What Wolbert and others in the bicycle industry really mean is that a mandatory bicycle helmet law would discourage people from buying a bicycle in the first place, and so reduce sales and income for them. I find such an attitude selfish and heartless. In other words, the bicycle industry is saying, if you believe Wolbert and his ilk, to hell with rider safety, let's just sell them bikes and let the riders risk injury or death without a helmet. Helmet laws do not reduce the number of motorcyclists on the road (check vehicle registrations, e.g.) and it won't reduce the number of bicyclists either. But if it's a choice between having to wear a helmet and riding a bicycle, my vote goes to the helmet law. Any trauma physician would agree, for obvious reasons.

I also teach bicycle safety to grade-school children. I can tell you that grade-school children resist wearing a bicycle helmet because they think it's "dorky" and silly. Well, that's what laws are for, to protect people despite themselves.

Since my letter, the Oregon legislature passed a law that requires bicyclists under the age of 16 to wear a helmet or face a $25 fine, which will be waived after the child (spell that "parent") buys a helmet. Given the increase in bicycle-related fatalities to adults over 25 (Table 2-2), I think helmet laws should apply to all ages. Table 2-3 is a recap of state helmet requirement laws for bicyclists at this writing.

A helmet should have a label inside that says it meets the Snell or A.N.S.I. Z90.4 standards, preferably both (Fig. 2-1).

TABLE 2-3: MANDATORY HELMET LAWS*

STATE, COUNTY, OR CITY	AGE REQUIRED TO WEAR HELMET
California	4 and under (trailer passenger)
California, cities of Chico and Bidwell Park	All ages
Georgia	Under 16
Maryland, Allegheny County	Under 16
Maryland, Howard County	Under 16
Maryland, Montgomery County	Under 18
Massachusetts	Under 5
New Jersey	Under 14
New York	Under 5
New York, city of Guilderland	Under 14
New York, Rockland County	All ages
Ohio, city of Beachwood	Under 16
Oregon	Under 16
Pennsylvania	5 and under
Tennessee, city of Clarksville	All ages
Washington, King County	All ages
Washington, city of Port Angeles	All ages

* From data supplied by The National Safe Kids Campaign, March 1993. For information on this organization phone 1-202-939-4993.

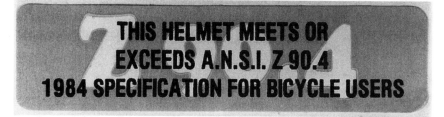

FIG. 2-1: Look for this label inside any helmet you buy for best-quality protection.

Helmet Fit

A bicycle helmet should equally protect the back of the head and the fore-head. Unfortunately, I see at least as many unsafely worn helmets as I do properly worn ones, particularly on children. A helmet tipped back leaves the forehead unprotected. The safest way to wear a helmet is with the front of the helmet no higher than one inch above the eyebrows (Fig. 2-2).

Some helmets come with little Velcro-attached pads to tailor the inside of the helmet more closely to the configuration of your head. I worry about these pads because they are soft and on impact they let the helmet move around so it could be dislodged. It's better to have the helmet fit you exactly and closely, and to adjust the retention straps so the helmet does not move around on your head. Remember, if on a severe impact the helmet pops off your head, your now helmetless head could be hit again in the same acci-dent. Headway, an Australian helmet manufacturer, for example, offers hel-mets in 10 sizes (Table 2-4).

Fit a helmet to your child or yourself this way. Put a tape measure around the head, about a half inch to an inch above the eyebrows. Read off the size where the tape meets itself. Use Table 2-4 as a guide in helmet selection. Run the tape measure around the inside of the helmet, match the measure-ment you made to the helmet that comes closest to this dimension. The first three columns in Table 2-4 give sizes that fit kids from ages one to nine. The last seven columns give sizes for ages seven to adult. By age seven, for ex-ample, some children can be better fitted with an adult model. The bottom sizes are in centimeters.

TABLE 2-4: HELMET SIZE SELECTION

AGES ONE TO NINE (APPROXIMATELY)			AGES SEVEN TO ADULT						
S	M	L	XSS	XS	S	M	L	XL	XXL
5⅜″	6⅛″–6⅜″	6½″–6¾″	6½″	6¾″	7″	7¼″	7½″	7¾″	8″
45–48 cm	49–51 cm	52–54 cm	52 cm	54 cm	56 cm	58 cm	60 cm	62 cm	64 cm

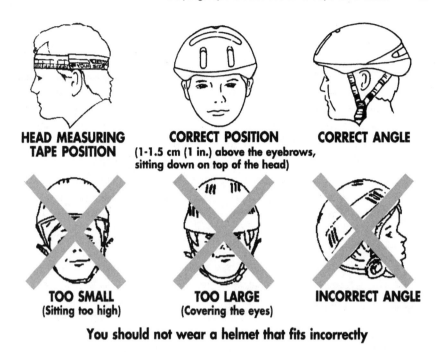

HEAD MEASURING
TAPE POSITION

CORRECT POSITION
(1-1.5 cm (1 in.) above the eyebrows,
sitting down on top of the head)

CORRECT ANGLE

TOO SMALL
(Sitting too high)

TOO LARGE
(Covering the eyes)

INCORRECT ANGLE

You should not wear a helmet that fits incorrectly

FIG. 2-2: Make sure your helmet fits snugly and squarely atop your head and comes to just over your eyebrows. This drawing shows how to measure your head for a helmet, and safe and unsafe ways to wear a helmet. Adjust straps so helmet won't move as you pedal.

A few words of warning about head impacts. No helmet can protect you against a severe top-of-the-head impact, as when you go over the handlebars and land headfirst on the top of your head. This type of impact can result in a compression fracture of the spinal cord that can turn you into a paraplegic or a quadriplegic. I say this not to scare you but to let you know that a helmet is no guarantee against severe bodily injury, so don't rely on the helmet alone. Follow the survival safety tips in this chapter. Be aware that although a helmet can protect against head damage, such damage in varying degrees of severity can still occur. The medical profession recognizes three basic types of concussions, and offers this advice about them:

1. With a *mild concussion,* you stay conscious. You may be confused for a short time, have some ringing in your ears, or be dizzy for a while, but you won't be unsteady on your feet or suffer poor coordination. You recover fast.
2. *Moderate concussion* involves a brief loss of consciousness, some confusion and mild amnesia (which is why cyclists in an accident seldom

remember much about the events just before a fall), some ear ringing and unsteadiness. You recover in about five minutes.

3. *Severe concussion* involves loss of consciousness for over five minutes, mental confusion, prolonged amnesia, severe ear ringing, and obvious unsteadiness. It usually takes five minutes or longer to recover. If these symptoms do occur get yourself to a hospital as soon as possible because there could be hidden damage of a more serious nature. For example, even if you recover from a concussion quickly, you may have a hemorrhage inside your skull that quickly builds up to pressure that could be fatal. Such internal pressure in your skull should be relieved by a competent physician. Symptoms of such pressure can occur at any time, even months after a severe impact. Have someone close to you watch for such symptoms as headaches, nausea and vomiting, different-size pupils of your eyes, dizziness and confusion, gradual loss of consciousness, a rise in blood pressure, and a slower pulse rate. If any of these symptoms occur, you must get to a hospital fast for an X-ray, diagnosis, and possibly a skull tap to relieve internal pressure.

A final observation about helmets. I have tried various types and colors of visors on helmets. Most are fastened by Velcro tabs. Visors are a safety measure that keeps the sun out of your eyes (particularly when cycling into the rising or setting sun) and so promotes forward vision. If you find, however, that a visor forces you to keep your head tilted uncomfortably upward to prevent the visor from physically interfering with forward vision, you might try repositioning the visor. If in the new position the visor still obscures vision unless you strain to keep your head up, I suggest you remove the visor and switch to Polaroid sunglasses.

FIG. 2-3: Look for designated bike routes and bicycle lane crossing signs for a safe place to pedal.

A guide sign used for marking officially designated Bikeways.

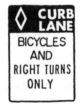

The "diamond lane" gives preference to certain vehicles such as bicycles.

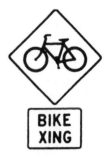

Used to warn motorists of a midblock bike path crossing.

City Street Smarts: Your Route to Safety

On any street, road, trail, or lane, keep in mind Sloane's first rule of bicycle safety: Always be alert, never assume anything, and above all give the right of way to anyone who asks for it. Never argue, do not give the finger to anyone, for you know not what fury you might unleash. Do not even fight for the right of way with a pedestrian. Let 'em go their way, you go yours when it's safe.

The bike boom started around 1970. That's when the first edition of this book hit the market. Since that time bicycle traffic experts have entered most big- and medium-size city transportation departments and have laid out bike trails and lanes and selected safe streets for you. Check to see if your transportation department has a map detailing recommended streets for you to pedal on. Or ask your local bike shop for such a map, or your local bicycle club. Use this map to select your urban route. Look for designated bicycle lanes on city streets, marked by signs such as those shown in Fig. 2-3. Ride only on such designated routes wherever possible in your city.

Watch for escape areas: On any city street, be aware that you may have to veer away from a traffic hazard such as a city bus that comes too close to you. You need some place to go, which could be a driveway, a yard, or a sidewalk, or even shelter between parked cars.

Use a rearview mirror: Keep tabs on traffic coming from behind, as well as from the front. If, for example, you come up to a parked car and somebody opens a door in front of you, you could be in for some dental work. So be not only aware of this possibility, but also ready to evade other hazards such as a car going from a parked position, or from a driveway, out into the road. You need to know, always, if it is safe for you to veer farther out into the car lane to escape such hazards. You could glance back over your left shoulder, but that interferes with forward vision, so this is not a safe practice. The solution: Install a rearview mirror on your handlebar end. I recommend a mirror that goes directly into your bar end, because the kind that is on a stalk wobbles too much and distorts your vision. Or use a rearview mirror attached to your glasses or to your helmet. *Caution:* Use any rearview mirror only to see what is behind you. *Do not rely on the rearview mirror to tell you how far behind a vehicle is or how fast it is coming up to you.* Be aware that a rearview mirror gives you only monocular vision, and that it takes two eyes, binocular vision, to sense speed and distance of an approaching object. I learned this the hard way on a city street in Chicago, many years ago. My bike mirror told me there was a car behind me. The car looked small, even for the VW it was. So I assumed it was safe to veer out into the street to avoid a pothole. Within a second that little car also had to veer out into the street to avoid hitting me, and it passed with much honking and screaming from the driver. Look at Table 2-1. You will see that a car moving at the moderate speed of 35 mph covers 51.3 feet *a second!* In just one or two seconds that car could be right on top of you. Again, never trust your rearview mirror for anything but object identification, not for its speed or distance from you.

More about parked cars: Do not cycle a city street where parked cars are *not* allowed, unless that street has a striped and dedicated bike lane at least four feet wide to keep traffic away from you. Bike-enlightened communities go further. They install free-standing cone-shaped concrete bumps about eight feet apart that cars would have to hump painfully over or, better and safer, a continuous concrete berm (like a free-standing curb) that really does bar all but the very drunk or insane driver from your safe lane.

Watch for road hazards that could dump you off your bicycle: Look out for open drains, usually near the curb (Fig. 2-4), that can swallow your front tire and cause you to pitch head first over the handlebars (bikers call this an "endo"). Your city should weld bars over these open grates so your wheel won't sink into these traps. By now most cities have safety-welded these openings. However, don't count on it. If you see a grated opening in the street ahead don't wait until you are right on it to steer around it. Even if there are bars welded across the grate, the sudden uneven bumps could still dump you, especially on a rainy day; steer away from all grates.

FIG. 2-4: Always scan the road ahead so you can avoid storm drain grates near curbs. They can trap your front wheel, bring you to a sudden stop, and propel you over the handlebars.

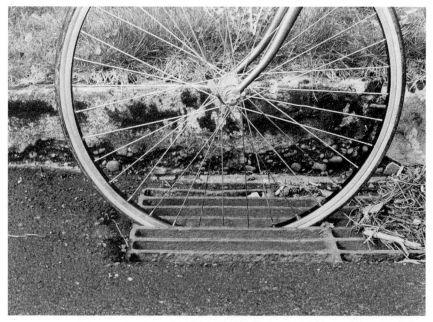

Other road hazards include snow, ice, and wet leaves in the fall. Snow is not as slippery as ice. You get a bit more traction on it than on sheet ice. Wet leaves are hazardous because you may not see them in time or may dismiss them as a danger. If you must ride on snow, use bicycle tire chains, available from your bike shop.

You can't avoid every bump. Learn how to take a bump with maximum comfort to you and minimum harm to your tires. If you watch the road, you know when a bump is coming up that you can't avoid. As you approach the bump, have both pedals flat, so cranks are parallel to the ground, as shown in Fig. 2-5. Here the rider has his weight off the saddle and is absorbing the

FIG. 2-5: Keep both pedals flat and your weight over the rear wheel on fast down-hill runs.

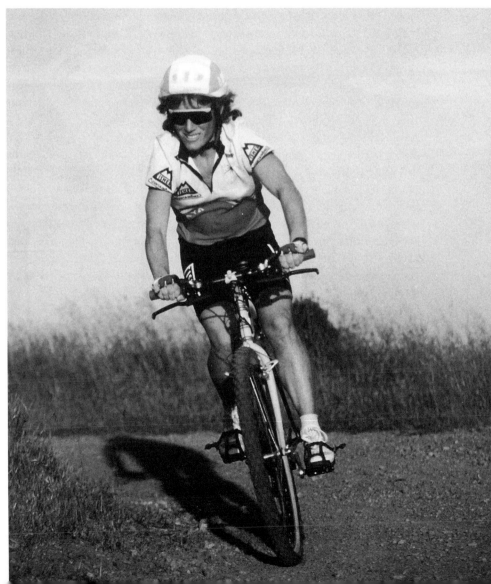

road shock with his legs and arms. The bike in this picture is an all-terrain model, so the posture is more exaggerated than what you'd do on a road bike.

Cross railroad tracks and bridge expansion joints and enter the inch- to two-inch rise of a driveway at as close to a right angle as safety permits. If you hit these objects at a shallow angle your front wheel can be twisted out of your grip and the bike, or you, can fall. If, to avoid traffic, you have to steer off the road and drop down an inch or two onto a shoulder, particularly a gravel shoulder, slow down and steer at a right angle toward the pavement before you venture back onto the road, after first, of course, checking vehicle traffic. As you hit the dropoff, apply lots of muscle power as you clamber back onto the pavement. It would be a tad unhealthy to get stuck halfway up the lip of the pavement, come to a stop, and fall over into traffic.

Make yourself visible to motorists at any time of the day or night! The U.S. Consumer Products Safety Commission requires that bicycles be equipped with reflectors in four different places: on the pedals, on the front and rear of the bicycle, and on each wheel. Do not remove these reflectors. They shine brightly from the lights of a car at night and tell the driver a bike is out there.

However, do not depend on reflectors alone to make you visible to motorists at night. Excellent blinking and solid rear lights are made by VistaLite (Fig. 2-6), NiteRider, and Turbo-Cat, to name a few. These firms also make powerful halogen beam headlights with clamps for mounting on your handlebars. The lights are powered by a rechargeable battery, which either fits in a water bottle cage or is frame-suspended. Most have a light time of three hours on the high beam and six hours on the low beam. Jogalite makes a tiny but highly visible little light that screws down over your tire valve. As the wheel turns this light becomes a highly visible circular light. These lights are available from your bicycle shop. Most states require bicyclists to have rear and front lights on their bicycle when out riding in reduced visibility, such as at dawn or dusk and at night. However, and you will find this out fairly quickly for yourself, motorists seem to take more risks on their hurried way to work and on the way home. So be extra careful during the rush hours. As for dense fog, I have only four words to say to you, *don't ride in it!* If your bike shop does not have these products, contact the manufacturer directly for a dealer near you. VistaLite is at 2950 Old Tree Drive, Lancaster, PA 17603-1287; NiteRider at 8151 Balboa Ave., San Diego, CA 92111; Turbo-Cat at 2669 Castillo Circle, Thousand Oaks, CA 91360-1302, phone 1-800-869-7618; Jogalite at P.O. Box 125, Silver Lake, NH 03875 (also for defensive dog sprays and the Dog Dazer electronic dog repeller, and reflective safety vests).

As an aside, here's a funny story. I used to think that you could not be too visible at night. Well, I was right, except at the Christmas holiday season. I had moved the brilliant little quartz blinking lights from the front to the back of a road worker's safety vest. As I pedaled through Chicago's busy shopping

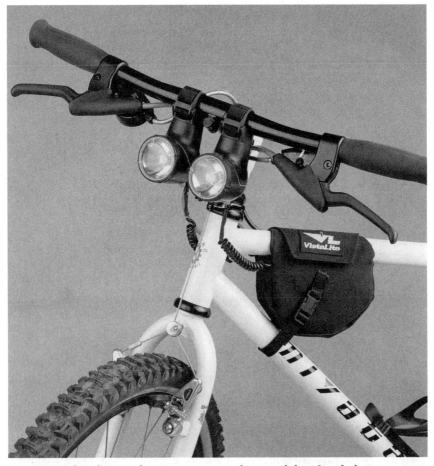

FIG. 2-6: Lights, front and rear, are a must when you bike after dark. Many states and most European countries require them. You can switch these VistaLites from powerful quartz, when you need more light, to a battery-saving but still highly visible beam. Rechargeable batteries are shown here strapped to the top and down tubes.

districts one Christmas weeknight with the vest blinking brightly away, I wondered why motorists zoomed up and drove too close to me for comfort. Suddenly it came to me. They wondered why on earth a Christmas tree was riding a bicycle. I did get a lot of comments. At any other time of the year I would have been just another visible guy on a bike.

Day and night wear a reflective vest (Fig. 2-7). Excellent vests of this kind are made by Jogalite. Friends who see me on the road wearing this vest tell me I am much more visible than bikers who do not wear one. After all, you see road workers and crossing guards so equipped, so you should be too. In addition to the lights and the vest, you can stick little self-adhering reflective

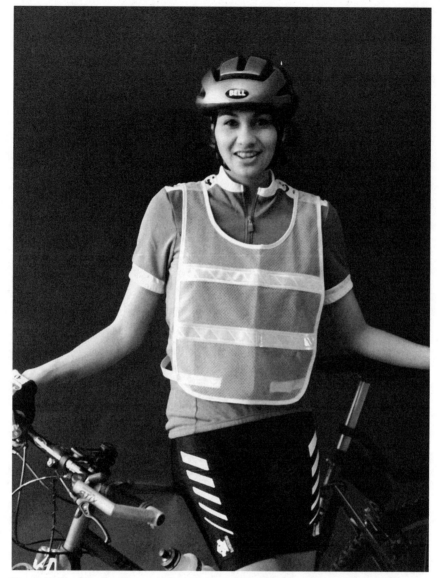

FIG. 2-7: Road workers wear reflective vests for a good reason. So they can be seen. You should wear one, like this Jogalite version, during the day and especially at night.

dots on your helmet, bike pack, water bottle, and clothes. They are made by Jogalite, so should be available from your bike shop. Reflective wear is also made by Nathan & Company, 7 North St., Pittsfield, MA 01202.

Obey all traffic regulations, because they apply equally to bicycles and to motor vehicles. Wait until the traffic light has turned in your favor before crossing an intersection, but watch out for a driver trying to beat the yellow or red light. Some of the newer traffic light signals have more sensitive sensors embedded in the road, so that even a bicycle can trigger the light to turn green.

Use conventional hand signals (Fig. 2-8). These were in use before motor vehicles were equipped with turn signals, and all drivers were required to use them. Your hand signals warn motorists, other cyclists, and pedestrians that you are going to change direction, slow, or stop. Teach your children to use these signals.

City Street Smarts: Coping with Traffic

As long as you obey traffic regulations, you have as much right to the road as any other vehicle, motorized or not. Sure, you are more vulnerable without three or four thousand pounds of nonrenewable fossil fuel guzzler to protect you. But otherwise, the road belongs to you as much as it does to the Rolls-Royce, BMW, Chevy, or pickup truck that competes with you for space. Keep this adjuration in mind as we go into city street survival competition. Drivers can be aggressive, but they can also be quite considerate. Use these nonverbal communication techniques to tame folks in four-wheeled beasties:

1. Make eye contact, nod, and smile.
2. If the motorist waits while you cross in front of the car at an intersection, wave your thank-you. That driver will feel better about cyclists in the future. And you'll feel better, too.
3. Never get into an argument with a driver. Keep calm. Do nothing to anger any motorist or anyone else. Life is short enough as it is. Don't risk it to massage your ego. Engulf drivers with your charm.

FIG. 2-8: Signal your intentions so other cyclists and car drivers know what you are about to do. Left hand out for a left turn; left hand up for a right turn; left hand down for slowing or stopping.

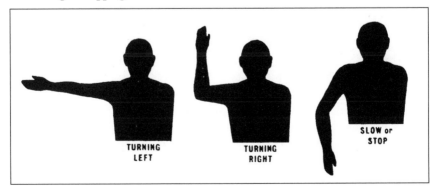

Safe Street Crossing and Turning Techniques

Two-Lane Road, at a Stoplight

To go straight ahead to cross the intersection when the light turns green, move to the center of the traffic lane (Fig. 2-9). That way you will be visible to drivers from all directions. You can accelerate across the intersection about as fast as a car. Once across, move back into the right side of the road (A), where it is safest. If you hug the curb at a stoplight and take off from that position you will be in a driver's blind spot. If the car turns right when you move straight ahead from the curb location, you could be hit, if not by that car then by the next right-turning vehicle. If you wait until all the cars behind you have turned right, the stoplight could by then have turned green.

To turn left at a two-lane intersection: Stay in the center of the right vehicle lane and make your left turn when you have the green, as if you were a car (B in Fig. 2-9). Get back to the right side of the road as soon as possible.

Four-Lane Turns

To turn left from a four-lane road or a dedicated "must turn left" lane: Get into the left lane, as a car would (Fig. 2-10). When you have the green, barrel across and cut to the right side of the new road.

On City Bike Trails: A Mix of Traffic

Various civil engineering, road, and bike trail designers have very specific recommendations regarding warning signs and trail widths. *Be aware that the lack of such signage does not necessarily mean that no hazard exists. All too often this simply means that the trail designers and trail maintenance authorities were negligent.* Here are a few of the types and locations of signs, and other trail design criteria.

From the International City Management Association, 1140 Connecticut Ave., Washington, DC 20036, "Management Information Service Report," April 1973, vol. 5, page 21, "Recommendations Regarding Bike Way Signage: "Warning signs informing bicyclists of potential hazards require the following specifications: Along bike paths and for all hazardous conditions on bike lanes or bike routes for which there are no existing signs, specific bicycle directed warning signs should be erected. In order to provide specific response time, these should be positioned not less than 50 feet in advance of the condition toward which they are directed."

From the 1988 *Bicycle Forum,* published by BikeCentennial, P.O. Box

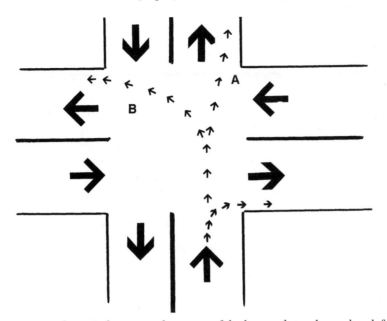

FIG. 2-9: On a two-lane road, move to the center of the lane and signal to make a left or right turn. Be bold about this. Remember, you can scoot across these turns about as fast as a car and you have just as much right to be in the center of the lane as a car does.

FIG. 2-10: On a four-lane road or from a designated left-turn-only lane, again, get into the center of the lane, make your turn quickly, and get back to the right of a two-lane road as soon as possible.

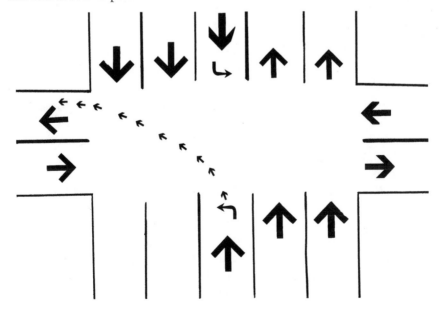

8308, Missoula, MT 59807: "Let's say a bicyclist is riding on a newly finished recreational bike path. The path has an asphalt surface and follows an abandoned railroad right-of-way. It's late in the day and the bicyclist is trying to get to the nearest town before darkness sets in. As he approaches an intersection with a crossroad, he collides with a barrier. The barrier had been placed across the path to keep unauthorized motor vehicles out; it has a three-foot-wide opening to allow bikes to get through. The barrier is painted dark brown, which blends with the dark background of the asphalt. When the path was built the 1981 AASHTO Guide gave this advice: 'bicycle paths need some form of physical barrier at highway intersections to prevent unauthorized motor vehicles from using the facilities. The barriers should be permanently reflectorized for nighttime visibility and painted a bright color for improved daytime visibility.' "

From the "Manual on Uniform Traffic Control Devices" (MUTC) published by the Federal Highway Administration: "Signs should be used more extensively to alert bicyclists to the presence of hazards that might cause loss of control, such as bridge grates, rough pavement or manholes." The MUTC provides for a Hazardous Condition Sign (W8-10), a yellow on black warning sign and supplemental plaques which describe the hazards.

If you ride on an off-road city-designed bike trail, in a city park, be aware that these trails may have danger spots because they may have been designed by noncyclist engineers. A degree in civil engineering does not necessarily translate to hands-on bicycle experience. *If you ride on any trail that you consider hazardous, you should notify the responsible public agency.* Here is what to look for:

1. *Sudden changes in trail width without posted warning signs:* Be careful when you go down a hill, especially where the trail makes a turn at the bottom. As an expert witness I had one tragic case in which the trail designer did not post signs warning that the trail narrowed from 12 to 8 feet at the bottom of a steep hill. The cyclist could not make the turn where the trail narrowed, veered too far to the right, struck the steel uprights of a guard rail, and lost the use of her right arm.

2. *Impeded visibility around curves, without posted warning signs for both directions:* I have cycled on bike trails on which visibility on a turn was blocked by shrubbery or trees. As I approached one such turn, in Cape Cod National Park, a group of kids came tearing around the bend, occupying the full width of the lane. We would have collided if I had not been cautious enough to stay on the last right-hand inch of the trail so I could squeeze by them. Collisions with other bicyclists, skaters, and pedestrians are not unusual on such poorly designed trails.

3. *A trail intersecting a highway:* There should be signs warning motorists of this trail crossing, but don't count on the signs being present or drivers observing them.

4. *A gravel trail crossing a paved sidewalk:* Go slow where such a trail crosses a paved path. You could spill on the pavement if, as often happens, rain and wind blow gravel over the sidewalk. Loose gravel on a paved surface can cause you to skid, especially if you have to make a turn at that point.

5. *Other bicyclists, particularly children or reckless teenagers, pedestrians, and skaters:* A well-designed trail, shared by bicyclists, skaters, runners, and pedestrians, should have a double yellow stripe down its middle that warns trail users to stay to their right of that line. The trail should be at least four feet on both sides of the line. Places where a clifflike dropoff exists should be fenced. Use a tinkle bell or other horn, such as Jogalite's Megahorn, to alert others of your presence. As you come up to the trail user shout "Passing on your left." But be aware that, as often happens to me, well-meaning people can abruptly move to the left as you pass. Slow until you are sure that they have moved out of your way before you pass them.

Group Riding Precautions

Keep at least one full bike length between you and the riders in front and to your rear. The reason: The bike ahead may make a sudden stop, brake to avoid a road hazard, or just decide to slow down for no reason. I've had kids behind me run their front wheel into my rear derailleur, which totaled it. At worst two or more of you could lose control and fall. So keep your distance. I know, I know, you have watched bicycle racers following within inches of each other and seen and heard an explanation of "drafting," which is where the rider up front serves as a windbreaker for the following rider and so makes it easier for that rider. Wind resistance is the second-greatest force resisting forward movement on a bicycle. The greatest resistance is gravity on uphill climbs. But don't draft unless you are an experienced cyclist willing to risk a crash, *and the cyclist in front of you knows you are drafting.*

Country Roads

Whether you are just out for a day ride or on a long-distance trip, be careful about the roads you select. Ideally they should have a yellow or white fog line separating the vehicle lane from the breakdown lane. The breakdown lane should be at least four feet wide, which gives vehicles room to clear and pass you safely. Cycle on the breakdown lane, of course.

Unfortunately, very few rural roads have such a breakdown lane. Most have a narrow, inches-wide strip on which you can ride and pray passing traffic sees and goes around you. If there is a shoulder, it is most likely to be gravel. The paved roadbed itself is often an inch or two higher than the gravel shoulder. This "lip" of an inch or two or even more is where you can come to grief, particularly if your bike has skinny, high-pressure road tires. The knobby tread on a mountain bike will grip the dropoff from pavement to gravel more firmly, but you still have to be careful. Go off the road onto the gravel at as close to a right angle to the lip as possible. As you descend onto the gravel, apply moderate braking power to slow without skidding. If the lip is an inch or less, get back on the road when traffic is clear by powering up to the lip at a right angle. As you approach it pull up hard on the handlebars and bunny hop back onto the paved road. Stop and walk the bike onto the road if the lip is higher than an inch. You will be coming off slippery gravel and you could fall over into traffic.

Hill Safety

On a hill climb, stay as far to the right of the road as possible as you approach the top. A vehicle coming up the other side of the hill toward you cannot see you coming up the hill any more than you can see it coming toward you. The reverse holds true on a downhill run. As you start down a hill also stay to the right because a car driver behind you, speeding over the crest, cannot see you going down the hill in front. Approaches to a hill crest, and going over it, are two danger points for cyclists on any road.

Safe braking: Keep speed under control as you descend, particularly when the road ahead twists and turns. It is hazardous to round a curve at 40-plus mph and come upon a stalled logging truck, or hit a serious pothole before you can swerve or stop. Apply the rear brake first, then the front brake. That way you avoid locking up the front wheel, which could dump you over the handlebars or cause you to skid to one side or the other. Make this brake test while you are safely at home. Place a book flat on the table. Put one hand in front of the book so it can't slide. Then push the book with your other hand. You will see that the end you push tends to rise off the table, while the end you are holding tends to dig into it. Keep this little scenario in mind as you brake your bike. If you grab the front brake first your rear wheel tends to rise off the ground. The front brake gives you some 80 percent of the braking power of both brakes. So on a downhill run move your body back over the rear wheel as far as possible to keep your rear wheel on the ground. Use your rear brake first, or for a longer time, before you apply the front brake. In a panic stop, always apply both brakes simultaneously, don't rely solely on the rear brake. On any road, remember that if it's raining or you are riding over snow, water on your wheel rims is a lubricant that cuts your braking power drastically. Practice braking on a rainy day so you see for yourself how seriously water reduces your ability to stop. Brake well before you would on a dry day, so you can stop in time at a street crossing, stop light, or stop sign. Be especially cautious about braking on a tandem. Tandems, with two aboard, are a lot heavier than a single bike. Gravity can speed your tandem up to 50 mph or even faster. Modern tandems have better brakes than single bikes, but even so, keep speed under control when you are breezing downhill. Use bicycle tire chains on both wheels of any bicycle if you have to cycle over snow or ice.

On a downhill run, keep your bike from wobbling by gripping the top tube between your knees. This may prevent wheel shimmy if your bike is so inclined. (There is more about the causes and cures of wheel shimmy later in this chapter.)

As you approach a hill, shift to a lower gear before starting your climb. If you delay shifting until the going is hard, you may find it difficult or impossible to shift to a more favorable gear. You may either have to ease off pedaling pressure by steering from one side of the road to the other and back again (not the safest of procedures) or stop, lift the back wheel, twirl the pedals, shift down, and start up again. Manufacturers of the latest wide-range derailleur systems claim you can shift while climbing steep hills. My experience tells me otherwise.

One hazard of shifting while hill climbing is that the chain may not shift accurately, so it lies partly on one gear and partly on another. In such a case the chain may not grab the teeth of the rear or front cogs and may slip. If the chain slips while you are exerting pedal pressure, the pedal may slip forward and you could very well lose your balance and fall off the bike, or inadvertently steer into another cyclist or into a vehicle.

Mount a Bike Safely

The best way to take off on a bike is to straddle the bike, put one foot on a pedal, into the pedal clips (keep the strap loose), or into the shoe lock on a clipless pedal. Then pull the pedal up to about the two-o'clock position. Push down hard on that pedal and at the same time shove the bike forward with your other foot, which will get you up into the saddle and get the bike moving forward. Once you get moving, coast for a second, move the other pedal to around the six-o'clock position, slip your foot into or onto the other pedal, and take off. *Keep your eye peeled for traffic while you are in the takeoff mode.* If you mount "macho" style, by standing next to the bike, putting one foot on a pedal to take off, and, while coasting ahead, swing the other leg and your body up over the top tube, you will be poorly balanced as you start off, and could lose control.

"Slick" Tires

"Slick" or totally bald tires come in sizes to fit both road and all-terrain bicycles. Manufacturers claim that because the tires have no tread at all, but instead have a smooth layer of rubber, they grip the road better than tires with tread, because there's more rubber on the road. I'm not sure where this story will end. All I can say right now is that at least one serious injury has occurred to a cyclist whose bike slid sideways on his first ride with the slicks. He had changed from knobby tires on his mountain bike to the bald tires. On his first sharp turn, the rear wheel skidded and the bike fell. He had been making the same turn, on the same road, with the same bike, but equipped with knobby tires, for years.

Try Not to Use Your Brakes as You Make a Turn

On a turn, your bike will be at more of an angle to the ground than it was when you were going straight. There will be greater side forces on the tire's contact patch with the ground. If the ground is at all slippery (gravel, wet leaves, and so forth) and you brake, these side forces could dump the bike on its side. Be especially wary of braking around sharp curves at high speed. Slow before you come to the turn if you're not sure of the slipperiness of the ground or what is around the curve.

Keep the pedal opposite the turn at the 6-o'clock position, or keep both pedals parallel to the top tube (see Fig. 2-5). It is easy to dump your bike if the pedal closest to the ground becomes a lever that takes you airborne on a sharp turn. Make this automatic. If you have to think about it, it could be too late.

Sideview Mirrors Can Hit You!

Keep an eye out for Winnebagos and other recreational vehicles and trucks with extended sideview mirrors projecting from their right side (Fig. 2-11). Cyclists have been killed or seriously injured when struck by these mirrors as the RV passes by. A huge 40-plus-foot-long recreational vehicle (RV) may be driven by an older driver without any qualifying training to steer these monsters. Truck drivers who drive semis have to take special training and pass rigorous driving exams. I worry about the depth perception and reaction time of older drivers at all times when I am out

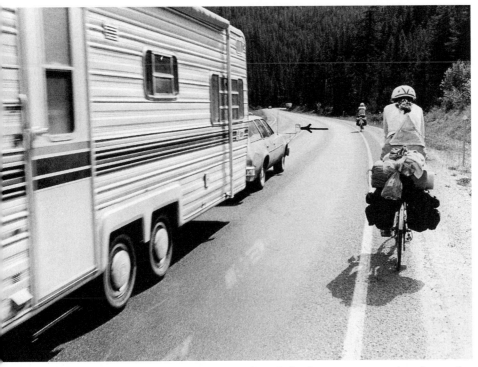

FIG. 2-11: Watch out for RVs coming from behind you. Be aware that their right-side projecting sideview mirror could hit you.

on a bike, and especially worry when I see a fat, wide, road-hogging RV coming up behind me.

Look for Escape Routes

Keep your eyes peeled at all times, on any road or trail, for an escape route. You never know when you may need to take it.

Practice Using Toe Clips and Clipless Pedals

A few years ago I was asked to write an owner's manual for a well-known European manufacturer of pedal toe clips and straps. It seems that new cyclists did not know how to get their feet into and out of pedals with clips and straps and were getting hurt. It happened to me way back in 1968 when I was a novice bike commuter in Detroit. I did what so many novices do even today, pulled the toe straps tight and took off. At the very first stoplight, on one of Detroit's busiest downtown intersections, I braked, came to a stop, tried to remove my locked feet from the pedals, could not, and fell ingloriously and embarrassingly over to the side. After that I kept the toe straps loose when on city streets, tightened them only on country rides.

Toe clips are a safety device because they keep your feet on the pedals even with the straps loose, so your feet won't slip forward off the pedals when pushing hard for speed or on a hill climb. They let you *pull* the pedal up from the six-o'clock position to the top of the pedal stroke while, at the same time, you can *push* the other pedal down with the other foot from the top to the bottom of the pedal stroke. So clips and straps can add as much as 30 percent to your pedaling efficiency, because you can apply power to the pedals through 360 degrees. If you are turned off by the idea of clamping your feet onto pedals, use a clipless pedal attachment such as that made by Campagnolo, which with a platform (flat plate) can be installed on all but clipless pedals.

Using Toe Clips and Straps

1. Straddle your bike. Move one pedal to the seven-o'clock position. Put your foot on that pedal, into the toe clip, with toe straps loose. Pull that pedal up to the two-o'clock position. Now do three things at once: Push down hard on that pedal and at the same time, with your other foot still on the ground, push forward so both actions get the bike moving. As you do so, hoist yourself onto the saddle.
2. Move the other pedal to the seven-o'clock position and insert the toe of your other foot into it, just as you did as you took off. Now you are moving the bike forward and can use both pedals.
3. To remove your foot from one pedal, tilt your heel upward. Your toe should be pointing down. The toe strap should be loose. Pull your foot up and back with a quick snappy motion. Once your foot is off the pedal, brake, extend the free foot toward the ground, and come to a safe stop. After stopping, pull your other foot off the pedal, out of the toe clips, the same way.

Using Clipless Pedals

If you have clipless pedals, adjust the shoe retention and disengagement force with an Allen wrench so it is the same for both ends of both pedals. Make adjustments on both ends of the pedal (Fig. 2-12—see Chapter 6 for more instructions). Otherwise your foot on the weaker engagement pedal could come off that pedal, with possible loss of control. *Be sure to use shoes, shoe cleats, and pedals that are compatible. Shoes, cleats, and pedals of different makes, for example, may not match, and your foot may come out of or off the pedal unexpectedly.* Practice using these pedals in two steps:

1. Straddle the bicycle. Keep one foot on the ground. Press the shoe cleat of your other foot into the clipless pedal while you apply the brakes (Fig. 2-13). Remove that foot from the pedal by twisting your heel to the outside, away from the bicycle (Fig. 2-14). Repeat this until you are sure you know how to get your foot into and out of these pedals. Do it with your other foot, and keep practicing until foot (shoe) insertion and removal become second nature.
2. Now ride on a safe, level place, such as an empty school playground, and again insert and remove each foot, one at a time, until this step becomes easy, natural, and automatic.

Adjust the spring tension as noted above so you can get your foot onto and off the pedals easily. If you ride where you need to stop and start a lot, use less spring tension. On rural roads or off-road, you can keep more spring tension. (See Chapter 6 for cleat adjustments for your clipless pedal shoes.)

"Float" means lateral rotation, which gives you some free-floating movement of your foot. Road-racing cyclists don't want any because float wastes energy. However, the rest of us do need some float because the foot moves a bit laterally as the pedal rotates. At one part of pedal rotation your foot may,

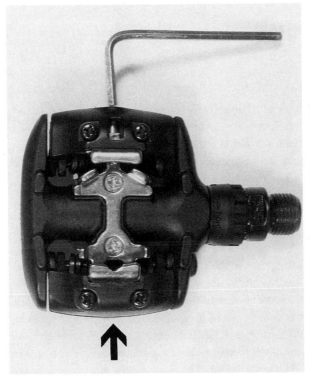

FIG. 2-12: On clipless pedals, adjust the shoe retention force with an Allen wrench, as shown, so you can get your feet easily out of and into these pedals.

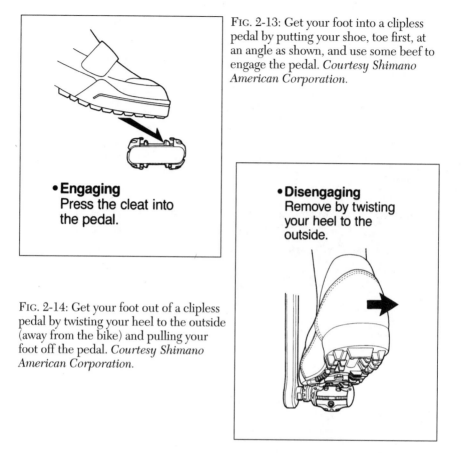

FIG. 2-13: Get your foot into a clipless pedal by putting your shoe, toe first, at an angle as shown, and use some beef to engage the pedal. *Courtesy Shimano American Corporation.*

• **Engaging**
Press the cleat into the pedal.

• **Disengaging**
Remove by twisting your heel to the outside.

FIG. 2-14: Get your foot out of a clipless pedal by twisting your heel to the outside (away from the bike) and pulling your foot off the pedal. *Courtesy Shimano American Corporation.*

for example, want to move a bit toward the bike frame. In another position, it may want to move away from the bike frame. If your foot can't do this, you could develop knee problems because a rigid, nonfloating pedal system forces your knees to move laterally instead. Float is the nonadjustable part of clipless pedal design. Pedals with float include those made by Shimano, Time, and Look.

Take Your Kids Along Safely

There are two ways to transport your small children on a bike trip.

First, you can use a sturdy child seat attached to the back of your bicycle (Fig. 2-15). The seat should have restraining straps to hold the child safely and side guards to keep little feet out of turning spokes. These seats are OK for short trips, but for longer rides a trailer is more comfortable for both rider and child, and much safer. A child seat puts the load up high, which makes the bicycle harder to balance and steer. The load will be unbalanced, over

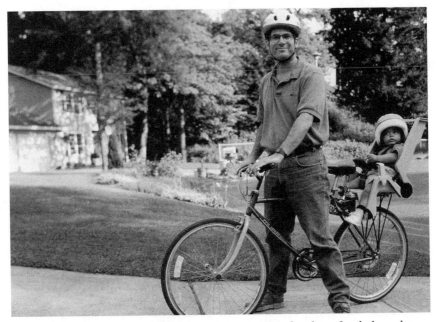

FIG. 2-15: Carry a child in a sturdy child carrier equipped with a safety belt, as shown, made by Rhode.

the rear wheel, which reduces the load on the front wheel and creates the possibility of front-wheel shimmy, as noted elsewhere in this chapter. Also, a child seat puts the passenger up high and in a fall the kiddie could hit hard.

A safer way is to carry children in a bicycle trailer. This way the load is off the bicycle and down closer to the ground. You can also carry camping gear in the trailer, along with the child, or carry two children.

Use care making turns when towing a trailer. Turn as wide as safety permits, go slow while you do it. Here are trailers I have checked and can recommend.

CycleTote (Fig. 2-16) makes an excellent trailer. It hitches to the seat post and has an inert-gas-welded frame of sturdy aluminum tubing, roll bars, and a well-designed five-point harness for a child from infancy to age five. See-through plastic panels let your child see the surrounding world and keep little fingers away from spokes. The CycleTote also comes with a nylon canopy for rainy days and a window with nylon netting that keeps insects from bugging your passengers. I like the CycleTote's low center of gravity, about four inches below the wheel axles, which reduces the likelihood of a pitchover on a sharp turn. Possibly best of all, the CycleTote has optional drum brakes, which are automatically actuated when you apply your bike brakes. When you brake, the forward momentum of the trailer pushes a rod on the trailer hitch backward, which then actuates the trailer brakes through brake cables.

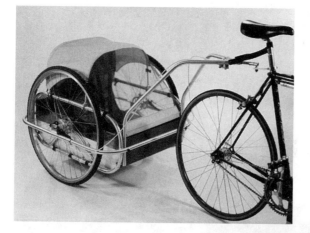

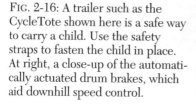

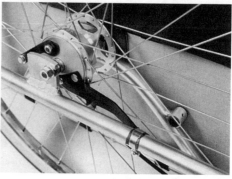

FIG. 2-16: A trailer such as the CycleTote shown here is a safe way to carry a child. Use the safety straps to fasten the child in place. At right, a close-up of the automatically actuated drum brakes, which aid downhill speed control.

These brakes are a major safety feature because they help you keep speed under control on downhill runs and when coming to an emergency stop. The wheels use the same size 700C tires and tubes as your road bike, so you won't need one size of spare tubes for the trailer and another size for your bike. The CycleTote lists for $380. Add $210 for the brakes, an investment in safety which I highly recommend. Contact CycleTote directly, at 1-303-482-2401, FAX 1-303-482-2402 or write them at 517 North Link Lane, Fort Collins, CO 80524.

The Burley trailer has inside pockets, an optional cover ($20), a three-point harness, and reflective tape along the back and sides. This trailer has an optional attachment for running with the trailer detached from the bicycle. It comes with a 40-inch-high flag on a plastic rod with a flag on top for highway visibility. The Burley lists for around $400. See your bike shop or contact Burley at 1-503-687-1644.

Another good trailer is the Winchester, which sports 20 by 1.75 quickly removable wheels canted inward five degrees, which reduces the possibility of rollover on a high-speed turn. The Winchester seats children facing each other, rather than side by side, which, according to Winchester, reduces bickering between the kids. It comes with a four-window canopy and is narrower than the other trailers. The Winchester lists for around $360. See your bike shop or contact Winchester at 1-714-738-4973.

Bicycling on Interstate Highways

Your first reaction to biking on interstate highways or freeways would be the same as mine, the first time I contemplated doing it. "No way!" Until, that is, you want to cross the mountains of the west United States, or travel in the western states. In these parts of this country noninterstate highways (state or county roads) may not go where you want to go, or may be snow-covered and unplowed at high altitudes. Or, if there are roads, they may be too narrow to be safe, with no shoulders for cyclists to escape passing cars, pickup trucks, logging trucks, or camp trailers. To cross the mountains of the West, an interstate highway may be the only route, or the safest one.

In many states, cycling on the shoulder of an interstate highway is illegal. In some states, such as California, Oregon, and Washington, it is legal to ride on the shoulder of many interstate highways, except near big cities, where there are alternative roads. The traffic on interstate highways near cities such as Portland or Seattle is too dense for safety.

Given a choice between bicycling on narrow roads shared by kids driving pickup trucks and bicycling on the shoulder of an interstate, I prefer the interstate. I see many bicyclists on Washington and Oregon interstate routes I-205 and I-5 (Figs. 2-17 and 2-18), for example, going both north and south, headed for Canada or California or someplace in between. The shoulder of many interstate highways is a nice, comfortable 10 feet wide. It's paved and usually smooth and free of debris. If you ride on the right side of the shoulder you have a good eight feet between you and the nearest vehicle. The hills of interstate highways are usually far less steep than those on two-lane side roads. There are reasonably spaced rest stops for calls of nature, and there are generous, landscaped places to stop to lunch without leaving the highway.

Here are a few safety tips for cycling on interstate highways.

Never ride on freeways at night! Bright lights and reflectors and a good taillight do not mean a fatigue-dulled driver won't wander onto the shoulder where you are. That could happen during the day, too, of course, but if you keep a careful watch for traffic behind you, you can see a meandering driver and ride off the shoulder onto the landscaping, if necessary, to escape. In some five years of cycling on interstate highways I have yet to come nearly as close to being hit by a vehicle as I have been when cycling on other roads.

Be aware of the push-pull effect of big trucks! Big trucks push a bubble of air in front of them, which tends to push you to the right as the truck ap-

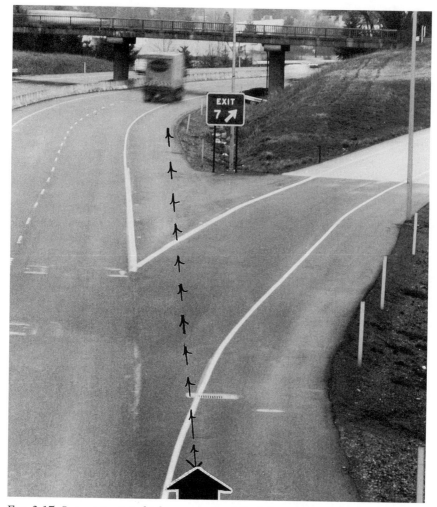

FIG. 2-17: Some interstate highways are legal for bikers. If you ride on one, watch out for cars behind you that want to use the exit ramp. Stop at the arrow (bottom) before the exit ramp, as shown here. When traffic has cleared, get across the exit area as fast as you can.

proaches you. The truck then creates a partial vacuum behind it as it displaces air, which pulls you to the left. Such displacement is known in physics as the "Bernoulli effect." Once aware of this effect, which is usually quite mild, I found it easy to counteract by leaning a bit to the left as the truck approached and a bit to the right after it passed. This push-pull effect, however, can dump you if it's compounded by high winds from any direction. Still, I have found that the suction effect of big trucks actually pulled me along no matter which way the wind was blowing. When I was cycling into a stiff headwind, big trucks always turned the wind around or reduced its in-

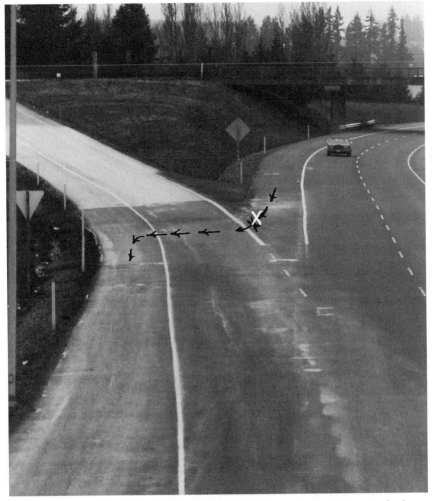

FIG. 2-18: *Stop* at the white X in this photo, before you cross an interstate highway on-ramp. When there is no traffic coming up the on-ramp, pedal fast across it and proceed down the shoulder as before.

tensity as they passed. There are so many trucks on the highway that I nearly always found my way eased by them when the wind was not going my way. This push-pull effect isn't limited to trucks on interstate highways; it applies to any big truck or camper on any road.

Be especially cautious as you approach on- and off-ramps! As you come to an off-ramp, where traffic on your left may exit and cross in front of you, you *must* stop. Do *not* depend on a rearview mirror to check how far away or how fast traffic is coming up from behind you. Traffic is *always* going faster than you think it is. Take a look at Table 2-1. You can see that from a block away a vehicle traveling 75 miles per hour takes only 2.5 seconds to reach you. You could never get out of the way fast enough if you decided to beat it across the intersecting off-ramp. Even if you were pushing 20 mph, it would still take you two full seconds to go 15 feet, and that's just cutting it too darned close. Wait, you're worth it.

As you approach an exit ramp (Fig. 2-17), stop (arrow), and look back. *Only* when you are positive that traffic coming in the right lane is not going to exit should you proceed across the ramp. If you see an oncoming vehicle with right turn signal blinking, of course you know enough to stop and let it turn off before you cross the ramp. It's the cars that exit from the freeway without a turn signal I worry about. Hundreds of times I have looked back at five miles of straight road, on a clear day, to see a car three or four blocks away. By the time I counted off 10 seconds, that car would be right next to me. Even a quarter of a mile away, a car going 70 miles per hour will be next to me in 13 seconds. Practice counting the seconds it takes for a car that you think is far enough away so you can cross the exit ramp safely to reach you, should that car exit as you cross the ramp. It won't take long until you can estimate, with a comfortable margin of safety, how long you have to get across that ramp before a vehicle that's coming down the highway would be in the exit ramp.

Interstate highway on-ramps (Fig. 2-18) are a little safer for the bicyclist than exit ramps. This is because you don't have to cross an exit ramp the long way, parallel to the traffic, and because vehicles will be moving more slowly than if they were on the highway. As Fig. 2-18 shows, what you do is stop at the point where the on-ramp merges with the highway (at the white X). When the on-ramp is clear (when you see no cars on the ramp), simply take a straight cut to the right, across the ramp, and turn left down the ramp's shoulder. You can then safely merge with the highway shoulder, at the base of the on-ramp.

One final note about interstate highways. If you plan to use them, it's advisable to check with your state Department of Transportation to make sure you can legally do so. Then, check again with the state highway patrol. I was stopped by a Washington state highway patrol officer recently and told I had to get off Interstate Highway 205, because "it was illegal for me to be cycling on the shoulder of that road." I did not argue. The next day I called the Washington State Department of Transportation, which assured me that it was legal. At my request they sent me correspondence between the DOT and the state police headquarters, together with a bicycle map of the entire state interstate road system, showing where bicycling was legal and where not on these highways. Then I wrote a letter to the chief of the Washington state highway patrol, and sent copies to the governor, my state senator, the officer that stopped me, and his boss, the lieutenant of his barracks, together with copies of this correspondence from the DOT to his department, plus my own background in bicycling. In about a week I had letters from all these people, plus a visit from the lieutenant, who was very nice about all this. As was the chief. The lieutenant said he asked his officers if they knew that it was OK for cyclists to ride on the shoulder of some 90 percent of the state's interstate highways. Half of them said it was their understanding that it is illegal to bicycle on the shoulder of any interstate highway, which documented the stories I had been getting from local bike shops and bicyclists. Seems the police had been routinely stopping and ordering cyclists off the freeways. I am sure many long-distance cyclists had their plans cut short by such police action, because convenient side roads are not always available. And I have found that such side roads as are available at many off-ramps are narrow, have high-speed local traffic, have no shoulders, and are far more hazardous than the interstate highway. As I noted, however, the Washington state patrol people were most cooperative once they understood the situation. Now, here are a few specific safety tips on spills, wheel shimmy, quick-releases, dealing with combative animals, and other threatening situations.

How to Fall

Don't practice falls, but if you see you are losing control and have a split-second interval between this realization and the actual fall, you might think about how you are going to land. For example, experienced cyclists try to do a "tuck." That is, they try assume a sort of fetal (that's *f-e-t-a-l, not f-a-t-a-l*) position, with head tucked, so they land on their shoulders, absorbing road shock as a forward roll. If you land stiff-armed, with arms straight out to absorb road shock, which seems instinctive with most people, you're heading for a bad wrist sprain or a broken arm. If you aren't wearing padded bike gloves (see Chapter 9) you may lose a little skin as the palms of your hands slide on the pavement. In any event, it's vital that the one part of your body you don't want to hit the pavement first is your head!—even with a helmet. A helmet protects against abrasion and offers impact resistance. But no helmet can protect against a really hard shock.

Wheel Shimmy—How It Starts, How to Keep It from Starting

It happened to me in the Austrian Alps, halfway between Graz and Vienna. I was leading 40 Americans on a bicycle tour. We were beginning the descent of a steep mountainside. The road was long and straight, with two lanes. Coming toward us was a loaded Mercedes logging truck. On the right was an unprotected dropoff of about 1,200 feet. At about 30 miles per hour, my handlebars and front wheel suddenly began to move violently from side to side. With every turn of my wheels, the shimmy increased in amplitude (width) and frequency. Within a few seconds after the shimmy started I realized it was only going to get worse. Nothing I could do, neither gripping the handlebars nor braking nor both, could stop the shimmy from increasing in intensity. I realized I was losing control, and that the bike was going to fall over to one side or the other. I did not want to hit the logging truck. Falling 1,200 feet did not appeal to me, either. So I shifted my weight until the bike fell over, with me on top of it, and slid down my side of the road. It all happened so suddenly that the cyclists behind me had no chance to take evasive action, until after three or four of them had fallen on top of me and each other. Fortunately no one was hurt, beyond losing a little skin, here and there, which is a hazard you learn to ignore. The endorphins you earn as a hard-pedaling cyclist, however, are themselves a mild form of anesthesia. Cuts and bruises never seem to hurt as much at the time they occur as they do later on, as you soak in a hot bath or shower.

Back to wheel shimmy. At the camp, we went over my bike minutely, but could find nothing obvious that would have caused the shimmy. Finally I checked the fork blade alignment. Sure enough, one blade was slightly bent, but not enough to be noticeable. The fork blade had been bent in shipment from the United States to Austria, by the airline. I had neglected to brace the fork dropouts with a dummy axle or piece of wood to keep them from being bent in transit. I should also have braced the rear dropouts. Front-wheel shimmy is not unusual but it certainly is avoidable. Here are causes of wheel shimmy. Correcting these causes will avoid a wheel shimmy accident.

As an expert witness on bicycle accidents I have had many cases involving accidents and injuries caused by front-wheel shimmy. First, the front wheel hits a bump in the road. Then the front wheel starts to shimmy. My investigation of the causes of these accidents revealed several possible reasons for wheel shimmy.

Loose headset bearings that let the fork move erratically from side to side.

Loose wheel bearings that let the wheel move erratically from side to side.

Unevenly tensioned spokes that permit wheel wobble under load.

Unbalanced weight distribution. Heavily loaded panniers, for example, when carried over the rear wheel, reduce front-wheel ground contact, so wheel shimmy can start. To avoid this cause of wheel shimmy simply distribute the load evenly between front and rear panniers. (Please refer to Chapter 9 for data on pannier mounting, safety, and load balancing, and to the data below on practice riding with loaded panniers.) Panniers should also be securely tied down to carriers. If panniers flop around loose, the forces exerted by such flop could cause or contribute to front-wheel shimmy. If the panniers are on tight but the carriers are loose, the same thing could happen. If carrier mounting bolts are loose, a carrier strut could come loose, catch in the spokes, lock the wheel, and cause loss of control and an accident.

Every one of these hazardous situations has happened to cyclists. Check all carrier mounting bolts before every trip, and on the road, each day. Keep the load evenly balanced, with about as much weight over the rear wheel as over the front wheel.

An unbalanced front wheel. If your auto steering wheel suddenly begins to vibrate and turn a bit rapidly in one direction and then in another, you have experienced wheel shimmy. You also know that your tire dealer can remove the wheels, put them on a balancing machine, and attach weights to them, which balances the wheels and solves the shimmy problem. In a car you can slow until the shimmy stops. In a car the shimmy won't dump you out. On a bike, as I said above, a shimmy can be hazardous to life and limb. An engineer friend, Frank Branzuela of Anchorage, Alaska, writes that he suffered a violent front-wheel shimmy caused by an unbalanced front wheel. Frank noted that "front-wheel imbalance, as opposed to rear-wheel imbalance, is the more likely cause of high-speed shimmy. An imbalanced front wheel feeds cyclic forces into the fork dropouts. The fork is not part of a structural triangle, and on better road bikes, the fork can be quite springy, which will allow ever-increasing oscillations at higher speed. There is a concept called the natural frequency of a spring. If the vibration due to imbalance happens to hit the natural frequency of the fork blades, things get wild very quickly once the tire loses contact with the pavement. A slight bump is all that is required for the wheel to be free to begin oscillating. At 40 mph a 27-inch wheel rotates eight times every second, smaller wheels even faster. The point is that just one-eighth of a second off the pavement is all that is needed for the wheel to make a full free-spinning revolution. Lighter-alloy wheels are more sensitive to imbalances and so require an extra measure of precision balancing."

I have not found any machine that will detect a bicycle wheel imbalance. However, you can make your own empirical test. Check your wheel balance this way: Hang the bicycle in a repair stand or by the top tube from the ceiling. Leave the handlebars free to turn. Spin the front wheel hard. Watch the fork blades and the handlebars for movement. If you see any movement the wheel is not balanced. Spin the wheel hard again. Feel the fork blades near the dropouts. If you feel vibration there the wheel is unbalanced. Correct the imbalance by moving a reflector to the opposite side of the wheel from the valve stem. If there is a cyclometer magnet sensor attached to the spokes, move it to where it counterbalances the reflector and valve stem. On repeated spins the wheel should show no preference about where it stops. If the wheel is severely imbalanced, try moving the reflector or cyclocomputer magnet or both to a different spoke or spokes.

Frank also notes that the bicycle retailer should check wheel balance, because neither the rim nor the tire manufacturer can do so because of manufacturing sequence. The rim producer can't control the tire or tube weight imbalance nor can the tire or tube producer control the rim imbalance.

Load-Carrying Bicycles

Be aware that a fully loaded bicycle handles a lot differently than a bike that is not loaded! Steering will be sluggish. You won't be able to make quick, sharp turns. Balance will be off. The bike will seem to have a will of its own, despite your attempts at balance. Get used to this new way your bike handles by practicing riding your fully loaded bicycle before taking off down the road. (If you're a woman, and you've had a child, you know what I mean by an unbalanced situation along about the seventh or eighth month of your pregnancy.) After the first 25 miles or so you'll learn how to handle the bike, how to get on it, start off, and stop. *Be aware that braking power is drastically reduced as you load up the bike.* You'll need to get used to the greater pressure you need to exert on brake levers to control speed, and to be especially careful at speed control downhill. Keep the load as low as possible, and use low-rider carriers over the front wheel, as shown in Chapter 9.

What to Do if You Get Hurt

If you should fall off your bike and get hurt, here's what to do.

Don't be a hero and try to ride home. A friend of mine, an attorney, fell off his bike, got up, and rode home. In an hour his neck began to hurt unbearably, so his wife drove him to a hospital emergency room. X-rays revealed that he had broken his neck. This man was a weightlifter as well as a bicyclist, so he had excellent musculature, which supported his head, in a fashion, after his accident. But, had he wiggled his head the wrong way just once, his spinal column could easily have been severed and he would have been an instant paraplegic or quadriplegic. He's fine today, but it was a close call.

If you dump and fall off your bike, don't assume you're OK. You may be fine, but you can't be sure. A hard impact on an unyielding surface such as cement can shake up the best of minds. You may very well be seriously injured and not know it. If you're in the line of traffic, crawl out of it if you can. Better, have someone help you. If you're not in a traffic lane, lie still until the paramedics come and take you to the hospital.

Try to get the names, addresses, and phone numbers of witnesses. Or have someone else do it for you.

Have someone call the police so an accident report can be filed.

Sequester your bicycle. Put it away. Do not ride it, do not get it repaired, do not let anyone else ride it. Your bicycle may very well be your star witness if there was something wrong with it that caused or contributed to the accident. Until an expert examines the bike, you can't be sure that there was nothing wrong with it.

Lock up the original owner's manual that came with the bike, your bill of sale or receipt for payment for the bike, and all subsequent repair receipts and have them ready for your attorney.

Keep the clothes you were wearing at the time of the accident. Wrap them up, including your helmet if you were wearing one, and your shoes. They could be important later on.

As soon as possible, have someone go out to the exact scene of the accident and photograph and videotape the roadbed and surrounding scenery.

Consult a good personal injury attorney. As you check the attorney's references, try to find out if he or she has had any experience with bicycle accident cases and what was the disposition of the litigation. After you review the case with the attorney, find out if he or she will take your case on a contingency basis. That means that the attorney will not charge you for preparing your case. In exchange for this investment of professional time, he or she gets 30 percent of whatever amount is recovered for you. However, you may have to pay certain out-of-pocket expenses, such as the fee of an expert witness, and any laboratory work, such as a metallurgical analysis of the bicycle or its components. If the attorney won't take your case on a contingency basis, that tells you what that counselor thinks of it. You could then discuss the case with other attorneys.

How to Keep a Quick-Release from Quick-Releasing!

I note a lot of accidents in which the rider claims that he or she hit a bump and the front wheel came off the bike, thereby causing loss of control and serious personal injury. The type of wheel-retention device involved in most of these accidents is the quick-release mechanism (Fig. 2-19). This device is easily opened by accident, or not safely tightened in the first place, so I am going to spend a lot of time describing its hazards and correct use. Bear with me here, because your life can depend on preventing wheel dislodgement, on keeping the front wheel safely locked in place. Your quick-release may hold your front wheel in place as you pedal over smooth surfaces, but if you hit a bump or a pothole, the front wheel may rebound upward and the wheel may fall out of the fork.

Make this check. With one hand on the handlebar stem, lift the front wheel. Pound down hard on the front-wheel tire with the clenched fist of your other hand. If the wheel falls out, read on. But even this pounding is not the acid test of wheel-retention safety. The quick-release may not be safely tight because your owner's manual did not show you how to check for quick-release tightness or even how to adjust and use the quick-release.

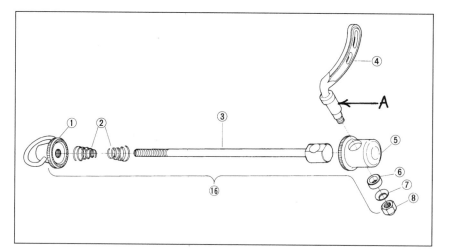

FIG. 2-19: Exploded view of a typical quick-release mechanism. Adjust tension on a quick-release by holding lever A with one hand while you tighten the locknut (1) at left, as shown. *Courtesy Shimano American Corporation.*

Someone else may have played with and loosened this mechanism without your knowledge. Let's review, first, how to use the quick-release mechanism.

Look closely at part 4 in Fig. 2-19, where I have added a line and an arrow labeled A. The arrow points to a fat part of the quick-release lever shaft. This is called a cam. The quick-release skewer (3) goes through the hub's hollow axle. The cam is part of the quick-release lever, so when the lever is turned toward the tightening position, its cam also turns. When it turns, it forces the nut (1) and the cam lever body (5) together. This cam action then squeezes the fork blades together to hold the hub (and wheel) securely in the dropouts (where the wheel axle fits). Please note that the small end of the springs (2) should face toward the hub.

Adjusting the quick-release mechanism is simple, once you understand that it is a cam-action device and not a nut-and-bolt mechanism. Make sure your quick-release is correctly adjusted so the wheel will be safely tightened in place.

Adjust the quick release this way:

1. Turn the quick-release lever so it is perpendicular (straight out) to the dropouts. Hold this lever with your hand and turn the adjusting nut (1 in Fig. 2-19) clockwise with your other hand until you feel it tighten and you can turn it no farther. *Do not use pliers or a wrench on the adjustment cone-shaped nut (1 in Fig. 2-19).*
2. Turn the quick-release lever toward the rear of the bicycle. You should begin to feel a lot of turning resistance as you force this lever past the

90-degree position, all the way to the closed position (Fig. 2-20). In fact, if you use the heel of your hand to close the lever it should leave a slightly red indent on your hand. Don't overtighten the lever because you could stretch the skewer and it could break, even as you ride. The curved lever should face inward, toward the bike frame, and the word "close" should face toward you (Fig. 2-20). The quick-release lever should always face toward the rear of the bicycle to avoid accidental opening of the quick-release should the lever catch on an obstruction, such as a tree branch. It should take about 30 pounds of closing force on this lever to tighten the wheel safely so it won't fall out of the dropouts when you hit a bump or pull up on the handlebars to bunny hop over an obstruction on the road or trail.

Follow these steps to make sure the wheel will stay in place under all conditions:

1. As noted above, with the front wheel up off the ground, punch down hard on the tire with your fist. The wheel should stay in place.
2. A better and more definitive test is to remove the wheel and look for "bite" marks on *both* sides of the dropouts (Fig. 2-21). You may see overlapping bite marks if the wheel has been removed several times. In this case apply fingernail polish or other quick-drying lacquer to both

Fig. 2-20: Turn the quick-release lever until the word "close" appears and the lever is pointing toward the rear of the bicycle. See text for further explanation.

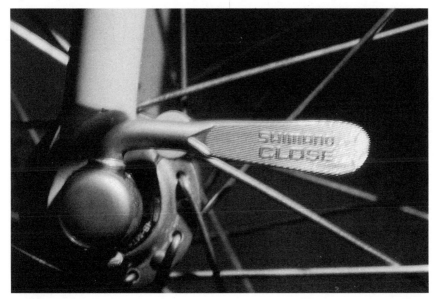

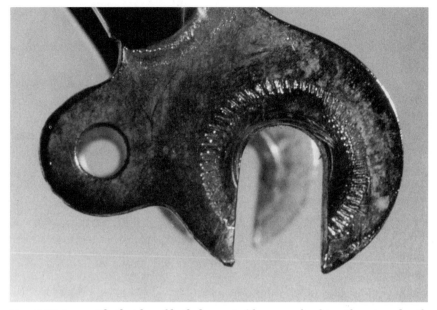

Fig. 2-21: Inspect *both* sides of *both* dropouts (the rear wheel too if equipped with a quick-release) for indentations like those shown. If you do not see them, readjust the quick-release (see text), remove the wheel, and inspect again. Repeat until "bite" marks are evident.

sides of both dropouts. When the paint has dried, replace the wheel, tighten the quick-release lever, remove the wheel, and look for *your* fresh bite marks. If they are weak or nonexistent, readjust the quick-release as above and try again until you do have fresh bite marks. These bite mark indentations are made by the sawtooth-like serrations on the quick-release lever on the *outside* of the left dropout (remember, a dropout is the slot the hub axle fits into), by the hub axle locknut on the *inside* of both dropouts, and by the quick-release adjusting nut (Fig. 2-19). Inspect dropouts on both wheels. First, remove the wheel by turning the quick-release lever all the way to the front of the bike, until the word "open" appears. On a mountain bike, squeeze brake pads together and pull the crossover cable out of the open side of the brake arm (see Fig. 3-9). The brake pads on a road bike will probably be far enough from the rim so you can pull the wheel out without the tire catching in the brake pads. If you have a bit fatter road bike tire and can't squeeze the tire out of the brake pads, look for a brake release lever, either on the brake lever or on the brake itself, where the cable is attached to the brake arm, and turn that lever to the open position. Remove the wheel and check for bite mark indents as noted above.

It should take a *lot* of force to pull a wheel out of the dropouts when the quick-release is safely tightened. Tests made by major bicycle manufacturers in this country and in Japan, for example, prove that it takes from 800 to 1,000 pounds of pull before such a wheel could be pulled out. That's a lot of energy! I can illustrate this situation by the three accidents that I had (over a span of 12 years). In one case, my front wheel caught in the expansion joint of a bridge. I was going at about 15 miles per hour. My tour-laden bike and I together weighed about 225 pounds maximum. The force that gripped my front wheel as it fell into the crevice of the expansion joint was great enough to throw me forward off the bike and to buckle the fork and top and down tubes. But the wheel did not come out of the fork dropouts. I have also smacked into two cars that stopped suddenly in front of me, both times buckling the fork and top and down tubes. Still the wheel did not come out of the dropouts. Moreover, the front wheel remained true both laterally and concentrically.

To conclude the quick-release data: Play it safe. Inspect the quick-release of both wheels every time you get on the bike. Be sure no one has tampered with it. Never assume that because it was safely tightened on your last ride, it is OK now. If your hub is equipped with retention rings (see Fig. 1-14), be sure they are in place so your wheel won't drop out if the quick-release is for some reason too loose for safety. These little retention units will (or should if properly designed) at least hold the wheel in place, although the wheel will wobble around and alert you to the immediate need to stop and take remedial action to the quick-release. All solid-axle, bolt-on hubs must have these retention devices by mandate of the Consumer Products Safety Commission.

I worry about using suspension front forks with quick-release hubs. These hubs have hollow axles, which are much weaker than the solid axles of bolt-on hubs. If you have installed a suspension fork (see Chapter 8) I recommend you replace the hollow axle with a high-quality solid axle, which is easy to do (see Chapter 6 or your bike shop). Then tighten the solid-axle bolt to at least 300 in./lbs. of torque. (See Chapter 3 for a definition of torque.) A suspension fork masks the myriad bumps the bicycle is subjected to. With such a fork you are likely to hit more bumps and contact them harder, because you won't feel them as you did before you installed the suspension unit. So you will tend to put much greater stress on the front-wheel axle, and if it's hollow, it could break and cause an accident. Suspension forks have been around for a few years, but more and more mountain bikes are coming with them already installed, and more cyclists are installing them on existing bikes.

As the number of mountain bikes with suspension forks proliferate I think (but hope I'm wrong) more axles will break and there will be more accidents as a result. If you have a dual-suspension, articulated mountain bike frame, I recommend a solid rear hub axle as well.

Radios Are a No-No

Listening to a radio while cycling is a safety hazard. First, it prevents you from hearing traffic noises around you. You can't hear the sirens of emergency vehicles clearly until they are right on top of you, let alone engine noises of other vehicles. Second, a radio distracts you from the traffic around you, keeps you from being as alert as you need to be to avoid an accident. Third, a radio masks warning noises from your bicycle of conditions that could cause an accident, such as a chain dragging on spokes. Some states recognize the hazards of radios on bicycles and have make them illegal. With a radio blaring in your ears, you also miss the music of the wind, the rustle of leaves, the rippling sound of waves, the songs of birds, in short, all the auditory glory of the outdoors.

Dogs and Other Animals

A dog may be a man's best friend when he's on foot, but a dog can be man's worst enemy when the man is on a bicycle. To a dog, a person on a bike seems to be an absolutely infuriating sight. It may be territoriality. The dog may think you're an intruder who needs scaring off. I've had dogs go out of their way to chase me, from blocks away. I think perhaps a bike may make a noise that dogs hate. More likely, it's the sight of a human being finally at a disadvantage, atop a machine that it can attack with impunity.

For whatever reason, dogs of any size or shape may attack a cyclist. I've had otherwise timid little poodles tear at me from a front yard, yelping an annoying high-pitched bark. I just glare and they retreat. But don't do that to any other breed of dog. In particular, be *very* suspicious of Doberman pinschers, bulldogs, weimaraners, and German shepherds. The friendliest of family pets can turn into an attack animal as you cycle past. Friends who have been bitten tell me that the owner usually says, "Why, I can't understand why Fido would bite you. You must have aggravated him terribly. The children all love him, he's so gentle and friendly!" So is a mother grizzly bear, to her cubs.

Dogs often attack silently, from behind. If you hear hard breathing and the patter of rapidly moving feet from the rear, it's going to be a dog on the attack. Dogs cheat, too. They will wait until you start a hill climb and then chase after you. Or, if they're in a farmyard, they'll cheat and cut at an angle across the large front yard to get to you.

Here's how to prevent being bitten, or knocked off your bike, by a dog:

Stop and dismount, putting your bike between you and the dog. Analyze the dog's body language. If the dog avoids eye contact, looks to one side, exposes its body by lying upside down, seems to grin at you, and keeps its body close to the ground and its tail down, chances are the dog intends to be friendly—until you get back on the bike, after which the chase may start again. Most dogs can run at speeds up to 15 miles per hour or a bit more, but they don't run long, either because you have left their territory or because they have run out of breath. If a dog comes at you and you're on a downhill run, you should be able to outspeed the animal.

However, if you have stopped, again, watch the body language. Never look the animal straight in the eye. If its body is tense, ears up, teeth bared in a snarl, and it growls, urinates, and paws the ground with a front foot, this animal is after blood, yours. You might try easing the tension by speaking softly, in a friendly manner. Don't extend your hand, though, unless you don't want it back. Be submissive, even though that thought is anathema to all cyclists. If the beast wants to come up and sniff you, let it do so. Don't sniff back. Keep your voice down, don't wave your arms about, because the dog may consider such an action threatening and an invitation to attack.

If you are convinced the dog will attack you, and you feel you won't be able to outrun him, use one of these excellent animal repellents:

1. Knockout pepper spray, a relatively harmless dog repellent carried by postal carriers, meter readers, and delivery people. It is a finely ground pepper substance in a pressurized can, available from bike stores and pet shops for around $5 in the half-ounce size. *Note:* Liquid sprays are illegal in California and Wisconsin. Check with your local police department for current city, county, and state regulations.
2. Liquid Bullet spray, like Mace but fortified with pepper, for the tougher, meaner dogs and other beasts both animal and human. Costs $10, comes in a leather holder.
3. Dog Dazer, an ultrasonic dog deterrent. It costs about $17.50. Makes the dog wince in pain and turn away, but does no harm to the animal. It is a nonchemical dog repellent, a small hand-held electronic sound generator that emits a high-frequency sound that causes extreme discomfort to the attacking dog. Dogs simply cannot stand the high-pitched sound. The closer to the Dog Dazer the greater the degree of temporary pain. I think that this gadget, if widely used by cyclists, would soon train dogs to keep away. If you can't find these animal repellents in your bike shop or pet store, contact the distributor/manu-

facturer, Jogalite, Silver Lake, NH 03875, phone 603-367-4741 or FAX 1-603-367-8098.

I believe Liquid Bullet is the most effective animal and people stopper. The Mace ingredients create pain, the pepper constricts the nasal passages. Very angry animals and drug-crazed humans shrug off Mace-only-type sprays, but not the pepper-spray-Mace combination. It is an effective defense against four- and two-legged beasties, even grizzlies.

Use sprays with caution. Be aware that the fine droplets of spray can be airborne for a short time, long enough to affect the cyclist behind you as well as yourself. For example, when I discharged some Liquid Bullet at a large aggressive dog coming at me from the front, I rode into my own spray. The droplets felt as though they were burning holes in my cheeks. Boy, that hurt! Fortunately I was near a friend's house where I could go and wash the spray off my face. Took about an hour before the pain subsided, though. (If you carry and use a chemical spray, be aware that if any of the spray falls on someone else, especially on a nearby child, you could be in for a lawsuit.)

Another way to stop an attacking dog is to club it with your tire pump. Personally, I don't want to let a dog get close enough to me so I can hit it, and I value my pump too much to break it over a dog's nose. Some cyclists carry a short piece of flexible metal electrical cable. If you use that, though, you're in for a real snarling encounter between man and beast, and the odds could be against you.

If you are bitten, try to track the dog home so it can be checked for rabies. Treatment for rabies these days is much less painful than it used to be, but you do need to know whether you have been exposed to the virus. You should notify the city or county health authorities as soon as possible, so they can hold the dog for as long as it takes to check it for rabies. If you are badly hurt, you also need a good attorney who can instigate litigation on your behalf. I urge you to take such action, because dog owners are reluctant to restrain their animals, and further attacks are very likely. More important, you should receive compensation for medical costs and time lost from work now, or in the future.

Other animals may also carry rabies. If a squirrel, woodchuck, possum, or raccoon, which are wild animals, comes up to you slowly, and seems friendly, it's more than likely to be infected with rabies. Mistrust any seemingly friendly wild animal.

The Bambi syndrome has been responsible for many animal-inflicted injuries to humans. Do not approach elk, deer, bears, and other large wild animals to offer them a snack or pet them. Those sweet little deer and other animals can chew your arm off or butt you off your bike and stomp on you if they think you are a threat. I recall all too clearly the time I saw some children cycling up to grazing elk near a campground in California. A ranger came running at full speed to shoo the kids away. He pointed at a warning sign, which said the elk can be dangerous.

Mountain bikers who travel on trails face a few special hazards from animals. Carry a snakebite kit and know how to use it. I'll never forget one time I was on a narrow, twisting mountain trail. Around one sharp corner, there right on the trail, in front of me, was a rattlesnake, sunning itself. I had no chance to avoid it, the trail was too narrow. So I pulled my front wheel up and bunny hopped over the snake. My rear wheel did not go over it, but the snake had no chance to bite me, or I don't think it did. I did not wait to find out what the snake would do.

Larger mammals, such as black and grizzly bears, can be a hazard to cyclists, particularly if your silent approach scares them or if the animal is a female with cubs. Rangers and large-mammal authorities say that if you can outrun a bear that's the safest action. But, they warn, a bear can run at a speed up to 30 miles an hour for a short distance. A black bear may simply walk away if you wait patiently. But it can climb trees, so that's no out for you. A grizzly bear, however, can't climb a tree, so if you can, do so in an attack situation. These authorities also say you could lie down and pretend to be dead, an action that with its implications leaves me somewhat less than enthusiastic. But if that's your only recourse, so be it. For more data on wilderness trail survival, read my book *Sloane's Complete Book of All-Terrain Bicycles*.

How to Ride Your Mountain Bike Safely

Going downhill, you need to keep speed under control so you can corner safely and not slide out on slippery surfaces such as loose gravel, sand, or snow. Do not exceed your off-road riding experience and training. Keep rear-wheel traction by extending your weight back as far as possible, your elbows out for steering control, both pedals and cranks about parallel to the ground, and hold your feet firmly on the pedals for good balance. Before embarking on a long downhill run, shift the chain to an intermediate rear cog and the center or largest chainwheel to keep the chain from bouncing off either cog, jamming, and locking up the rear wheel.

Going uphill, shift to a lower gear before you start the climb. Ease pedal pressure as you shift. Do not wait until you are straining and gasping for breath to shift because by then you may be going so slowly it may be safer simply to stop, lift up the rear wheel, twirl the pedals and shift down that way. But on startup, be sure you follow the mounting techniques mentioned earlier in this chapter, and do it with as much strength as you can muster. If you still can't get going even in the lowest gear, just walk the bike up to where the hill eases off enough to get riding again. If the trail or road is wide enough, you could go from one side to the other, much the way a skier keeps speed under control downhill by slaloming. This technique reduces the road gradient because you are going to the side and back again. But if you use it, be doubly sure traffic permits this sideways movement. Keep your weight about evenly balanced between the wheels so you have both rear-wheel traction and front-wheel steering control.

On slippery surfaces, such as snow and ice, use bike tire chains. On sand, gravel, and mud, think about riding over eggshells. The idea is to ride gingerly and carefully, not to shift your weight about, and to keep your body weight as far back as possible. Remember, wet leaves on pavement are also very slippery. Try to ride around the leaves if you can do so safely.

Jumps and Bunny Hops

A jump is a trail maneuver to be avoided if possible, unless you are highly skilled. A bunny hop is a maneuver that gets you over small obstacles on the trail such as logs, small rocks, depressions, and on the road, a curb to escape a maniac driver. Lets start with jumps.

A jump is a hazardous move for most mountain bike riders. It is very stressful on your body and on your bike frame. It is safer to slow and let your wheels roll down the incline. If, however, you become unexpectedly airborne when going down a small hillock or sudden depression on the trail, try to follow these survival steps:

1. Get your weight back as far as possible.
2. Keep pedals and cranks parallel to the top tube and absorb the landing shock with your legs.
3. Land rear wheel first, then move your weight forward to get the front wheel down quickly for steering control.
4. After you land, brake carefully to avoid locking up the rear wheel, which could, as a result, skid out and cause the bike to fall over.

Use a bunny hop to go over small logs and other trail obstructions. Here's how.

1. As you approach the obstruction, lean forward and press down on the handlebars, then quickly and with vigor pull up on the handlebars so your front wheel goes over the obstruction.
2. After the front wheel goes over the obstruction, immediately push your body forward so the rear wheel clears it.

Fording a Stream

First make sure the stream is fordable (not even mountain bikes can go *over* water). A foot is about the maximum depth you can pedal through, but if you are strong enough, try deeper. I know I said, earlier in this chapter, that air is the greatest resistance you face on the road, but on the trail water is it. Once you know the depth, go back away from the stream far enough so you can get up to full speed. Hit the water with your front wheel straight and *keep pedaling.* If you try to coast, I guarantee you will fall over in the middle of the stream before you can make it to the other side.

Follow These Rules of the Trail

The International Mountain Bicycle Association has rules of the trail, which add not only to your own safety but also to the safety of those who share the trail with you.

1. *Ride only on open trails.* Do not ride on trails and roads that are posted with a "Closed" sign or a "Bicycles Not Permitted" sign. These trails may be closed because of sensitive environmental concerns. Obtain permission of the owner if you wish to cycle over private land. Remember that (at this writing) federal and state wilderness areas are closed to cycling.
2. *Leave no trace.* Be sensitive to the ground beneath you. Even on open trails, do not ride where you will leave evidence of your passing, such as on sensitive soils right after a rain. Be aware of the different types of soils and trail construction and practice low-impact cycling. Stay on the trail. Do not create any new trails. Do not cut switchbacks. A switchback is a zig-zag trail that reduces a steep grade to a manageable one, sort of like an uphill slalom. On a downhill run I know it is tempting to shortcut over these zig-zags, but don't do it because then you will be cutting a new trail, which destroys the ecosystem where you ride. Pack out everything you pack in. This includes empty containers, soiled paper, and so forth.
3. *Be generous, share the trail.* Use a bell to let others ahead know you're approaching. Do not startle those who share the trail. A gentle, warm "Hi" or other friendly greeting will make trail life easier for all of us. Respect trail sharers by slowing to a walk as you pass, or stop and walk your bike if the trail is narrow. Anticipate that other trail users may be coming toward you around blind corners and other blind spots. Stay as far to the right of the trail as possible and be ready to stop if necessary.

4. *Do not spook animals.* Announce your presence as you come up to equestrians so as not to frighten the horse. Remember, if you scare the animal and the rider is thrown and injured as a result, you could be sued and could well lose the case. Do not startle any animal by a loud noise. Do not run or chase cattle or disturb any animal. If you have to open a gate to proceed, be sure to close it behind you, or leave it in the same position as you found it. For your own safety try to avoid slippery new cow flops, which could cause you to do the same.

5. *Be self-sufficient.* Know how to make minor repairs such as fixing flats, readjusting derailleurs, retruing rims, replacing a broken spoke or chain. Remember, you may be miles from a bicycle shop, so you will need to know how to care for your bike yourself. On long trips carry wet- and cold-weather clothing, food, a first-aid kit, and other supplies. Always file a trip itinerary with a friend, so if you don't arrive when and where you planned to, someone can come look for you. I suggest you review Table 2-5 for periodic maintenance data and refer to the appropriate chapter for details.

TABLE 2-5: PERIODIC MAINTENANCE SCHEDULE

PART	SERVICE	FREQUENCY	CHAPTER
Axle nuts	Check tightness	Monthly	2
Bottom bracket	Disassemble, clean, lube, replace worn bearings, adjust	Yearly	6
Brake cables	Remove cable stretch slack, check for worn, frayed strands, replace as needed	Six months	3
Brake levers	Check mounting bolt tightness	Six months	3
Brake pivot nut	Check tightness	Two months	3
Brake shoes	Check wear, alignment, toe-in, mounting nut tightness	Four months	3
Carriers	Check tightness of mounting bolts and nuts	Four months	9
Chain	Remove, clean, lubricate, replace if worn	Two months	4
Chainwheels	Clean, check wear, check tightness of binder bolts	Two months	4 and 5
Cranks	Tighten binder bolt to spindle	Four months	6
Derailleur cables	Remove cable stretch slack, replace frayed or worn cables	Four months	5
Derailleurs	Check and adjust limit bolts for accurate shifting	Four months	5
Fenders	Check mounting bolts (tightness)	Four months	9
Freewheel	Clean, lubricate, check cog wear, replace worn cogs as needed	Four months	5
Handlebars	Check binder bolt on stem	Four months	1
Headset bearings	Remove, clean, relube, replace worn bearings, readjust	Four months	8

TABLE 2-5: PERIODIC MAINTENANCE SCHEDULE (continued)

PART	SERVICE	FREQUENCY	CHAPTER
Hubs	Remove bearings, clean, relube, replace worn bearings	Six months	6
Pedals	Remove bearings, clean, relube, replace worn bearings	Six months	6
Quick-release	Check adjustment	Before every ride	2
Seat post	Check binder bolt or quick-release	Four months	2
Shift levers	Check mounting bolt tightness	Six months	5
Spokes	Check tightness, replace worn or abraded spokes	Four months	7
Stem bolt	Check tightness	Four months	1
Tires	Check air pressure, inspect for wear, cuts, gouges	Weekly	7
Wheels	Check alignment, retrue as needed	Four months	7

Finally, if you do not feel comfortable about any of the data on bicycle maintenance in this book, I urge you to take your bicycle to a bike shop and have their mechanic do the work.

Now let's get into the mechanics of your braking system, in Chapter 3.

References

1. Lewiston, Diana. *Two Year Bicycle Accident Survey, July, 1981, Through June, 1983.* Palo Alto, CA.
2. Karlson, Trudy A., M.S. *The Incidence of Hospital-Treated Facial Injuries from Vehicles.* Madison, WI: Center for Health Systems, University of Wisconsin.
3. Hodgson, V.R., Director, Gurdjian-Lissner Biomechanics Laboratory, Department of Neurosurgery, Wayne State University, Detroit, MI. *Improving Head Crash Protection.*
4. Fife, Daniel, M.D., et al. "Fatal Injuries to Bicyclists: The Experience of Dade County, Florida." *The Journal of Trauma,* vol. 23, no. 8.
5. The National Safety Council of Dade, *Accident Facts,* 1993 ed.

CHAPTER THREE

HOW TO BE SURE YOUR BRAKES WILL STOP YOU IN TIME

You need to keep your brakes in tip-top operating condition at all times, for these reasons and more:

1. A child may run out into the street in front of your bike.
2. A truck may run a red light just as you're entering the intersection.
3. You may build up dangerous speed down a steep hill.

Your brakes may work very well when you know in advance that you will have to stop, but will your brakes work in an emergency? Will they always stop you? Are they near failure right now? In this chapter you will learn how to tell when your brakes need attention and how to keep them in safe operating condition.

The U.S. Consumer Products Safety Commission requires that your brakes be able to bring you (and your bike) to a complete, controlled, safe stop within about 15 feet on a dry, level surface from an initial speed of around 15 miles per hour if you weigh 150 pounds. If you are heavier than that it may take a foot or so more to stop. If you weigh less than 150 pounds you should be able to stop a foot or so sooner. If your brakes do not meet this criterion or exhibit other problems, use the information that follows to keep them in safe condition. Preventive maintenance is the key to longevity both for your bicycle and for yourself.

Mountain Bike Handlebars and Brakes

Caution: If the front brake cable is routed through the stem, and you *raise* the handlebars of a bike equipped with a cantilever cam, you will, in effect, shorten the front brake cable. This causes the front brake shoes to be positioned closer to the rim. You may raise the handlebars so far that the brake shoes will rub on the rim. That makes pedaling a great deal harder, of course, and wears out brake shoes much faster. To readjust the brake if you do raise handlebars, see instructions below on cantilever brake shoe clearance adjustments.

If you *lower* the handlebars of a bike with cantilever brakes, you in effect lengthen the brake cable. In this case the front brake shoes will be farther away from the rim, reducing braking response time and efficiency. If you lower the handlebars, follow the steps for brake shoe adjustment that follow.

Quickie Brake Safety Check

Make these basic brake checks, then follow the procedures below to correct any problems you find:

1. *Ride brake check:* Test braking ability on a dry, flat surface, where there is little or no traffic, such as a school yard or playground on a weekend. Speed up to around 15 miles per hour. Apply the brakes, first the rear brake lever, then a second later, the front brake lever. You should be able to stop within about 15 feet from the point where you first began to apply the brakes. If you can't stop within this distance, your brakes are unsafe. Read on.
2. *Brake cable stretch check:* Straddle the bicycle with both feet on the ground. Squeeze the main brake levers as hard as you can. Do the levers come within a half-inch of the handlebars? Are brake shoes more than one-eighth inch away from the rim when you let go of the brake levers? If so, brake cables have stretched or brake shoes are worn. See brake shoe and brake cable stretch removal instructions below.
3. *Brake cable slip check:* Squeeze each brake lever as hard as you can. Does the brake cable slip so one or both brakes won't stop your bike? If so, the offending brake cable must be pulled taut and tightened in the cable binder bolt as shown below. Otherwise your brakes are definitely a hazard to your health. See brake shoe binder bolt tightening data below.
4. *Do brakes squeal* when you brake? If so, you need to adjust brake shoe toe-in as described below, for the type of brakes on your bike.
5. *Extension lever check:* Do you have extension safety levers (See Fig. 1-12) on your road bike, in addition to main levers? If so, apply these levers as hard as you can. You can see that they come a lot closer to the handlebars than your main levers. These levers simply do not have the same travel distance as the main levers. If the cables stretch (and they

will), your extension levers could come all the way to the handlebars and still not stop you! You may be able to bring your bike to a halt on a planned stop where you have lots of time and distance to do so. But too often these so-called safety levers will not let you make an emergency stop. The hazard of these levers is twofold. First, cable stretch is so gradual you may not notice it. Second, because the safety levers are much easier to reach you get into the habit of using them. Before making the other brake checks and adjustments below, I urge you to remove extension levers by following these steps (or have your bike shop do so):

a. Unscrew the extension lever binder bolt at the main brake lever and remove the lever.
b. Replace the brake lever shaft with a shorter one that does not protrude and won't hurt your hand.

6. *Brake Shoe Clearance:* Put your bike in a bike work stand or hold it off the ground so you can spin each wheel in turn. As the wheel spins, apply the brakes slowly until one brake shoe just touches the wheel rim. Both shoes should touch the wheel rim at about the same time. If not, readjust brake shoe clearance as shown below, or retrue the wheels, as shown below, or both.

To be sure we speak the same bicycle language, please study Figs. 1-1 and 1-2 until you are familiar with the names and locations of bicycle components, and refer again to these drawings as necessary for forthcoming chapters.

The Torque Wrench

Use a torque wrench to be sure you have tightened a particular bolt or nut to manufacturer's specifications for safety and function. See Table 3-1 for a list of recommended torques, given in inch/pounds (in./lbs.) of torque. Torque is the force of a rotating movement, as when you use a wrench to tighten a nut or a bolt. The torque specifications throughout this book ensure that each part is turned to the safest possible maximum tightness. If a nut or bolt is too loose, vibration from road shock could loosen it further and cause an accident. You can check the torque to which a nut has been tightened by turning it clockwise with the torque wrench until that nut or bolt just begins to move. The setting on the torque wrench will tell you what that torque was, at that point. Checking torque by turning a nut in the loosening direction (counterclockwise) will give you an inaccurate reading.

The torque wrench you buy should be calibrated in inch/pounds (in./lbs.).

Some torque wrenches are calibrated in foot/pounds, so you would have to multiply the reading by 12 to arrive at in./lbs. Also a foot/pound torque wrench is heftier and has a longer handle, which could snap the slimmer nuts and bolts on your bike. Let's leave the foot-pounder to truck mechanics.

TABLE 3-1: TIGHTENING TORQUE VALUES FOR BRAKES (IN IN./LBS.)

PART	CANTILEVER	SIDEPULL	CENTERPULL
Brake shoe binder bolt to brake arch	50–75	43–60	50–75
Cable binder nut—holds brake cable on brake arms and cable carrier where used	57–70	57–70	50–75
Brake mounting bolt or nut—holds brakes on frame and fork	44–60	70–88	50–70
Brake lever clamp bolt or nut—holds brake lever on handlebar	50–70	50–70	55–80

Other Tools You Will Need

You will need tools besides the torque wrench to work on your brakes. They will vary according to the brakes you have. You may not use all of those listed, but it's best to have them because you'll need them for other bike maintenance problems. These tools should be available from your bike shop. You will need:

1. *A Park Tool third hand:* Holds the brake shoes closed against the wheel rim while adjusting shoe clearance. You could also use a toe strap.
2. *A Park Tool fourth hand:* Holds cable tension while you tighten the cable binder bolt. Or you can use a pair of pliers.
3. *A set of 13, 14, 15, 16, and 17 open-end cone wrenches:* These (thin) wrenches are necessary for centering some brakes, and for conventional hub maintenance.
4. *A set of 2-, 4-, 5-, and 6-mm Allen wrenches.*
5. *A Set of 6-, 8-, 9-, 10-, and 12-mm metric sockets:* These fit the torque wrench. (Buy a complete metric socket set, because you'll need sizes from 2 to 12 mm. You'll be able to use them for other bicycle parts.)
6. *Wire cutter:* Electrician's wire cutters don't work on bike cables. A good wire cutter clips cable ends neatly. Attach an end cap or solder the clipped ends after tightening cable binder bolts, to keep ends from unraveling. Leave an inch or so in case you have to remove and install the same cable again.
7. *Folding bike stand:* No home bike workshop should be without one.
8. *A set of 8-, 9-, and 10-mm open-end and box wrenches.*

Brake Shoe Alignment

All brake shoes, regardless of brake type, should be aligned so the shoe is about 1/32 inch below the top of the rim, as shown in Fig. 3-1. If brake shoes are too far below the wheel rim, particularly on cantilever, centerpull, and U-brakes, the brake shoe may dive under the rim on hard braking, so they tangle in wheel spokes, causing loss of control and an accident.

All brake shoes, regardless of brake type, should be aligned so the clearance between the brake shoe and the wheel rim is from 1/32 to 1/8 of an inch. (Fig. 3-2 gives these dimensions in millimeters. Convert inches to millimeters by multiplying the millimeter measurement by .03937.) If brake shoes are too far away from the wheel rim, braking power can be reduced. Braking response time will also be reduced because the brake levers have to travel farther before the brake shoes impact the wheel rim. Brake shoes can become farther away from the rim because:

1. Brake cables stretch or even break.
2. Brake shoes wear below the wear mark (Fig. 3-3).
3. Brake shoes may be installed so the grooves or brake tread design is opposite to the direction of wheel rotation (Figs. 3-1 and 3-3). Note the

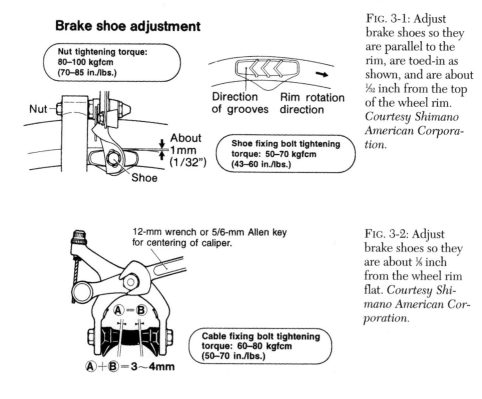

Brake shoe adjustment

Nut tightening torque:
80–100 kgfcm
(70–85 in./lbs.)

Nut

Direction of grooves   Rim rotation direction

About 1mm (1/32")

Shoe

Shoe fixing bolt tightening torque: 50–70 kgfcm (43–60 in./lbs.)

Fig. 3-1: Adjust brake shoes so they are parallel to the rim, are toed-in as shown, and are about $\frac{1}{32}$ inch from the top of the wheel rim. *Courtesy Shimano American Corporation.*

12-mm wrench or 5/6-mm Allen key for centering of caliper.

Ⓐ=Ⓑ

Ⓐ+Ⓑ=3~4mm

Cable fixing bolt tightening torque: 60–80 kgfcm (50–70 in./lbs.)

Fig. 3-2: Adjust brake shoes so they are about $\frac{1}{8}$ inch from the wheel rim flat. *Courtesy Shimano American Corporation.*

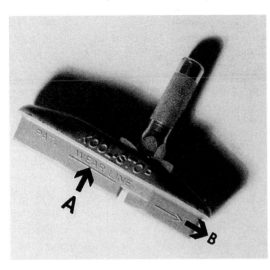

FIG. 3-3: This is a cantilever brake shoe, but is similar to road bike brake shoes. Replace the shoe when it wears down to the wear line (A) and point the new shoe in as shown by the arrow (B), in the direction of wheel rotation.

arrow embossed in the brake shoe in Fig. 3-3, which points in the direction of rim rotation.

4. Both brake shoes do not contact the wheel rim at the same time. One brake shoe may drag on the rim and make pedaling harder, the other brake shoe may be too far from the rim.

5. Brake shoes may not "toe-in" so the front part of the brake shoe contacts the wheel rim first (Fig. 3-4). Such toe-in also prevents brake shoes from squealing with hard braking.

All these clearances and adjustments will be discussed by type of brake—cantilever, centerpull, or sidepull. Let's start with cantilever brakes, used on mountain and some hybrid bicycles.

First, however, please note that brake cable stretch is one of the major causes of poor braking and reduced braking response time. Such cable stretch may be minor, in which case simple adjustments can bring brake

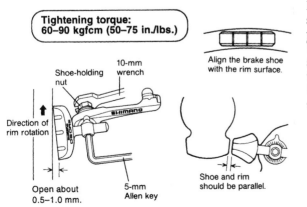

FIG. 3-4: Brake shoes should toe-in as shown to prevent squealing when brakes are applied. Shoes should also be parallel to the wheel rim. *Courtesy Shimano American Corporation.*

shoes back to the correct shoe-to-rim clearance. Or brake cables may have stretched so much that more basic steps must be taken to remove the stretch. Let's start with minor cable stretch, which is most frequent. Whether your cable stretch is minor or major, remember that the end result of your adjustment must be to bring brake shoes to within 1/32 to 1/8 inch from the wheel rim.

First Check Wheel Alignment

Before you make any adjustments to brake shoes, check to make sure the wheel itself is true both laterally and concentrically. Spin the wheel. Watch where the wheel rim passes by a brake shoe. If it moves closer to, then farther away from the brake shoe, the wheel must be retrued before taking any other steps to center the brake shoes. Please refer to Chapter 7 for wheel truing instructions.

Also make sure the wheel is correctly centered in the dropouts (see Figs. 1-1 and 1-2). Spin the wheel. If the wheel is consistently closer to one brake shoe than the other, the wheel is not centered in the dropouts. After retruing the wheel (Chapter 7), replace it in the dropouts and check with a ruler that the front wheel rim is the same distance from the fork blades or that the rear wheel is the same distance from the seat stays or chain stays (Figs. 1-1 and 1-2).

To Remove Minor Cable Stretch

On cantilever brakes, remove minor cable stretch at the shift levers (Fig. 3-5). Use a Park brake tool or a toe strap to hold the brake shoes tight against the rim. Turn the knurled nut (A) counterclockwise, just enough to loosen it. Then turn the cable stretch adjuster (B) counterclockwise until the cable slack is removed and tighten the knurled (A) clockwise as far as possible.

On centerpull brakes, strap brake shoes against the rim, loosen the knurled nut (A in Fig. 3-6) as above, remove the slack with nut B as above and tighten nut A.

On sidepull brakes, turn the cable slack adjuster (D in Fig. 3-7) until the slack is removed and the brake shoes are about 1/8 inch from the wheel rim.

To Remove Major Brake Stretch

On cantilever brakes, strap brake shoes tight against the rim, then turn the cable stretch locknut (A in Fig. 3-5) counterclockwise four or five turns. Then turn the slack adjuster (B) clockwise as far as possible so the cable is as loose as possible, and tighten the locknut. Now with 9- and 10-mm wrenches,

FIG. 3-5: A is the cable slack adjuster locknut. B is the cable slack adjuster. C shows the location of the cantilever brake cable position inside the brake lever. Note that A and B are aligned so the cable can be fitted into the brake lever. Use a 2-mm Allen wrench (D) to adjust brake lever "reach" to fit your finger length. To reposition the brake lever on the handlebars, loosen the clamp bolt (E).

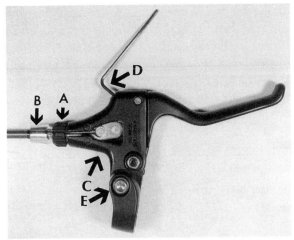

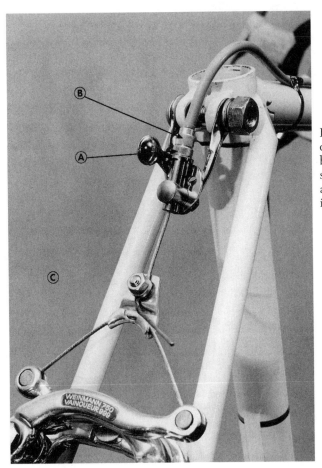

FIG. 3-6: Remove centerpull brake cable stretch at the stretch adjuster (A and B). See text for instructions.

loosen one end of the cable locknut (A) on the cable carrier (Fig. 3-8), while you hold the other end (R) with the other wrench. Pull all cable slack through the cable binder bolt, hold the cable taut with pliers, and tighten the cable binder bolt nut so the cable can be pulled tight through the cable holding bolt. Hold the cable tight with pliers while you tighten the cable binding bolt with the wrenches. If you have the round type of cable carrier shown in Fig. 3-9, loosen the cable binder bolt (B) and repeat the steps above for remov-

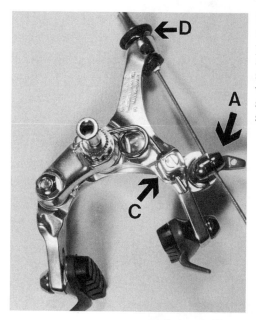

FIG. 3-7: Rear view of a sidepull road bike brake arch assembly. A points to the cable binder bolt and the quick-release lever, which spreads brake shoes apart for wheel removal. C is the brake tension adjuster and D is the cable slack adjuster.

FIG. 3-8: A cantilever cable carrier and crossover cable. This configuration is also used with centerpull brakes. H is the main brake cable. R is the cable binder bolt, with its locknut A. E is the cable carrier. L is the crossover cable, which fastens to the brake arches (not shown). M is a Park Tool fourth hand, which holds the crossover cable taut until you tighten the cable binder bolt.

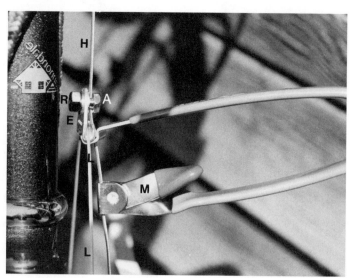

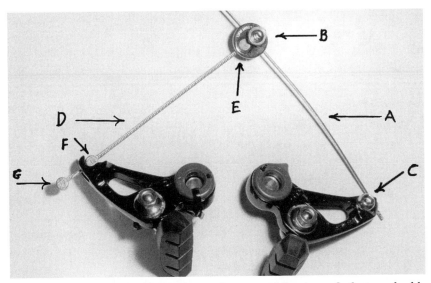

FIG. 3-9: This is a round cable carrier, used on some bikes instead of a tunnel cable carrier like the one in FIG. 3-8 (E). In this photo, A is the main brake cable from the brake lever. B is the crossover cable carrier. C is the brake arch binder bolt. D is the fixed-length cable. F is the fixed cable end in the brake arch, and G is its pull tab. To spread brake shoes for wheel removal, squeeze brake shoes onto the wheel rim, pull cable C out from the brake arch by the pull tab G.

ing major cable slack. Tighten cable binder bolts to 57 to 70 in./lbs. Remove the tool or toe strap holding the brake shoes against the rim.

On centerpull brakes, remove major cable stretch by first strapping brake shoes against the wheel rim. Then loosen cable adjuster lock (A in Fig. 3-6), so you can turn the minor cable slack adjuster (B in Fig. 3-6) clockwise as far as possible, then tighten A in Fig. 3-6. Now there should be even more cable slack. Now follow the same procedure as shown above, under cantilever brakes. (Cantilever and centerpull brakes have the same type of cable carrier and crossover cable.)

On sidepull brakes, turn the cable slack adjuster (D in Fig. 3-7) until the cable is as slack as possible. Loosen the cable binder bolt (A in Fig. 3-7), pull out cable slack, hold the cable taut with pliers, and tighten the cable binder bolt to 70 to 88 in./lbs.

Brake Shoe Replacement

Replace brake shoes when the tread is worn off or the shoe is worn down to about half its original thickness. Use original equipment brake shoes or a high-quality replacement such as the Kool-Stop shoes shown in Fig. 3-3. Be sure the tread faces in the direction of wheel rotation (Figs. 3-3 and 3-4) as specified by the brake shoe manufacturer. Check with your bike shop if you are not sure which way the tread should face. Replace all four brake shoes, not just one or two. They aren't that expensive, and with all-new shoes you can be assured of maximum braking power.

Cantilever Brakes

1. Pull the crossover cable out of the brake arch, by the leaded tab end (G in Fig. 3-9) to spread the brake shoes away from the wheel rim.
2. Hold the brake shoe axle nut at one end with an Allen wrench while you loosen the binder nut with a wrench at the other end, as shown in Fig. 3-4. Twist the brake shoe up if necessary, pull it out of the brake arch, and replace it with a new brake shoe.
3. Align the new brake shoe so it is 1/32 inch below the wheel rim top, parallel to the wheel rim, and angled so all of the shoe contacts the rim when the brake lever is depressed (Fig. 3-4).
4. Move the brake shoe until it is about 1/8 inch away from the wheel rim. This may seem to contradict the toe-in directions in the next paragraph, but it will give you room to make the shoe correctly angled to reduce squealing when braking.
5. Hold the locknut (Fig. 3-4) with the open-end or box wrench while you adjust the eccentric washer with the Allen wrench until the brake shoe is toed in as shown in Fig. 3-4. The part of the brake shoe facing in the direction of wheel rotation should just clear the wheel rim and the rear end of the brake shoe should be about 1/64 to 1/32 inch away from the wheel rim, as shown in Fig. 3-4.
6. Hold the binder bolt with the Allen wrench and tighten the locknut to 50 to 75 in./lbs.
7. Check brake shoe clearances on both sides of the wheel rim. Both shoes should be the same distance from the wheel rim. If not, use a 2-mm Allen wrench on one of the brake arches, as shown in Fig. 3-10, to even them out. If your brakes do not have a spring force tension adjustment, loosen the brake axle binder bolt as shown above, and move one or the

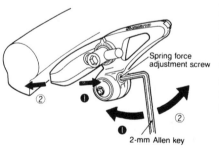

2-mm Allen key

FIG. 3-10: Some brakes, such as this cantilever brake arch, have a spring force tension screw. When turned one way or the other with a 2-mm Allen wrench it adjusts the brake arch so the shoes are the same distance from the wheel rim on both sides. *Courtesy Shimano American Corporation.*

other of the brake shoes toward or away from the rim, adjust toe-in as shown above, and tighten the brake shoe axle binder bolt to 50 to 75 in./lbs. *Caution!* If the brake shoe mounting nut is not sufficiently tightened, the brake shoe could become loose enough to dive under the rim when you squeeze the brake lever. In this case, the brake shoe could get caught in the spokes, or you could lose braking capacity. In either case, an accident could occur.

Centerpull Brakes

1. Squeeze brake shoes against the wheel rim and remove the crossover cable (L in Fig. 3-8) from the cable carrier (E in Fig. 3-8).
2. Remove the brake shoe binder bolt and replace the old brake shoe with a new one.
3. Adjust the brake shoe so it is flush with the wheel rim (Fig. 3-1).
4. Tighten the brake shoe binder bolt to 50 to 75 in./lbs.
5. Replace the crossover cable in the cable carrier (Fig. 3-8).
6. Readjust cable tension so the brake shoes are about 1/8 inch from the wheel rim, as shown above for cantilever brakes.

Sidepull Brakes

1. Unscrew the brake shoe mounting nut (Fig. 3-4), install a new brake shoe, and tighten that nut to 43 to 60 in./lbs. with the torque wrench.
2. Adjust sidepull brake shoe clearance to the top of the wheel rim by loosening the brake shoe nuts and sliding brake shoes up or down in the brake arch so the shoe is 1/32 inch from the top of the wheel rim. Then adjust brake shoe distance from the rim as shown above in the section on cable slack removal.
3. Adjust toe-in as shown in Fig. 3-11. If your sidepull brakes do not have an eccentric washer, simply grasp the brake arch just above the brake

■ How to use the abjustment washer The rim surface and the shoe surface can be made parallel by exchanging the positions of the adjustment washers.

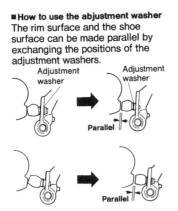

FIG. 3-11: Newer sidepull brakes have an eccentric washer so brake shoes can be evenly aligned, parallel to the wheel rim. *Courtesy Shimano American Corporation.*

shoe with an adjustable wrench and carefully and gently twist the arch to obtain toe-in.

4. Adjust brakes so both brake shoes are the same distance from the wheel rim when the brake levers are *not* applied. Loosen the nut that holds the brake assembly on the fork crown (Fig. 3-5) (front brake) or on the brake bridge (rear brake). Twist the brake unit until both brakes are equidistant from the wheel rim, and while you hold the brake unit in place, retighten the mounting nut to 50 to 70 in./lbs. You may have to repeat this procedure a few times until you get it right.

5. Center sidepull brakes as shown in Fig. 3-2.

Cable Replacement

All brake cables eventually fray and wear and need to be replaced. No matter what type of brake you have, the replacement procedure is essentially the same, with minor differences between sidepull handlebar brake levers and cantilever brake levers.

Brake cables can become frayed and even snap if not replaced. For safety, replace both brake cables yearly, less often if you are an infrequent cyclist. Also buy new spaghetti tubing for the new cable to ensure smooth cable function.

Follow these steps for cable replacement:

1. Use the correct type of replacement brake cable. Cable R in Fig. 3-12 is for sidepull and centerpull brakes, cable M is for cantilever brakes.
2. Before replacing any cable, add a light layer of grease, such as Lubriplate, on the new cable.

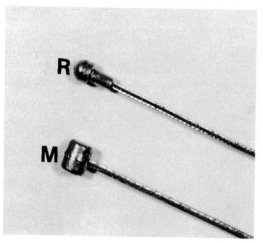

FIG. 3-12: R shows a sidepull road bike brake cable end. M is a mountain bike cable end.

Cantilever Brake Cables

1. Turn the brake cable binder bolt (A in Fig. 3-6) on the cable carrier (use two wrenches) to loosen the brake cable.
2. Turn the locknut and the cable slack adjuster (A and B in Fig. 3-5) so the cable channel is aligned with the channel in the brake lever body.
3. Lift the leaded end of the cable out of the brake lever body and pull the cable out, along with its spaghetti tubing.
4. Install a new brake cable and tubing by reversing the steps above.
5. Adjust brake shoe clearances as noted in cantilever data above.
6. Apply solder to the new brake cable about one inch below the binder bolt, then snip off extra cable.
7. Note: If your bike has a round cable carrier, loosen the cable binder bolt marked B in Fig. 3-9, then loosen the cable binder bolt marked C in Fig. 3-9 at the brake arch. When you install a new cable, be sure that the main brake cable, A in Fig. 3-9, is the same length from the carrier to the brake arch as the shorter cable, D in Fig. 3-9.

Centerpull Brake Cables

Follow steps for cantilever brakes, but adjust brake shoe clearances as noted in centerpull cable slack removal steps.

Sidepull Brake Cables

1. Loosen the cable binder bolt marked A in Fig. 3-7 and pull the cable out at the brake lever (Fig. 3-13).

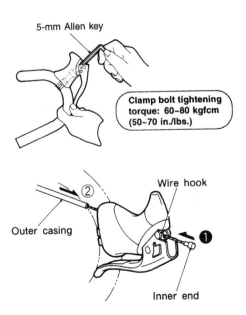

5-mm Allen key

Clamp bolt tightening torque: 60~80 kgfcm (50~70 in./lbs.)

Wire hook

Outer casing

Inner end

FIG. 3-13: Remove sidepull brake cable from the brake lever by pulling it out by the leaded bell end, as shown. To reposition a brake lever, loosen the clamp bolt, move the lever, and tighten the clamp bolt to 50 to 70 in./lbs. *Courtesy Shimano American Corporation.*

2. Insert a new cable, bell end last, into the slot in the brake lever (Fig. 3-13). Adjust brake shoe clearances as noted in the data on sidepull brakes above. On most road bike brake levers, the cable exits at the top of the brake lever. New designs allow the cable to exit from the base of the brake lever body (Fig. 3-14). The cable is routed under the handlebar tape for a clean, uncluttered look. Another nice feature of this design is that you can reach in and unscrew the brake lever mounting bolt (Fig. 3-15) without having to remove the cable, or depress the brake lever (which otherwise would be in the way) should you wish to move the brake levers to a more convenient position.

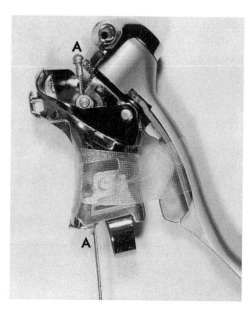

FIG. 3-14: Newer sidepull brake levers incorporate a shift lever. Tape holds the brake lever closed while the brake hood has been pulled back so you can see where the cable, A, is inserted in the lever handle.

FIG. 3-15: A set of Mathauser hydraulic brakes. M is the master cylinder, which mounts on the handlebars. S is the slave cylinders with their brake shoes.

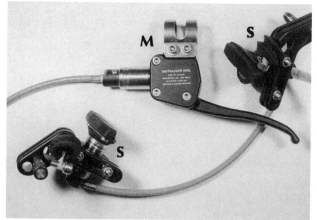

Important! Prestretch New Brake Cables

After you have installed new brake cables, squeeze both brake levers at least five times, as hard as you can. If the new cables stretch under this pressure (and they will), readjust brake clearances as noted above. This way brake shoe clearances and braking effectiveness will stay put longer. Now you may go for months or longer, depending on bicycle use, without having to readjust brake shoe clearances. The route to health and happiness on a bike is effective braking on demand 100 percent of the time.

Prestretching new cables is also a good way to tell if you have safely tightened brake cable binder bolts. As you press the brake levers, make sure the cables have not slipped out of their carriers or the brake arch of a sidepull brake. Such cable slippage instantly cuts braking power of the affected brake to zero. Since the front brake offers around 80 percent of total braking power of both brakes combined, cable slip on the front brake can lead to an accident.

Hydraulic Brakes

Mechanical brakes became obsolete on automobiles around 1932. Since then motorized vehicles have used hydraulic brakes, for a lot of excellent reasons. It's about time hydraulic brakes were more widely used on all bicycles. The reason they are not is simply that they cost more than mechanical brakes. However, they cost very little more. Hydraulic brakes offer much smoother and improved graduated braking control and much greater stopping power. They have no rods or cables that stretch or can break. Once adjusted, hydraulic brakes stay adjusted.

You can replace mechanical sidepull and cantilever brakes with Mathauser hydraulic brakes, which offer excellent graduated brake application control and fantastic stopping power, which is great for tandems. M in Fig. 3-15 shows the Mathauser master cylinder, which mounts on the handlebars, S shows the two slave cylinders, which replace your mechanical brakes.

At 118 grams (4.2 ounces) the Pro Model of these hydraulic brakes is lighter than leading mechanical brakes. Mathauser's brakes do not use a corrosive liquid. Suggested list price is $280 for mountain and road bikes, $325 for tandems. However, you won't need brake cables or have to make brake adjustments to compensate for cable stretch. Mathauser hydraulic brakes require only two basic adjustments. We have already discussed these adjustments above, but I'll repeat them just to make sure. The brake shoe should be about 1/32 inch below the top of the wheel rim, and parallel to it, and about 1/16 to 1/8 inch from the rim. These adjustments, once made, need never be redone except when you change brake blocks. Set brake clearance on Mathauser hydraulic brakes by loosening the two Allen bolts in the slave cylinder arrows (Fig. 3-15) and moving the brake shoes the correct 1/16- to 1/8-inch distance from the wheel rim. The Mathauser brakes come with an instruction manual. But if you are not sure about the installation procedure I urge you to have these brakes installed by your bike shop mechanic.

There are other hydraulic brakes on the market, such as the Dia-Compe disk brake, but they require special hubs and new rims and are more expensive.

Help Your Bicycle Stay Upright

It is downright annoying to have the front wheel move, the handlebars turn, and the bike fall over all by itself when you lean it against a tree or a wall. Prevent this paint-scratching situation. Install a little plastic brake holder (available from bike shops) in the space displayed when you depress the front brake lever. This locks the front brake and prevents the bike from rolling ahead on its own. Or simply pick up a twig from the ground and use it the same way. You could, of course, install a kickstand. The problem is that kickstands are heavy and they get loose. When you tighten them down again and again they squeeze and weaken the chainstays. More important, kickstands relegate your light, efficient bicycle to the level of discount-store heavy bikes. Riding a bike with a kickstand is like going to a prom in dungarees. It's inelegant.

Before I get into the remaining basics of bicycle maintenance in Chapters 4 through 8, let me tell you about an excellent combination of advanced bike mechanic training program and vacation. The school is in Ashland, Oregon, home of the famous Shakespeare Festival event where you can attend plays every night and on weekends. The school is the United Bicycle Institute, which holds a two-week training course covering every aspect of bicycle assembly and overhaul, for $875. UBI also offers a one-week advanced mechanics course for $525 and a frame-building course for $1,600. Reach United Bicycle Institute at P.O. Box 128, Ashland, OR 97520; phone 1-503-488-1121; or FAX 1-503-488-3485. You can stay at a nearby guest house for $15 a night or camp at a nearby state park.

Now, let's get into the transmission system of your bicycle.

CHAPTER FOUR

ALL ABOUT YOUR BICYCLE CHAIN

Here's how to make your bicycle chain run smooth as silk, shift like lightning, and live out the many miles and long life designed into it. This chapter will make bicycling easier, more economical (parts will last longer and be more reliable), and a lot more fun. You will avoid mechanical problems that can arise on the trail or on a remote country lane, far from the madding crowd and the nearest bike shop. The confidence you gain from knowing you can fix just about anything on your bike except a broken frame is basic to cycling happiness. There are a lot of truly brilliant engineers behind all the moving parts of your bike's transmission system, usually miles from where you happen to be. I am sure they wish you all the best when it comes to keeping these components up to the performance they have designed into them. My job is to help you do just that.

These are the tools and parts you need to maintain your chain:
1. A chain tool to remove the chain rivet and reinstall it (Fig. 4-1).
2. A Quick-Link tool (Fig. 4-2) to hold the chain while you remove or re-install the chain. Unless you have four or five hands, this little gadget will make chain work a lot easier.
3. Needlenose pliers.
4. Chain lubricants, for both wet and dry conditions. Two types, made by Sachs Sedis, are available from your bike shop.
5. Chain cleaner kerosene.

More than any other part of your bike, the chain is exposed not only to abrasives such as dirt, sand, and mud, but to water as well, which washes

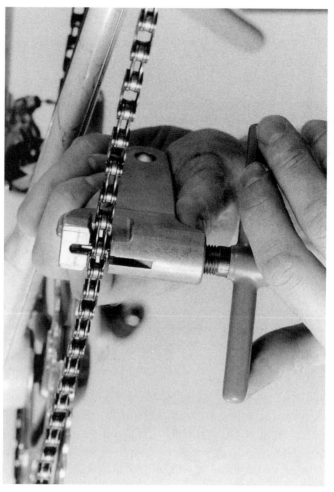

Fig. 4-1: Use this chain tool to remove and install a chain.

Fig. 4-2: This Quick-Link tool is a good way to hold the chain together while you remove or press in a chain rivet.

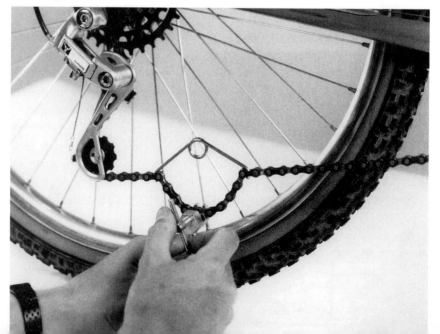

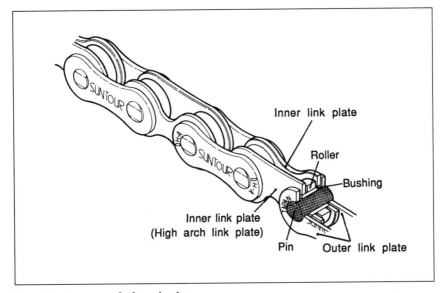

Fig. 4-3: Anatomy of a bicycle chain.

away protective lubricants. When these metal-eating particles work their scratchy way into, around, and between chain pins, rollers, and bushings (Fig. 4-3), or when water washes away lubricant, the chain wears out fast. Sometimes the chain succumbs to an early death and breaks apart, or as it wears, becomes a bit longer and jumps off cogs or jams. If you treat your chain with respect, however, by cleaning it often and keeping it well oiled, it can last up to 3,000 miles. If not, it can wear out within 500 miles.

Wear causes the chain to stretch. When the chain stretches, the pitch of the chain becomes greater than the pitch of the teeth of the freewheel cog and the teeth of the chainwheel. The pitch of the chain and the pitch of the cogs are mismatched. The load is carried by fewer cog teeth, instead of by as many cog teeth as the chain is on (a function of chain "wrap-around" —discussed in Chapter 5). This concentrated wear puts additional stress on the chain and further accelerates chain wear. In addition, if the cogs carrying the chain are worn (Fig. 4-4), the chain is prone to hang up on that cog, which causes the chain to slip and jump to the next cog. Such chain skip and jump can cause erratic pedaling, a distraction the rider does not need, especially in traffic. Chain slippage while straining uphill, off the saddle, may also cause the rider to come down suddenly on the top tube, a painful occurrence for either sex. It may also cause loss of control and an accident.

Clean your chain anytime it looks dirty and before every long trip. A dirty chain not only wears out faster, it also wears down the teeth of your freewheel and chainwheels as noted above, and their replacement costs a bun-

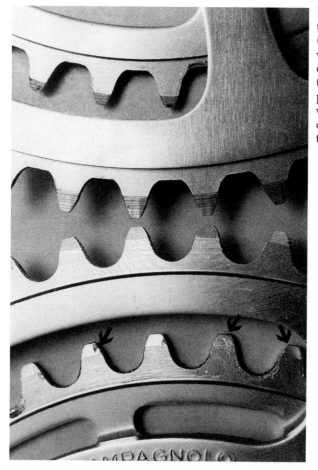

FIG. 4-4: Worn cog teeth on chainwheels (arrows) and on freewheels can cause chain jump, stressing the chain and causing premature chain wear. On top, a newer chainwheel has pristine teeth.

dle. Clean your chain while it's on the bike, or remove it for a more thorough cleaning.

On the bike, clean it with a chain cleaner, such as the Park Tool unit. The chain passes through kerosene and over brushes as you turn the crank counterclockwise. The cleaners are small and light enough to carry along on your trip. If your cookstove uses kerosene you can use the same fluid in the cleaner. Remove the cleaner, dump the kerosene in an ecologically kind place, and relube the chain. Or remove the chain (see steps below) and dunk and steer it around in a pan of kerosene until clean.

After you clean the chain, use a stiff-bristle brush or an old toothbrush to remove accumulated gunk and dried-on grease and dirt from freewheel and rear derailleur cogs and chainwheels. Relube the chain with the correct lubricant that matches where you ride. For example, there are now wet-weather chain lubricants with tenacity that stick to chain parts through rain, hail, snow, and other forms of water. But a lubricant that stubbornly refuses to let water wash it off also attracts and holds sand, dirt, and other abrasives with equal stubbornness. So if you are not riding through liquid, and the weather is delightful outside, use a lubricant designed for dry weather.

How often should you clean your chain? Sometimes every day if you have pedaled miles along a sandy beach or have forded shallow streams four or five times. Sometimes every one or two months if you have been riding on pavement and it's been dry outside. There are no hard and fast rules here. Just let your good common sense prevail and remember that a clean chain lasts longer and is safer than a dirty one.

Follow these steps to remove the chain from the bike for a more thorough cleaning job, or to replace it with a new chain:

Use a chain breaker tool (aka rivet remover—Fig. 4-1) to take the chain apart. Always carry this tool with you on a trip. If the chain breaks on the road, you will need the tool to remove the broken link and put the chain back together. (The day I left my chain tool home was, of course, the day the chain broke on a rural road in Wisconsin. I pounded the broken link pin out with an old nail and a rock I found nearby. I removed the broken link and pounded the pin back into the now shorter chain, using the nail and the rock.) Also carry a couple of spare links removed from an extra chain. If you are on a safari, take the entire extra chain. If you carry a few links, they *must* be the same make and model as the chain on your bike. Just being the same make won't do; busy R&D types are always developing new chain configurations, such as bowed-out sideplates and narrower chains. Links between the same makes but different model years of chains are not necessarily compatible.

1. Shift the chain to the small rear and front cogs. Better yet, lift the chain off the small chainwheel and drop it down onto the bottom bracket shell, to the left of the small chainwheel. This reduces chain tension and makes it easier to use the chain tool.
2. Remove the chain by using the chain tool to push a rivet out of the chain link. Using the tool with caution, turn its handle until about 1/64 inch of the rivet remains inside the chainplate. Six complete turns of the handle should work for 3/32-inch derailleur chains. Use 7 1/2 turns for single- and three-speed coaster brake hub chains. The protruding rivet will hold the chain together as you snap the links back, long enough to push the rivet back in.

3. Remove the chain. Before wasting time cleaning it, check it for wear by one of two methods:

   a. Lay the chain flat. Count off 24 links. Since link pins (rivets) are a half-inch apart (Fig. 4-5), 24 links should measure 12 inches. If they measure much more, say 12 1/16 inches, replace the chain.

   b. Or, bend the chain and compare it to a new chain, as shown in Fig. 4-6. The chain at the bottom is worn and should be replaced.

Replace a worn chain with an exact duplicate, especially if you have index shifting.

4. Relube a clean chain by laying it on newspapers, on the garage floor, side plates vertical. Spray the chain with the appropriate lubricant as discussed above. After spraying one side, turn the chain to the other

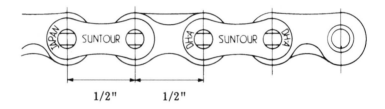

Fɪɢ. 4-5: Chain links should be a half-inch apart if the chain is not worn.

Fɪɢ. 4-6: Compare an old chain, A, with a new one, B, as shown here. Chain A is worn and should be replaced.

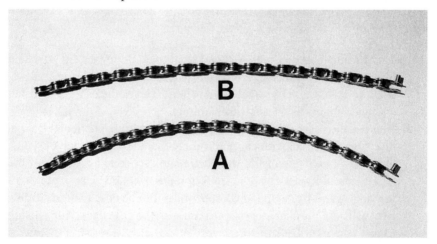

side and spray it. If possible, let the lubricant penetrate for a couple of hours, or overnight, before reinstalling the chain.

5. Wipe off excess lubricant to prevent drip. Replace it this way on the freewheel cogs, rear derailleur wheels, and chainwheel:

   a. Start with the end of the chain without the protruding rivet.
   b. Thread it through the front derailleur cage, then on *top* of the free-wheel cog, then in front of the derailleur upper (jockey) wheel, then behind the derailleur bottom (idler) wheel.
   c. So the chain will run the same way it was before you removed it, face it the way you pushed it out. If you pushed the rivet out toward the left side of the bike, push it back with the chain tool from the right side. It's a bit more difficult this way, but it's better for the chain be-cause it keeps the same wear pattern.

6. Chain riveting is easier if you hold the chain together with a tool such as the Quick-Link, Fig. 4-2. Snap the two ends of the chain together. If you had about 1/64 inch of the rivet left inside the side plate, you should be able to force (snap) that much of it into the chain.

7. Push the rivet the rest of the way in with the chain tool, until the same amount of the rivet shows on both sides.

8. The chain will most likely be stiff at this rivet you pushed in. Grasp the chain links on both sides of the section you riveted and twist the chain from side to side until it feels loose. If you don't free up this stiff link you will have chain jump.

New Chains

1. The new chain should be the same length and make as the old one.
2. Lay old and new chains side by side on the floor. Remove unneeded links with the chain tool. Install the new chain as shown above, except that here it makes no difference which side the rivet is on.
3. *Make this check to be sure the chain is the correct length.* Chains come in 112-, 116-, or 120-link sizes. The chain should be long enough that you can shift to the large freewheel cog, yet short enough so the chain won't skip or jump off a gear. If the chain is too long it will be too slack when it is on smaller gears and may jump off. If it is too short you may be able to shift to the big rear cog but not to the biggest chainwheel or even to the middle chainwheel.
4. Shift the chain so it's on the largest freewheel sprocket and the largest chainwheel. The rear derailleur should now be almost parallel to the

chain stay (Fig. 4-7). If you can't shift the chain to the biggest freewheel cog and to the largest chainwheel, you may have a super-low gear setup, such as a 34 or 38 rear cog, for which the chain is too short. In this case don't add links to the chain because if you do, the chain will be dangerously loose when you shift to the smallest freewheel sprocket, say on a downhill run where it could jump off a cog if you hit a bump. When you coast downhill, shift to the big rear cog and chainwheel to keep tension on the chain and back to an appropriate gear when you hit the flats. Console yourself that you have a super-low granny gear for steep hills. If, on the other hand, your biggest freewheel cog has 32 teeth or fewer, you should be able to shift so the chain is on that sprocket and on the large chainwheel. If not, add chain links as needed.

5. Shift the chain to the smallest freewheel sprocket and the smallest chainwheel. The rear derailleur should be about vertical to the ground (Fig. 4-8). If not, remove one or two links.

FIG. 4-7: A chain is the correct length when, on the big rear cog and the big chainwheel, the derailleur body is at the angle shown here.

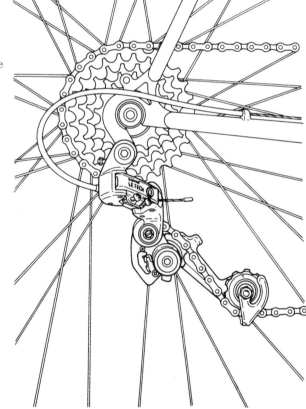

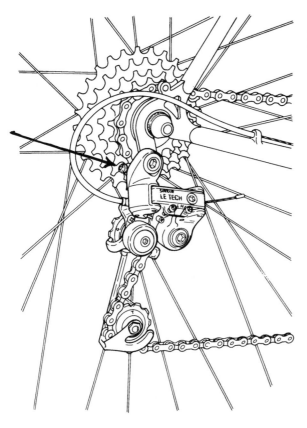

FIG. 4-8: The chain is also at the correct length when, on the smallest freewheel cog and on the smallest chainwheel, the derailleur body is at the angle shown here.

6. Shift the chain to the largest freewheel sprocket and the largest chainwheel.
7. Check and adjust chain wraparound as in the section on derailleurs in this chapter.

I recommend installing a plastic self-adhering chain guard on your chain stay, to prevent occasional chain rub from damaging its finish. Clean the stay before installing the guard.

New Chain Designs

New makes of chain require special installation consideration. SunTour Superbe Pro chains have "high arch" inner links (Fig. 4-9). When you replace the SunTour chain, be sure the arched part of the outer link goes over the gear teeth, as in Fig. 4-9. *For index systems,* it is especially important that you use the same make and model chain that came on the bike. Some chains

FIG. 4-9: If your chain has an arched side or link plate, be sure the arch side is on the gear cog as shown here.

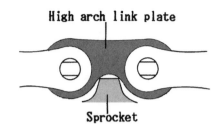

are narrower than others. For example, a seven-speed freewheel usually requires a narrow-design chain. A normal-width chain will just not work.

The Shimano Hyperglide ultra-narrow HG chain (Fig. 4-10), takes a special pin every time you take it apart. These pins are available in bike shops. I can report that my standard, garden-variety chain tool worked just fine with this chain. Do not cut (remove the rivet from) a new Hyperglide chain only

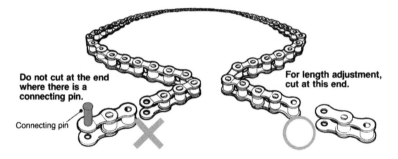

FIG. 4-10: Break a Shimano Hyperglide chain at the special reinforced black pin.

where you see a black rivet. Check instructions that come with your new chain. If you lengthen or shorten this chain, or remove it for cleaning, use the special reinforced pin to replace the pin (rivet) you removed. Break off the excess part of this pin with a pair of pliers, as shown in Fig. 4-11. Your bike shop should have a supply of these pins. I have tried to put this chain

FIG. 4-11: Use a new replacement pin when you replace a Hyperglide chain. Snap it off with pliers as shown.

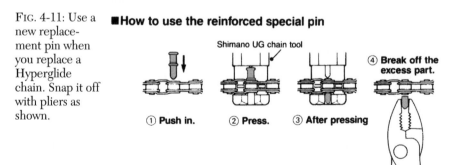

back together. It is not easy. You have to press the old pin all the way out of the chain. Then you have to fight to get the new, special pin back in the chain sideplate. You can do it, but it's a time-consuming task. Again, never remove the original black pin that connected the chain when the chain was brand-new. Push out any other pin but that one and use the special new pin instead. The Park Superchain tool (available from your bike shop) makes this job easier.

More About Chain "Jump" and Breaking

There are reasons for chain jump and chain break other than chain wear. I have had cases in which a new chain snapped apart within a few miles of the new bike owner's very first ride. In one of these cases the chainwheels were badly warped. The repeated right and left chainwheel movement puts severe strain on the relatively thin sideplates of the new chain. A chain is designed to withstand thousands of pounds of pressure in a rotating direction. But rapid left and right movements on a warped chainwheel can snap a brand-new chain very quickly. Check your chainwheels to make sure they run true. Shift the chain to the smallest chainwheel and to the smallest freewheel cog to remove as much chain tension as possible. Then pick the chain up off the small chainwheel and put it down onto the bottom bracket shell. Now spin the chainwheels and eyeball them for trueness. If all the chainwheels are bent in the same place it is most likely due to a bend of one or more of the arms of the chainwheel "spider" (A in Fig. 4-12). The spider is an integral part of the right crank. If the spider is bent, all the chainwheels attached to it will be bent at the same place. Such a bend should have been caught by the bike shop and corrected before sale or detected by the bicycle manufacturer in normal quality control during assembly at the factory. If all three chainwheels are bent in the same place, replace the crank with its spider, because the spider is almost impossible to bend back to true. I would also replace the chainwheels at the same time.

A bend or warp of just one chainwheel can be caused by impact due to mishandling of the bicycle by the owner, or by impact when the right side of the bicycle hits, say, a rock or a tree stump. You, or your bike shop, can correct minor single chainwheel bend by twisting the chainwheel back to true with an adjustable crescent wrench. Do any straightening slowly and precisely. Aluminum chainwheels can't take much side-to-side bending.

Another cause of chain break is a freewheel cog design introduced a few years ago to make index shifting easier and quicker. These cogs have so-called shifting gates in two places on each cog, as shown in Fig. 4-13. When you shift the chain from one rear cog to another, chain sideplates are sub-

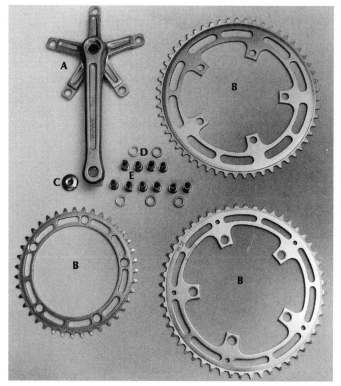

FIG. 4-12: Parts of a chainset. A is the "spider" to which the chainwheels, B, are attached by nuts, bolts, and washers, D and E. C is the dustcap that goes over the mounting bolt that holds the spider onto the bottom bracket spindle.

FIG. 4-13: Newer freewheel cogs have "gates" that ease the chain from one cog to another as you change rear gears. These gates can shorten chain life by imposing side forces for which the chain is not designed.

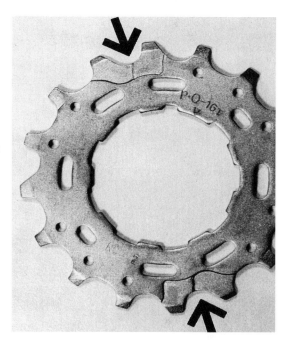

jected to twisting as they pass over these gates, leading to earlier chain demise. This is particularly true with narrow chains used on index shifting systems.

How to Shift Gears

Yet another cause of chain jam or short chain life has to do with how you shift gears. Follow these steps for foolproof shifting, whether or not you have indexed shifters:

1. Ease off on pedal pressure before you shift.
2. Shift to a lower gear before starting a hill climb. If you wait until you are straining uphill you may not be able to shift at all. In that case stop, get off the bike, lift up the rear wheel, twirl the pedals, and shift to a more favorable gear.
3. On non–index shifters (friction shifters) move the shift lever just enough to move the chain precisely to the gear of your choice. This goes for front and rear gears. If you hear noise after you shift you have not moved the chain so it is fully engaged.

Please see Chapter 5 for data on derailleur adjustment for the solution to chain overshift and undershift and chain skip. For example, if front or rear derailleurs are not correctly adjusted the chain may be overshifted to the left or to the right, causing chain jam or skip.

Older or less expensive bicycles will most likely have straight mechanical shifting. Most bicycles these days, however, come with some form of automatic precision shift mechanism (index shifters) integral in the shift lever. There is more information on index shifters in Chapter 5.

Coaster Brake Chains

Bicycles with coaster brake hubs use wider chains that won't fit derailleur bicycles. Remove the connecting link to take this chain apart. Be sure to face this link *with the open end facing toward the rear of the bicycle!*

CHAPTER FIVE

ALL ABOUT DERAILLEURS AND GEARING

As you know, your bicycle has two derailleurs. One moves the chain from one to the other of the freewheel gears. The other moves the chain from one to the other of the chainwheels up front.

You will, eventually, have to make adjustments to both of these derailleurs, if for no other reason than that the cable that connects them to the shift levers will stretch in time. When the cable stretches, you may not be able to shift up to the large (low-gear) rear cog or to the large (high-gear) chainwheel.

Here are the tools you will need to adjust derailleurs, and in Table 5-1, the correct tightening torques for them and their shifters.

1. Torque wrench (in./lbs. model) (see Chapters 1 and 3).
2. Small Phillips head screwdriver.
3. 4-, 6-, and 8-mm Allen sockets for torque wrench.
4. Park fourth-hand tool (optional) or pliers.
5. Cable cutter.
6. Workstand (optional). You could also hang your bike from ceiling hooks.

TABLE 5-1: TORQUE TABLE FOR DERAILLEURS, CHAINWHEELS, AND FREEWHEELS* (VALUES IN IN./LBS.)

Front and rear derailleur cable fixing bolts	35–53
Front derailleur clamp fixing bolt	53–65
Rear derailleur mounting bolt	70–85
Shift lever fixing (clamp) bolt	35–53
Shift lever fixing bolt (holds shift lever onto shift lever boss)	18–23
Jockey and idler wheel axle nuts	50–60
Chainwheel fixing bolts (hold chainwheels together)	70–95
Freehub lock ring	260–434
Freehub freewheel body fixing race	305–391
Freehub body fixing bolt	305–434

* See data on torque in Chapter 1 for use of torque wrench, and torque values as they relate to safety.

Rear Derailleur Problems, Causes, and Solutions

PROBLEM ONE: The chain overshifts to the right when you shift down from a larger to a smaller rear cog. The chain rubs noisily between the smallest rear cog and the chain stay (see Figs. 1-1 and 1-2 for chain-stay location), or falls off the small cog and jams between that cog and the chain stay (A in Fig. 5-1). A chain jam could lock up the chain and cause unexpected pedaling resistance, loss of control, and a fall. It's happened.

Cause One: High-gear derailleur adjuster lets the chain move too far to the right when you shift.

Solution: Put the chain back on the small rear cog. If the chain has jammed so you can't lift it, pry it from between the chain stay and that cog

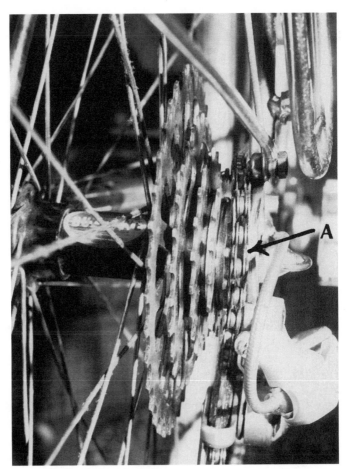

FIG. 5-1: A chain overshift to the right, arrow A, shows that the chain can jam between the chain stay and the small freewheel cog.

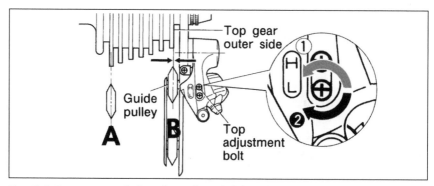

Fig. 5-2: Prevent overshift to the right or left by adjusting the derailleur high- and low-speed bolts to align the freewheel upper jockey wheel directly under the small and big cogs. *Courtesy Shimano American Corporation.*

with a screwdriver. Now turn the high-gear adjuster (H in Fig. 5-2) until the top derailleur pulley is just a tad to the right of the small cog (B). Check shifting again. If the chain still rubs on the chain stay, or does not move squarely onto the small cog, turn the high-gear adjuster to move the top derailleur pulley a bit more to the left.

Cause Two: Cog teeth are worn (Fig. 4-4).

Solution: Replace worn cogs.

Cause Three: Chain is worn and stretched, which lets the chain jump off the cog. Shifting may be inaccurate on all gears.

Solution: See Figs. 4-5, 4-6, 4-7, and 4-8 for instructions on checking chain wear and for replacing a worn chain with a new one.

Cause Four: The rear derailleur mount may have been bent, which changes the derailleur mounting angle with respect to the rear cogs.

Solution: Have your bike shop check the rear derailleur mounting bracket alignment (also called a "hangar") and straighten it as necessary. This alignment check requires a special tool.

Cause Five: Buildup of mud (or ice and snow) on rear cogs or cable routing guides located underneath the bottom bracket shell.

Solution: Remove accumulated mud, snow, or ice.

PROBLEM TWO: The chain overshifts to the left and falls down behind the big rear cog and the "pie plate" spoke protector. In this case the pedals could suddenly skip forward and cause loss of control and an accident. If a spoke protector is not installed, the chain can jam between the spokes and the large rear cog. The chain can also actually knife into and cut the spokes. In that situation the gouged spokes can snap later, or actually be severed as the chain jams. If one or more spokes are severed, the rear wheel will be misaligned, sometimes to the point of rubbing on a chain or seat stay (see Fig. 1-2 for seat-stay locations). In that case you can true up the wheel well enough so it at least won't rub on a stay, then get home or to a bike shop for spoke replacement (which requires removal of the freewheel or freehub cogs as shown in this chapter and in Chapter 6). Use the spoke wrench you are, of course, carrying in your emergency on-the-road repair tool kit (see Chapter 9 for a list of such tools) to change spoke tension as needed. Or use a pair of pliers to turn the appropriate spoke nipples to temporarily retrue the wheel. Please see Chapter 7 for wheel truing instructions. Replace cut or severed spokes as soon as possible.

Cause: The rear derailleur low-gear adjuster lets the chain move too far to the left as you shift up.

Solution: Turn the low-gear adjuster bolt (L in Fig. 5-2) until the top derailleur pulley is aligned directly under the big rear cog (A).

Note: Also see Causes Three, Four, and Five and their solutions in Problem One above.

PROBLEM THREE: Cannot shift up to the biggest (low-gear) rear cog.

Cause: The shift cable has stretched.

Solution One: Shift the chain down to the smallest rear cog. Check for cable stretch by lifting the cable with your finger where it passes over the down tube. If you can lift the cable 1/4 inch, it's minor stretch. If you can lift it more than that, it's major cable stretch. Remove minor cable stretch at the rear derailleur cable stretch adjuster (Fig. 5-3) or at a similar ad-

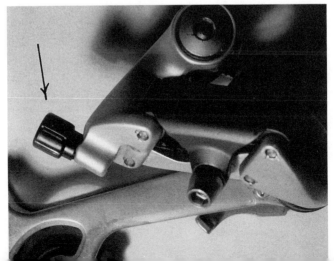

FIG. 5-3: Turn the slack adjuster (arrow) at the derailleur, if it has one, to remove minor cable slack.

juster on a mountain bike shift lever mounted on the handlebars. Make this adjustment by first loosening the adjuster lock barrel under the adjuster knob, turning the adjuster knob counterclockwise until the cable is taut, then tightening the adjuster lock barrel.

Solution Two: If you find that you cannot remove cable stretch at an adjusting barrel, follow these steps:

1. Shift the chain to the smallest rear cog.
2. Loosen cable stretch adjusters at the derailleur or shifters, or both, turn the adjusting barrel clockwise as far as possible, and retighten the adjuster lock barrel. Now the cable should be even looser.
3. Loosen the cable fixing bolt and pull the cable through it with a pair of pliers. Hold the cable tight while you tighten the fixing bolt. See Table 5-1 for tightening torque.

PROBLEM FOUR: Erratic shifting on all rear cogs.

Cause: Not enough chain wraparound. The upper rear derailleur wheel is too far away from the cogs, so the chain does not fall on about half of the cogs.

Solution: Shift the chain to the large (low-gear) rear cog. Turn the adjuster bolt, located just under the derailleur mounting bolt (Fig. 5-4), to move the chain closer to the cog teeth.

Note: Also see Causes Three, Four, and Five and their solutions in Problem One above.

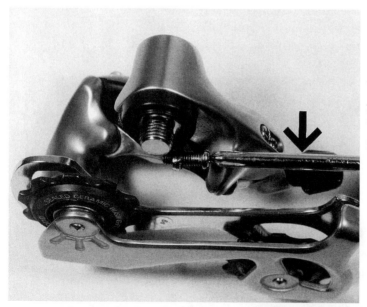

FIG. 5-4: Bring the derailleur wheel as close as possible to the biggest rear cog for maximum chain wraparound by adjusting the derailleur wheel adjuster bolt. The arrow points to a screwdriver in this bolt.

PROBLEM FIVE: Chain noise—you cannot seem to get the chain to fall accurately on a gear, but instead it seems to ride partly on two cogs.

Cause: Inaccurate shifting.

Solution One: If you have a manual (nonindex) rear shifter, the chain noise is telling you that you probably have not shifted accurately. Anytime you hear a grinding noise from the freewheel (or the chainwheel), remember you can quiet things down with a tiny adjustment of the shift lever one way or the other.

Solution Two: If you have an index shifting system and it has a friction mode, turn the shift lever indicator from index to manual mode. In the manual shift mode, simply shift, carefully, from one cog to another. Make sure that as you do, the chain falls squarely on the cog of your choice and is not noisy as you pedal. Make minor readjustments of the shift lever, as in the manual mode noted above, to move the chain precisely onto the cog you wish.

Solution Three: Some index shifters do not have a manual shift option. In this case either readjust the left and right limit bolts on the rear derailleur, as noted above in Problems One and Two, or wait until you get home or can get to a bike shop for this readjustment.

PROBLEM SIX: You can't shift to any rear cog.

Cause One: The shift cable has slipped out of the cable binder bolt on the derailleur, because that bolt was never tightened enough (See Table 5-1).

Solution: See Solution Two in Problem Three above.

Cause Two: The shifter cable has snapped.

Solution: Replace the shift cable. Here's how:

1. Loosen the cable binder bolt at the rear derailleur.
2. Remove the old cable (or the pieces of it), and note, as you do, where the leaded end of the cable comes out of the shift lever. Be sure you replace any shifter cable with the correct size and length. Your bike shop can tell you which cable you need. Be sure to buy new outer spaghetti tubing to go with your new shifter cable. Cut the spaghetti tubing so it is the same length as the old one. Install the new cable and tighten it in the derailleur cable binder bolt (see Table 5-1). Snip off

unneeded cable and install a cable end, or solder the cable *before* you cut it, to keep cable ends from becoming unraveled.

3. Where the shifter is part of the brake lever, move the small shift lever two or three times to align the cable hole in the shift levers. Push the new cable through and out the other side, as shown in Fig. 5-5. It may take time, but if you work at you will eventually get the new cable through.

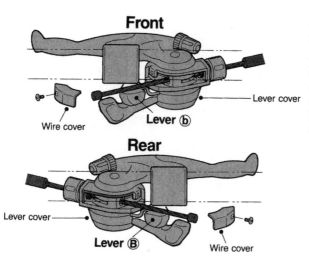

Front

Wire cover

Lever ⓑ

Lever cover

Rear

Lever cover

Lever Ⓑ

Wire cover

Fig. 5-5: This shift lever is attached to the brake lever body. B points to the leaded end of the shift lever cable, the unleaded end of which should be inserted first, of course.

PROBLEM SEVEN: The chain seems to shift by itself, without human intervention, on a nonindex (manual) shift system.

Cause: The wing nut that holds the shifter lever, usually on the down tube of a road bike, has worked loose.

Solution: Flip up the wing on the nut and tighten the nut by hand. If no wing is present, tighten the nut with a screwdriver or a coin.

Front Derailleur Problems, Causes, and Solutions

PROBLEM ONE: The chain overshifts to the left, falls off the small chainwheel and down onto the bottom bracket shell.

Cause One: Low-gear (small chainwheel) adjuster bolt lets the front derailleur cage move too far to the left, where it pushes the chain off the small freewheel.

Solution: If the derailleur is adjusted so the chain moves too far to the left, falls off the small chainwheel and onto the bottom bracket shell, the chain may get jammed between the fixed cup of the bottom bracket and the base of the chainwheel. Such sudden jamming can lock up or place considerable resistance to pedaling and cause you to lose balance and control. Or, the chain may simply rotate on the bracket shell, so you experience sudden zero resistance to pedaling. Adjust low-gear (left) travel. Lift the chain back up onto the small freewheel. While turning the cranks, shift the front derailleur so the small chainwheel (low gear) is close to, but not touching, the inner surface of the left chain guide plate, as shown in Fig. 5-6. Turn the low-gear adjuster bolt (Fig. 5-6) clockwise or counterclockwise, as necessary, to limit left movement of the derailleur to this location of the small chainwheel.

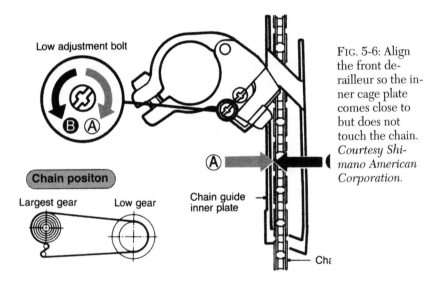

FIG. 5-6: Align the front derailleur so the inner cage plate comes close to but does not touch the chain. *Courtesy Shimano American Corporation.*

Cause Two: A bent chainwheel. Chainwheels are made of aluminum. They can be bent if the bike is dropped on them, if another bike runs into them, or for any of myriad similar impacts.

Solution: If you suspect a chainwheel is bent, remove the chain from it, spin the cranks, and eyeball the chainwheel from the rear. Mark any bent place with chalk. With a crescent wrench, *gently* force the chainwheel back to true. When you do this, remember that aluminum has a very limited modulus of elasticity, and it won't take many bends back and forth to break it. One such bend, back to true, is what you should aim for.

PROBLEM TWO: The chain falls to the right, off the big chainwheel, and down onto the crank arm.

Cause: The high-gear (big chainwheel) adjuster bolt lets the derailleur cage move too far to the right, so the derailleur cage pushes the chain off the big chainwheel. The hazard here is, again, unexpected zero pedaling resistance as the chain becomes disconnected from the chainwheel. The chain can also fall off the big chainwheel and tangle in the crank.

Solution: Adjust the front derailleur high-gear (right) travel. If necessary, lift and replace the chain on the big chainwheel. While turning the cranks, shift the front derailleur so the large chainwheel (high gear) is close to, but not touching, the inner surface of the right chain guide plate, as shown in Fig. 5-7. Turn the top adjustment bolt (Fig. 5-7) clockwise or counter-clockwise, as necessary, to limit right movement of the derailleur to this location of the large chainwheel.

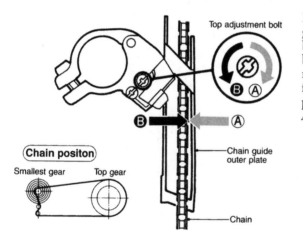

FIG. 5-7: Turn the high-gear adjuster bolt to bring the chain close to but not touching the right side of the inner front derailleur cage plate. *Courtesy Shimano American Corporation.*

PROBLEM THREE: The chain falls between chainwheels, where it can jam and lock up the chain.

Cause: The bolts and nuts that hold the chainwheels together are not tight. The chainwheels have spread farther apart, so the chain falls between them.

Solution: Tighten the chainwheel binder bolts (see D and E in Fig. 4-12) to the torque shown in Table 5-1. (I could give you the torque but I want you to get used to referring to this table. Tightening to the correct safe torque is vital to bicycle safety.)

PROBLEM FOUR: The chain cannot be shifted all the way to the biggest chainwheel.

Cause: The derailleur shift cable has stretched.

Solution:

1. Shift the chain to the smallest chainwheel.
2. Loosen the cable binder bolt at the derailleur (Fig. 5-8), and with a pair of pliers pull out the cable slack until the cable is taut.

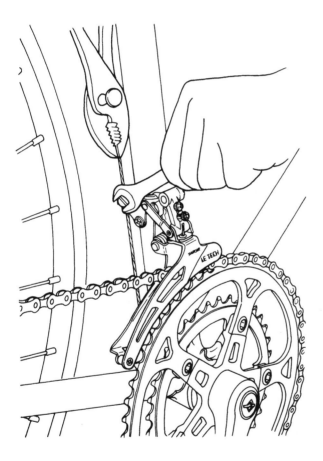

FIG. 5-8: Remove cable slack by loosening the cable binder bolt so you can pull the cable through it. *Courtesy Sun-Tour.*

PROBLEM FIVE: Grinding noise or chain rubbing sound from front derailleur.

Cause One: Sometimes you will hear a grinding noise coming from the front derailleur cage, after you have shifted to a higher or lower rear gear but have not shifted the front gear. This is because as you shift from one rear gear to another, the chain assumes an increasing angle with respect to the front derailleur cage. Try this for yourself. With the bike on a stand or suspended from the ceiling, shift the chain to the third gear of a five- or six-speed freewheel, or the fourth gear of a seven-speed freewheel. With the front shift lever, adjust the front derailleur until the chain is centered in the derailleur cage. Shift the chain to the smallest rear cog. You will see that the chain moves closer to the right front derailleur cage plate as you do so. Shift the chain to the largest rear cog. You will note that the chain moves closer to the left front derailleur cage plate. This change of chain angle in the front derailleur cage as you shift the chain from one rear cog to another explains why you can have chain rub and noise from the front derailleur.

Solution: The solution to this chain rub and noise is simple. Just be aware that you may have to move the front shift lever slightly to move the front derailleur cage enough one way or the other to keep the chain from rubbing on it as you shift to another rear cog, especially when you have shifted two or three cogs away from the original position. This problem of chain rub is particularly acute if you have a seven-speed freewheel and a three-speed chainwheel.

Cause Two: The front derailleur is positioned too low on the seat tube. In this position, the outer (right) side of the derailleur cage can strike and rub on the big chainwheel and the chain. Or the derailleur cage is not parallel to the big chainwheel.

Solution: Reposition the derailleur. Loosen the derailleur clamp bolt (Fig. 5-9) and move the front derailleur so the right side of the derailleur cage is between 3/64 and 1/8 inch above the big chainwheel (Fig. 5-10). The right side of the cage should also be parallel to the big chainwheel. Tighten the front derailleur clamp bolt to the torque specified in Table 5-1.

Dual-Lever Index Shifters

Dual-lever index shifters are now available for both mountain and road bicycles. They all work basically the same. The shifters all have a big lever and a small one. The big lever (I call it the power lever), A in Fig. 5-11 (a handlebar-mounted mountain bike shift system), moves the chain from a small to a larger gear. The shorter lever, B, moves the chain from a large gear to a smaller gear.

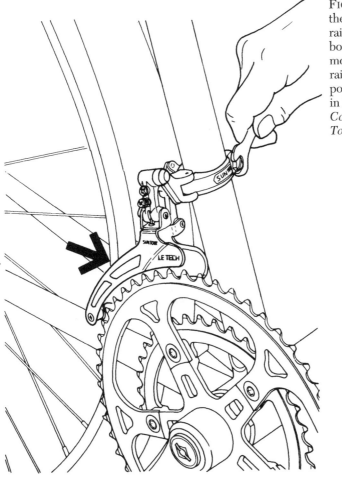

FIG. 5-9: Loosen the front derailleur clamp bolt so you can move the derailleur to the positions shown in FIG. 5-10. *Courtesy Sun-Tour.*

FIG. 5-10: Position the front derailleur cage so it is parallel to the big chainwheel and between 3/64 and 1/8 inch above it. *Courtesy Shimano American Corporation.*

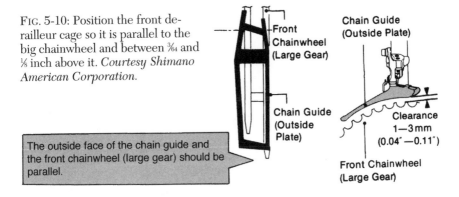

Front Chainwheel (Large Gear)

Chain Guide (Outside Plate)

Chain Guide (Outside Plate)

Clearance 1—3 mm (0.04″—0.11″)

Front Chainwheel (Large Gear)

The outside face of the chain guide and the front chainwheel (large gear) should be parallel.

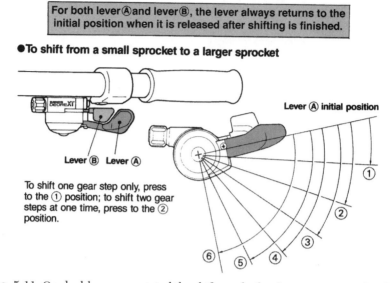

For both lever Ⓐ and lever Ⓑ, the lever always returns to the initial position when it is released after shifting is finished.

● **To shift from a small sprocket to a larger sprocket**

Lever Ⓑ   Lever Ⓐ

To shift one gear step only, press to the ① position; to shift two gear steps at one time, press to the ② position.

Lever Ⓐ initial position

FIG. 5-11: On dual-lever mountain bike shifters, the big lever, A, moves the chain from a small to a larger sprocket (cog). The small lever, B, moves the chain from a big to the next small cog. *Courtesy Shimano American Corporation.*

A combination brake and shift lever unit for road bikes (Fig. 5-12) uses a side movement of the brake lever to move the chain from a smaller to a larger freewheel cog or chainwheel and a side movement of the small lever, built into the brake lever (Fig. 5-12), to move the chain from a big to a smaller cog.

Do not disassemble any of these dual-lever shifters. This is a shop job, which requires special tools and training. About the only part you need re-

FIG. 5-12: This is a road bike front brake/shifter. Move the big lever sideways to move the chain to a larger cog. Depress this lever to brake. Move the smaller lever, recessed under the big lever, to move the chain from a bigger to a smaller cog. *Courtesy Shimano American Corporation.*

Downshift   Upshift   Brake

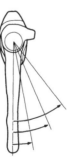

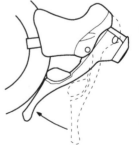

move is a shift lever wire cover, which should be removed when you install a new derailleur cable on the front or rear shift lever assembly.

Another word about shifting: As I noted earlier in this chapter, you should ease pedaling pressure while you shift, but keep pedaling. I also said that you should shift to a bigger rear freewheel cog or a smaller chainwheel *before* you start climbing a steep hill. Index shifter manufacturers state that you don't have to do this with their new freewheel, chainwheel, and shifter designs. You might check this out, but for myself I prefer to be on the safe side and get into a gear I know will get me up the hill before I start the climb.

Earlier models of index shifters worked only on the rear freewheel cogs. Current models work on both the freewheel cogs and the chainwheel up front. However, if you have the chain on the biggest rear cog and the smallest chainwheel, remember that you have put the chain at an extreme angle. At this angle the chain may rub on the front derailleur cage. If you hear noise when you shift to this gear combination, move the big shift lever a bit to move the chain away from the derailleur cage.

Gear Ratios

Back around 1968, the biggest rear freewheel cog you could buy had only 28 teeth and the smallest chainwheel had just 48 teeth. Mountain bikes, with wide-range gearing, had yet to be invented. Road bikes sold in the United States were mostly made in Europe and designed with extremely close ratio gearing for muscular road racers. I got the message on my first bike ride in hilly San Francisco. On my return to Detroit I said to Gene Portuesi, then the U.S. Olympic bicycle team coach and a bike shop owner, "Gene, I just got back from San Francisco. Do you have a 28-tooth . . ." That's as far as I got before he burst out laughing. He knew exactly what I meant, which was to please, please fix me up with wider-range gears—a set of gears that the bike industry today calls "granny gears."

If you are tired of straining up steep hills, or walking and pushing your bike up them, or if you are planning a long bike trip and want to carry camping gear, extra clothing, tools, and spare parts, you do need wide-ratio gears. You will rotate the cranks fast to crawl up steep hills in low gears, but the slowest such crawl is faster and a lot easier than walking alongside a loaded bike and pushing it up a steep hill. Wide-range gearing also reduces the temptation to reduce the grade of a hill by slaloming, a skiing term that means going from side to side on a hill. Cycling from one side of a steep road to the other side as you go up the grade is unsafe for two reasons. First, you will be working hard and concentrating on the climb, rather than looking out for motor vehicles. Second, car drivers won't expect you to be weaving around and may run into you.

Mountain bikes come with wide-range gearing because off-road trails can be steep, the terrain winding and sometimes slippery. But you can add even bigger gears to them. Road bikes typically have less favorable gearing for hill climbing, and their rear derailleur is not designed to accommodate these bigger gears. If you want to add bigger gears, either to your mountain or your road bike, here is how to do it.

Gear Availability and Compatibility

The biggest rear cog on the market has 34 teeth (Shimano). The smallest chainwheel up front has 24 teeth (except for a special triple chainwheel set available from SunTour, on which the smallest chainwheel has only 20 teeth). You should be able to find a 24-tooth chainwheel that is compatible with the triple chainwheel set you now have. In fact, since most mountain bike chainwheel sets have a 24-tooth chainwheel, you won't need to bother changing chainwheels. On a road bike you will have to install a new bottom bracket with a longer spindle (axle) so the wider triple chainwheel set you install will clear the chain stay. Well, you could replace a 34-tooth with a 24-tooth chainwheel on a double chainring set, but you would then find the jumps between gears so wide as to be virtually unusable. My advice is to consult your bicycle shop when you want to install wider-range gears on a road or mountain bike to make sure the parts you buy are compatible with the parts you now have.

Years ago SunTour made a 38-tooth freewheel cog, which I installed on a mountain bike and on a road bike. I just love that big old rear cog, because it lets me climb even a 15 percent grade with a camp-gear-laden bike sitting down, with the chain on the 38-tooth rear cog and on a 24-tooth chainwheel up front. My pedals are churning fast, the bike is moving at a pace that barely keeps me upright, but it's a lot easier than walking and pushing that bike up the hill. I can't, of course, have the chain on the 38-tooth cog and on the big chainwheel at the same time, because no rear derailleur on the market will handle that wide a gear range. But the sacrifice of that gear combination is worth the hill climbing ease from the 38-tooth cog. However, the Shimano 34-tooth cog, combined with a 24-tooth chainwheel, should be all the super-low gear you need to get up steep hills.

Gear Numbers

Before I get into the mechanics of installing bigger gears, you should know about gear ratios. This way you can select gear combinations that fit your athletic ability and cycling skills.

For the past 100 years or so the bicycle fraternity has referred to gear ratios in "inches" of gear. The gear-inch concept is a throwback to the high-wheel bicycle in use before 1900, (see Fig. 13-1), when the gear ratio of a bicycle was simply the diameter of the big front wheel in inches. These high-wheelers did not have gears. The pedals and cranks were attached to the front wheel. The bigger the wheel, the faster you could go. All you needed were legs long enough to reach the pedals. This concept was translated to modern multigeared bicycles by a leap of the imagination, a love of bicycle lore, and some simple math.

To arrive at the "inches" of gear for any combination of front chainwheel and rear freewheel cog, use this simple two-step formula. Count the number of teeth of the freewheel cog of your choice. Do the same for the chainwheel of your choice. Find the *gear ratio* between these two gears by dividing the number of teeth in the chainwheel by the number of teeth in the freewheel cog. For example, if you counted 48 teeth in the chainwheel and 32 teeth in the freewheel cog, $48 \div 32 = 1.5$, which is the *gear ratio of this combination*. The second step in finding the gear *inches* is to multiply this *gear ratio* by the diameter of the rear wheel, which on a mountain bike is 26 inches. For example, $26 \times 1.5 = 39$ inches, rounded off. That is the number of inches of this gear combination. For a road bike with 27-inch wheels (or 700-cm wheels), the above combination of freewheel and chainwheel teeth would give you $1.5 \times 27 =$ a gear inch of 40.5.

Let's go to the other extreme and find a super low, low gear, in the archaic "inch" terminology (we're stuck with it). Say you have a rear cog with 34 teeth (which is as big as they come) and a small chainwheel with 24 teeth (as small as they come). Put these two gears together and you have $24 \div 38 = .63$ (a negative gear ratio), and .63 × your 26-inch wheel diameter gives you an *inch* equivalent gear of 16.4, or, for a 27-inch (or 700-cm) wheel, $.63 \times 27 = 17$, truly a wall climber.

In any bicycle gear selection you are going to have duplication of gears. For an example, look at Table 5-2. You can arrive at a 54-inch gear by a combination of a 24-tooth chainwheel and a 12-tooth freewheel cog, a 26-tooth chainwheel and a 13-tooth freewheel cog, and many other combinations of chainwheel and freewheel cog teeth. Use the gear tables to avoid such useless gear combinations when you decide to add granny gears to your bicycle. Gear inch tables for 27-inch and 700-cm wheels are in Table 5-2, for 26-inch wheels in Table 5-3, for 24-inch wheels in Table 5-4.

TABLE 5-2: GEAR TABLE FOR 27-INCH AND 700-CM WHEELS

NUMBER OF TEETH IN CHAINWHEEL

GEAR INCHES

Rear \ Chainwheel	24	25	26	27	28	29	30	31	32	33	34	35	36	37	38	39	40	41	42	43	44	45	46	47	48	49	50	51	52	53	54
12	54	56	59	61	63	65	68	70	72	74	77	79	81	83	86	88	90	92	95	97	99	101	104	105	108	110	113	115	117	119	122
13	50	52	54	56	58	60	62	64	67	69	71	72	75	79	79	81	83	85	87	89	91	94	96	98	100	102	104	106	108	110	112
14	46	48	50	52	54	56	58	60	62	64	66	68	69	71	73	75	77	79	81	83	85	87	89	91	93	95	96	98	100	102	104
15	43	45	47	49	50	52	54	56	58	59	61	63	65	67	68	70	72	74	76	77	79	81	83	85	86	88	90	92	94	95	97
16	41	42	44	46	47	49	51	52	54	56	57	59	61	62	64	66	68	69	71	73	74	76	78	79	81	83	84	86	88	89	91
17	38	40	41	43	45	46	48	49	51	52	54	56	57	59	60	62	64	65	67	68	70	72	73	75	76	78	79	81	83	84	86
18	36	38	39	41	42	44	45	47	48	50	51	53	54	56	57	59	60	62	63	65	66	68	69	71	72	74	75	77	78	80	81
19	34	36	37	38	40	41	43	44	46	47	48	50	51	53	54	55	57	58	60	61	63	64	65	67	68	70	71	73	74	75	77
20	32	34	35	36	38	39	41	42	43	45	46	47	49	50	51	53	54	55	57	58	59	61	62	64	65	66	68	69	70	72	73
21	31	32	33	35	36	37	39	40	41	42	44	45	46	48	49	50	51	53	54	55	57	58	59	60	62	63	64	66	67	68	69
22	29	31	32	33	34	36	37	38	39	41	42	43	44	45	47	48	49	50	52	53	54	55	56	58	59	60	61	63	64	65	66
23	28	29	31	32	33	34	35	36	38	39	40	41	42	43	45	46	47	48	49	50	52	53	54	55	56	58	59	60	61	62	63
24	27	28	29	30	32	33	34	35	36	37	38	39	41	42	43	44	45	46	47	48	50	51	52	53	54	55	56	57	59	60	61
25	26	27	28	29	30	31	32	33	35	36	37	38	39	40	41	42	43	44	45	46	48	49	50	51	52	53	54	55	56	57	58
26	25	26	27	28	29	30	31	32	33	34	35	36	37	38	39	41	42	43	44	45	46	47	48	49	50	51	52	53	54	55	56
27	24	25	26	27	28	29	30	31	32	33	34	35	36	37	38	39	40	41	42	43	44	45	46	47	48	49	50	51	52	53	54
28	23	24	25	26	27	28	29	30	31	32	33	34	35	36	37	38	39	40	41	41	42	43	44	45	46	47	48	49	50	51	52
29	22	23	24	25	26	27	28	29	30	31	32	33	34	34	35	36	37	38	39	40	41	42	43	44	45	46	47	47	48	49	50
30	22	23	23	24	25	26	27	28	29	30	31	32	32	33	34	35	36	37	38	39	40	41	41	42	43	44	45	46	47	48	49
31	21	22	23	24	24	25	26	27	28	29	30	30	31	32	33	34	35	36	37	37	38	39	40	41	42	43	44	44	45	46	47
32	20	21	22	23	24	24	25	26	27	28	29	30	30	31	32	33	34	35	35	36	37	38	39	40	41	41	42	43	44	45	46
33	20	20	21	22	23	24	25	25	26	27	28	29	29	30	31	32	33	34	34	35	36	37	38	38	39	40	41	42	43	43	44
34	19	20	21	21	22	23	24	25	25	26	27	28	29	29	30	31	32	33	33	34	35	36	37	37	38	39	40	41	41	42	43

NUMBER OF TEETH IN REAR SPROCKET

TABLE 5-3: GEAR TABLE FOR MOUNTAIN BICYCLES WITH 26-INCH WHEELS*

NUMBER OF CHAINWHEEL TEETH

NUMBER OF FREEWHEEL TEETH	24	26	28	36	38	40	46	48	50	52
	GEAR INCHES									
13	48	52	56	72	76	80	92	96	100	104
14	45	48	52	67	71	74	85	89	93	97
15	42	45	49	62	66	69	80	83	87	90
16	39	42	46	59	62	65	75	78	81	85
17	37	40	43	55	58	61	70	73	76	80
18	35	38	40	52	55	58	66	69	72	75
19	33	36	38	49	52	55	63	66	68	71
21	30	32	35	45	47	50	57	59	62	64
22	28	31	33	43	45	47	54	57	59	61
23	27	30	32	41	43	45	52	54	57	59
24	26	28	30	39	41	43	50	52	54	56
28	22	24	26	33	35	37	43	45	46	48
30	21	23	24	31	33	35	40	42	43	45
32	20	21	23	29	31	33	37	39	41	42
34	18	20	21	28	29	31	35	37	38	40

* Gear tabulations are rounded off to the nearest whole number. Differences in the tire diameters of tire sizes 1.5-inch, 1.75-inch, and 2.125-inch have not been calculated because they are so small. Note the many gear duplications possible with various combinations of front and rear cogs. For example, you can get a 45-inch gear with 10 combinations of these cogs.

TABLE 5-4: GEAR TABLE FOR 24-INCH WHEELS*

NUMBER OF TEETH IN CHAINWHEEL

NUMBER OF TEETH IN FREEWHEEL	20	24	26	28	34	36	38	44	48	50	52	54
	GEAR INCHES											
12	40	48	52	56	68	72	76	88	96	100	104	108
13	37	44	48	52	63	66	70	81	89	92	96	100
14	34	41	45	48	58	62	65	75	82	86	89	93
15	32	38	42	45	54	58	61	70	77	80	83	86
16	30	36	39	42	51	54	57	66	72	75	78	81
17	28	34	37	40	48	51	54	62	68	71	73	76
18	27	32	35	37	45	48	51	59	64	67	69	72
19	25	30	33	34	41	43	46	53	58	60	62	65
21	23	27	30	32	39	41	43	50	55	57	59	62
23	21	25	27	29	35	38	40	46	50	52	54	56
25	19	23	25	27	33	35	36	42	46	48	50	52
26	18	22	24	26	31	33	35	41	44	46	48	50
28	17	21	22	24	29	31	33	38	41	43	45	46
30	16	19	21	22	27	29	30	35	38	40	42	43
32	15	18	20	21	26	27	29	33	36	38	39	41

If you know what gear you're in and how many crank arm rpm's you are pedaling, you can figure out how fast you are traveling from Fig. 5-13. A simple way to compute your own gear inches is to use a computer program developed by Brian Rosenthal of 1550 Olene Ave., Stillwater, MN 55082. All you do is enter the number of teeth in your cogs, front and rear, and your IBM-compatible computer will do the math for you in a split second.

FIG. 5-13: Compute your speed using this chart.

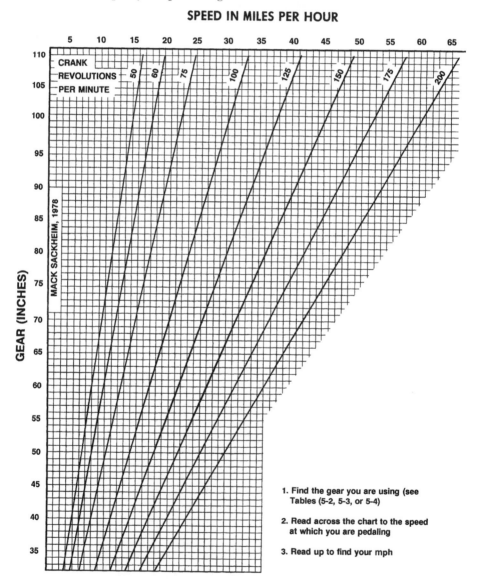

SPEED IN MILES PER HOUR

GEAR (INCHES)

MACK SACKHEIM, 1978

1. Find the gear you are using (see Tables (5-2, 5-3, or 5-4)

2. Read across the chart to the speed at which you are pedaling

3. Read up to find your mph

Derailleur Capacity

It's important to know how derailleur capacity is arrived at and what it means to you. For example, you may be unhappy with the gear ratios you now have. You want a lower gear, let's say, to ease your way when your bike is heavily laden and the hills are steep. To change to lower gears you will have to change your low freewheel gear to one with more teeth, or change the small chainwheel to one with fewer teeth, or both. Or change the chainwheel setup from a double to a triple chainwheel set with a smaller chainwheel at the low end. The problem here is that your old derailleur may not be able to handle the bigger gears. Any bike shop can show you a close-ratio derailleur and a wide-ratio derailleur. When you compare them you will see that the wide-ratio derailleur has a longer body that can handle the extra chain length involved with bigger gears. While you are in the bike shop, also compare the size of the cogs in a close-ratio rear freewheel gear cluster with a relatively wide-ratio gear cluster. You can see that the bigger cogs will require a longer chain.

Select front and rear derailleurs that have the capacity to handle the larger gears you plan to install on your bike. Derailleur manufacturers give you their capacity, but it needs some interpretation. Here's how to determine what derailleur capacity you need.

To compute derailleur capacity, simply subtract the number of teeth in the smallest rear cog from the number of teeth in the largest rear cog. Then subtract the number of teeth in the smallest chainwheel up front from the number of teeth in the largest chainwheel. Add these two numbers for the total capacity of the derailleur.

For example, my mountain bike has a super-granny freewheel gear of 13 teeth on the small cog and 38 on the big cog—38 minus 13 equals 25. The small chainwheel has 24 teeth and the big one has 48 teeth—48 minus 24 equals 24. Adding these, 25 plus 24 equals 49. That's the capacity of the rear derailleur I am supposed to be using. I say "supposed" because there is not a derailleur on the market rated at 49 teeth. Not, at least, the last time I looked. The penalty I pay for this wall-climbing set of gears is that I can't use the biggest (low-gear) freewheel cog and the biggest (high-speed) chainwheel at the same time. To me this is no penalty at all. I love the hill-climbing low gear I get with this combination. Sometimes I believe I could walk up hills faster than I can ride when my chain is on the 38-tooth freewheel and on the 24-tooth chainwheel, but when I try I soon discover that, slow as it seems, *riding* uphill is a whole lot easier and more comfortable than walking and shoving the bike along, especially when the bike is loaded with camping gear.

If you have index shifting on your bike I strongly recommend you consult your bicycle shop mechanic before investing in bigger gears. Any gears you select must be compatible with your index shifters. If you have straight friction shifting you should have no problem swapping smaller for bigger cogs, as long as you make sure your current derailleurs can handle the new gearing or you buy a derailleur than can do so. The single- and dual-lever index shifters are designed for a specific number of gears. A five-gear rear index shifter won't work on a six-gear setup, nor will a six-gear index shifter handle a seven-speed freewheel. The same goes for dual to triple chainwheel conversions. If you lust for a "granny" hill-climbing gear, you may either have to return to good old reliable friction shifting or install a new index shifting system that's compatible with your new gearing. For cassette-style freehubs, some rear gear clusters come riveted together in sets of six cogs. The more expensive clusters are bolted to a flange so individual gears (cogs) can be exchanged. In addition, rear cassette freehub gears are not interchangeable between makes of these hubs. Some chainwheels are interchangeable with other makes. For fixed freewheels, which come as a unit and thread onto the hub, you should have no problems switching cog sizes. Check with your bike shop before buying any parts.

Crank Lengths

Archimedes, an ancient Greek mathematician, said "Give me a long enough lever and a place to stand and I can move the world." Well, a crank is simply a lever. The longer the crank, the easier it is to pedal; the shorter it is, the harder. But that's a gross oversimplification. The following data were contributed by Frank M. Branzuela, a brilliant engineer who lives in Anchorage, Alaska, and who is also an ardent bicyclist. Frank says: "After researching 'women's' bicycles, I realized that many manufacturers (and bicycle shops) think nothing of installing shorter cranks *while leaving everything else as it is.* At first glance this seems perfectly acceptable. But a little thought will tell you that shorter cranks mean less leverage and that this less leverage requires more force. So petite women have to pedal *harder* (but not faster) than someone riding a standard bicycle with 170-mm cranks.

"How much difference can 5 mm make? Well, unless the gearing is changed to bigger rear cogs, women riding bikes with 165-mm cranks have to work harder to keep the same pace as those of us with 170-mm cranks. Look at it this way: The pedal axle goes around in a circle. I think we can all agree about that. With a 170-mm crank, this circle has a circumference of 42.03 inches (170 mm = 6.69; 6.69 × 2 = a diameter of 13.38 inches, which, multiplied by pi of 3.14159 = 42.03 inches). So the rider's foot moves 42.03 inches for each crank rotation. For this example, let's say the rider's bike has a 52-tooth chainring.

"Let's see what happens when that same rider's bike has a 165-mm crank with the same 52-tooth chainwheel. Now the rider's foot moves through a smaller circle. The 165-mm crank is $6.49605 \times 2 = 12.992 \times 3.14159 = 40.815851$ inches. But one revolution of this 165-mm crank with a 52-tooth chainwheel still only moves the 52-tooth chainring one revolution, and the rider's foot moves through a smaller circle. Now here's the problem. One revolution of the 170-mm crank moves the 52-tooth chainwheel 42.03 inches. But one revolution of the same 52-tooth chainwheel with a 165-mm crank only moves the chainwheel 40.815851 inches. The 52-tooth chainring on the bike with 165-mm cranks should be changed to a 50-tooth chainring to compensate for this loss of leverage. And the rider with the 165-mm crank must spin faster to keep up with the rider with the 170-mm crank."

Table 5-5 shows the relationship between crank length and gearing. It was computed by Frank Branzuela.

You don't need to go to the trouble and expense of changing crank lengths (you'd be looking at upward of $150 just for the new cranks). Individual chain-

TABLE 5-5: THE EFFECT OF CRANK LENGTH ON GEARING

CRANK ARM LENGTH

CHAINRING	160 MM	165 MM	170 MM	172.5 MM	175 MM	180 MM
54	57.4/50.8	55.6/52.4	54.0/54.0	53.2/54.8	52.5/55.6	51.0/57.2
53	56.3/49.9	54.6/51.4	53.0/53.0	52.2/53.8	51.5/54.6	50.1/56.1
52	55.2/48.9	53.6/50.5	52.0/52.0	51.2/52.8	50.5/53.5	49.1/55.1
51	54.2/48.0	52.5/49.5	51.0/51.0	50.3/51.8	49.5/52.5	48.2/54.0
50	53.1/47.1	51.5/48.5	50.0/50.0	49.3/50.7	48.6/51.5	47.2/52.9
49	52.1/46.1	50.5/47.6	49.0/49.0	48.3/49.7	47.6/50.4	46.3/51.9
48	51.0/45.2	49.5/46.6	48.0/48.0	47.3/48.7	46.6/49.4	45.3/50.8
47	49.9/44.2	48.4/45.6	47.0/47.0	46.3/47.7	45.7/48.4	44.4/49.8
46	48.9/43.3	47.4/44.6	46.0/46.0	45.3/46.7	44.7/47.4	43.4/48.7
45	47.8/42.4	46.4/43.7	45.0/45.0	44.3/45.7	43.7/46.3	42.5/47.6
44	46.7/41.4	45.3/42.7	44.0/44.0	43.4/44.6	42.7/45.3	41.6/46.6
43	45.7/40.5	44.3/41.7	43.0/43.0	42.4/43.6	41.8/44.3	40.6/45.5
42	44.6/39.5	43.0/40.8	42.0/42.0	41.4/42.6	40.8/43.2	39.7/44.5
41	43.6/38.6	42.2/39.8	41.0/41.0	40.4/41.6	39.8/42.2	38.7/43.4
40	42.5/37.6	41.2/38.8	40.0/40.0	39.4/40.6	38.9/41.2	37.8/42.4
39	41.4/36.7	40.2/37.9	39.0/39.0	38.4/39.6	37.9/40.1	36.8/41.3
38	40.4/35.8	39.2/36.9	38.0/38.0	37.4/38.6	36.9/39.1	35.9/40.2
37	39.3/34.8	38.1/35.9	37.0/37.0	36.5/37.5	35.9/38.1	34.9/39.2
36	38.2/33.9	37.1/34.9	36.0/36.0	35.5/36.5	35.0/37.1	34.0/38.1
35	37.2/32.9	36.1/34.0	35.0/35.0	34.5/35.5	34.0/36.0	33.1/37.1
34	36.1/32.0	35.0/33.0	34.0/34.0	33.5/34.5	33.0/35.0	32.1/36.0
33	35.1/31.1	34.0/32.0	33.0/33.0	32.5/33.5	32.1/34.0	31.2/34.9
32	34.0/30.1	33.0/31.1	32.0/32.0	31.5/32.5	31.1/32.9	30.2/33.9
31	32.9/29.2	31.9/30.1	31.0/31.0	30.6/31.5	30.1/31.9	29.3/32.8
30	31.9/28.2	30.9/29.1	30.0/30.0	29.6/30.4	29.1/30.9	28.3/31.8
29	30.8/27.3	29.9/28.1	29.0/29.0	28.6/29.4	28.2/29.9	27.4/30.7
28	29.7/26.4	28.8/27.2	28.0/28.0	27.6/28.4	27.2/28.8	26.4/29.6

wheels and freewheel cogs are a lot less expensive. Just change chainwheel or freewheel *cogs.* Here's how to do it. First, these are the tools you will need for swapping chainwheels, and while I'm at it, for changing freewheel cogs on both conventional and freehub freewheels. These tools should be available from your bike shop. If not, send for the Third Hand catalog, Box 212, Mt. Shasta, CA 96067, or phone 1-800-926-9904 at any time day or night.

1. Five-millimeter Allen wrench for chainwheel binder bolts.
2. L wrench to hold chainwheel binder nuts.
3. Special bottom bracket spindle bolt wrench (B in Fig. 5-14) or a 14-, 15-, or 16-mm thin wall socket wrench, or a 5-mm Allen wrench (depending on make and model of bottom bracket) (A in Fig. 5-14).
4. Crank puller tool (C in Fig. 5-14).

FIG. 5-14: To remove a crank, remove the crank lockbolt with wrench, B, or a 14-, 15-, or 16-mm thin wall-socket wrench. Then insert the threaded end of the steel crank-tool, C, *carefully* into the aluminum dust-cap threads. Turn the crank tool clockwise with an adjustable crescent wrench until the crank is loose. Use an Allen wrench, A, and the tool, D, to remove individual chainwheels either to replace worn chainwheels or to change chainwheel sizes (and gear ratios).

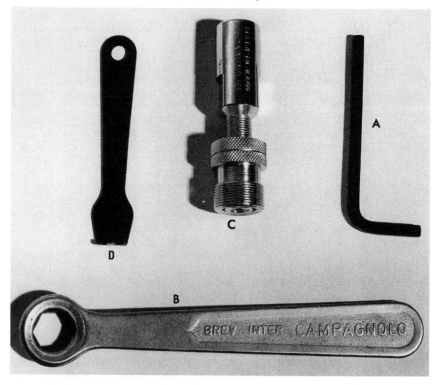

5. Freewheel remover for conventional freewheels, which thread onto the hub. Every freewheel model or make seems to take its own individual tool. There is about as much industry standardization in the bike business as there are identical snowflakes.
6. Freewheel cog tool for conventional freewheels.
7. Lock ring tool for freehub cassettes. Each of the three Shimano lock rings takes a different tool, so be sure to buy the correct tool from your bike shop.

Changing Chainwheels

The only reason to change a chainwheel would be to go down to a smaller third chainwheel, say from 28 to 24 teeth. Or you could replace worn chainwheels the same way. Do it like this:

1. Shift to the small chainwheel. Lift the chain off the chainwheel and place it on the bottom bracket shell.
2. Remove the right crank arm dustcap.
3. With a 14-, 15-, or 16-mm socket wrench, or a crankbolt wrench (B in Fig. 5-14), remove the binder bolt that holds the right crank arm onto the bottom bracket spindle.
4. Insert the crank puller (C in Fig. 5-14), into the dustcap threads of the crank arm (Fig. 5-15). Be careful not to strip the crank arm aluminum threads! If this tool will not thread all the way into the dustcap threads, turn the outer section of the tool counterclockwise as far as possible.
5. With a wrench (Fig. 5-15), turn the outer section of the crank puller clockwise until the crank arm is loose from the bottom bracket axle and can be pulled free. If you can't get the crank loose without danger of stripping the dustcap threads, tap the end of the crank puller with a hammer a few times.
6. With the Allen wrench and tool D (Fig. 5-14), loosen the bolts that hold the chainwheels onto the crank spider.
7. Replace the chainwheel(s) with the sizes that meet your gearing needs. Be sure the new chainwheels are compatible with your crankset. Also, replace any chainwheels with worn teeth (see Fig. 4-4). For semi-elliptical BioPace chainwheels, be sure the high point of these chainwheels is aligned along the centerline of the crank arm and that these high sectors all face the same direction.
8. Tighten the chainwheel binder bolts and the crank arm binder bolt (see Table 5-1 for torques) onto the bottom bracket spindle (axle).

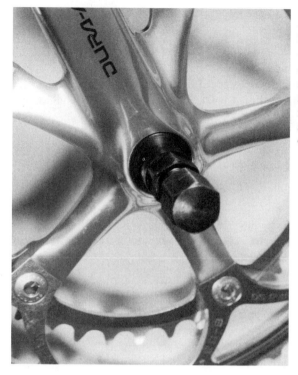

Fig. 5-15: Use the crank-puller tool, C (Fig. 5-14), to remove a crank from the bottom bracket spindle. (A similar tool is available from your bike shop for the lock ring from freehub freewheels so you can remove their cogs.)

Changing Freewheel Cogs

If you want bigger granny gears that ease hill climbing, or closer-ratio gears for the flats or for racing, here's how to change freewheel cogs. Since there are more bikes out there with conventional freewheels—the kind that thread onto a rear hub—I will start with them. First, make sure the cogs you choose will fit and be compatible with your hub, your chain, and your shifting system. Talk to your bike shop about this first. While you're at it, replace any worn cogs (Fig. 4-4).

Steps to Remove Freewheel

1. Remove the wheel from the bicycle.
2. Remove the quick-release unit or, if your bike has a solid axle, the axle bolt on the freewheel side.
3. Insert the correct size freewheel remover (Fig. 5-16) in the freewheel. Tighten the quick-release, as shown in Fig. 5-17, or axle bolt, so it holds the freewheel remover in place. Turn the bolt clockwise to remove the freewheel unit. The quick-release or bolt should not be tightened down all the way. Set it just close enough that it will let you

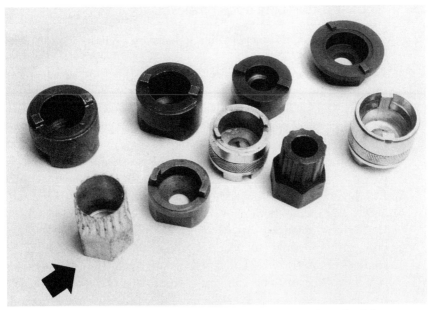

FIG. 5-16: Insert one of these freewheel tools to remove the freewheel from a conventional (nonfreehub) hub body.

FIG. 5-17: Use the quick-release or axle bolt to hold the freewheel tool in place while you turn it counterclockwise to remove the freewheel from the hub.

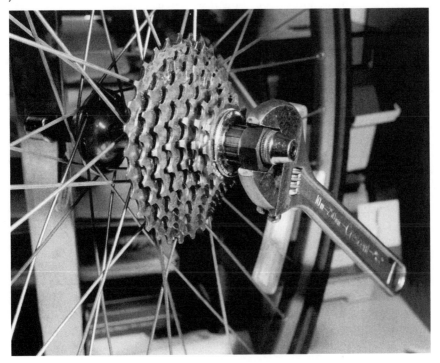

turn the freewheel remover counterclockwise a half to one turn with a wrench (Fig. 5-17).

4. When the freewheel breaks loose from the hub, remove the quick-release or the axle bolt.

5. Finish removing the freewheel by turning the freewheel tool by hand. As the freewheel approaches the last few threads, hold it firmly so it comes off the hub without harming the softer aluminum hub threads.

6. Agitate the freewheel in kerosene. With a brush and rag clean each cog.

7. Dry the freewheel with an air hose, if available, to remove the solvent.

8. Squirt *light* oil into both sides of the freewheel.

9. Resist the temptation to take the freewheel unit itself apart. There are dozens of minuscule ball bearings inside, which, once free from the confines of the freewheel, flee pell-mell to the floor and hide themselves away, never to be seen again. Not to mention the teensy little springs and pawls. If you need a new freewheel, just take it to your bike shop for a replacement. If you have any form of index shifting you will need an exact replacement freewheel.

10. If the chain has slipped off the big rear cog at any time it may have cut into one or more spokes. With the freewheel removed, look for spoke gouges that foretell spoke breakage. See Chapter 7 for spoke replacement and wheel truing instructions.

Replacing (Conventional) Freewheel Cogs

1. Remove the freewheel as shown above.

2. Drill two holes in your wood workbench to hold two bolts, spaced to fit the holes in the large freewheel cog. Use the cog remover (Fig. 5-18) to turn the small freewheel cog counterclockwise. Remove it. On most freewheels only the small cog is threaded on. If the second cog is also threaded on, remove it the same way. Now you can slide off the remaining cogs and their spacers. As you remove these parts, make a note of which spacers go where, because some may be thinner than others. If the space between any two cogs is too wide or too narrow, the chain may slip when you shift and cause an accident.

3. Replace worn cog(s) and/or install cogs with different number of teeth. For example, if you want a lower, hill-climbing granny gear, replace the big cog with a 32- or 34-tooth cog. Years ago SunTour made a 38-tooth cog. If you call enough bike shops you may find such a super-low-gear cog on a freewheel board. Before you go this route, please review the

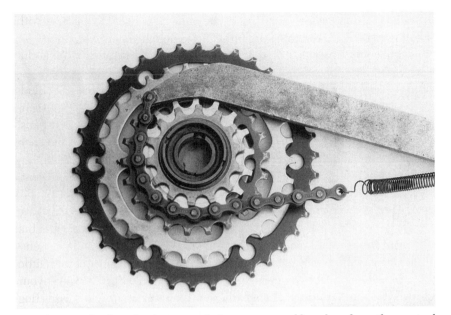

FIG. 5-18: Fit the freewheel over two bolts on your workbench and use the cog tool (counterclockwise) to remove the first cog. Cogs behind it should slide off, along with spacing washers.

data earlier in this chapter on gears and gearing, especially the data on rear derailleur capacity. Any cogs you replace must also be compatible with the old cogs and with whatever shift system and chain you use. See your bike shop for specific fit help. Note also that if you go to a bigger rear cog you will probably have to install a longer chain. Don't just add new links to your old chain. They won't be worn the same way as the old links, so you could have chain skip. Review Chapter 4 for more data on chains.

4. Replace the freewheel on the hub. Again, be absolutely certain that the threads in the freewheel go evenly onto the hub threads. If you cross threads, you are very likely going to strip the softer aluminum hub threads and will have to replace the hub (see Chapter 7 for wheel building and truing). If you started cross-threaded, insert the freewheel tool (Fig. 5-17), remove the freewheel carefully, and start again. If you did strip some of the threads on the hub, take the wheel to your bike shop and see if the hub freewheel threads can be recut. Replace the wheel in the bike.

Note: If on a bike ride you suddenly find that your freewheel works in both rotations, so your cranks don't move the bike but spin freely, a piece of dirt is holding up a freewheel pawl. Just squirt some kerosene into the freewheel, spin the freewheel, and that little bit of dirt should be knocked loose. If not, repeat this procedure. But do not get any solvent on the tire, brake shoes, or wheel rim.

Removing Freewheel Cogs on Freehubs

Freewheel cogs on freehubs are a lot easier to remove and replace than cogs on conventional hubs. Here's how:

1. Remove the wheel.
2. *On older freehub freewheels* use two cog tools. One cog tool is the same type as that shown in Fig. 5-18. Use the cog tool that fits your freehub and remove the small cog.
3. *On newer freehub cassette freewheels* use the cog chain tool to hold the freewheel, insert the correct size lock ring tool (Fig. 5-16—see your bike shop) into the lock ring and turn the tool counterclockwise to remove the lock ring.

FIG. 5-19: On a cassette freehub, turn the lock ring tool counterclockwise to remove the ring, then pull the cogs off the freewheel body.

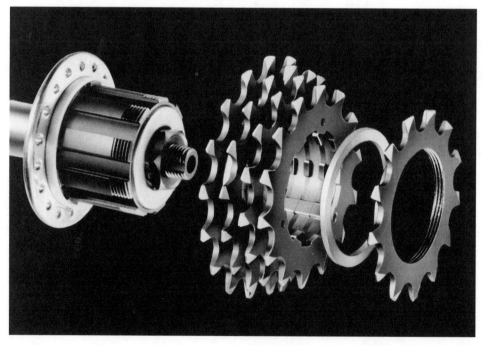

4. Pull the first four cogs and one spacer (Fig. 5-19) from the freewheel body.

5. To replace the bigger cogs, unscrew the bolts that hold them on the freewheel spider. Remove each cog and as you do note how each of the spacer washers between them is aligned. When replacing cogs, be sure the projections on the surface of the spacers face toward the smaller cogs. Replacement cogs must be compatible with the freewheel.

6. Replace all cogs and tighten the lock ring (see Table 5-1 for correct torque). Note, too, that cogs will only fit back on the splines of the freewheel when the one widest groove is aligned with the one widest spline.

The next chapter will cover the maintenance of the bottom bracket bearings and pedals.

CHAPTER SIX

HUBS, BOTTOM BRACKETS, AND PEDALS

In this chapter you will learn how to care for your hubs, bottom brackets, and pedals. I will start with hubs.

HUB MAINTENANCE

This chapter will include both standard and sealed-bearing hub maintenance, beginning with the standard design. First, though, please review the section on the adjustment and use of the hub quick-release mechanism in Chapters 1 and 2. Be sure you understand how to adjust the quick-release mechanism to keep the wheel safely held in the fork and chain-stay dropouts.

Hub Disassembly

Clean and relube conventional non-sealed-bearing hubs after every extensive trip or every two weeks on a road or trail trip if you have biked through water or over sand. This two-week maintenance frequency for non-sealed-bearing hubs may seem excessive. If so, here's a suggestion, based on my experience. I was on a road trip in Vermont. I had pedaled over dirt and sandy roads to get into state parks at night. One evening, after dinner, I decided to check my hubs. Spinning a bike wheel, I heard a grinding noise coming from my precision-machined, costly Campagnolo rear hub, a gritty sound that penetrated to the very depths of my wallet. Sand had worked its destructive way into the bearings. Fortunately I had a set of hub wrenches along. When I disassembled the hub I did indeed find sand, but no damage. I was lucky. So my suggestion is to make the following daily hub check on a bike trip, or make it at least monthly if you do more casual day riding: Turn the bike upside down. Spin each wheel. Feel for grinding with your fingertips on the hub body (careful, don't catch your fingers in the spokes), listen for grating sounds from the hub. Relube by following the instructions below. If all seems OK you may be able to get by for a longer period. But if you have forded streams or cycled over sand a lot, I urge you to increase the relube frequency. These instructions apply to freehubs (with an integral freewheel) as well as to conventional hubs.

First, here are the tools you will need to work on your hubs, bottom bracket, and pedals:

1. Crank puller (C in Fig. 5-14).
2. Socket wrenches, 14 or 15 mm, for the bottom bracket axle (aka spindle) bolt, usually 14 or 15 mm. If you have a Shimano bottom bracket with an Allen bolt, you need a 5-mm Allen wrench and won't need the crank puller.
3. Bottom bracket lockring wrench (Fig. 6-1). Be sure to buy the one that fits the indents on your lockring.

FIG. 6-1: Use this tool to remove and install a bottom bracket lockring.

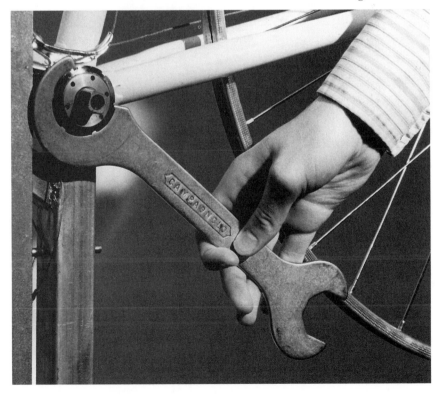

4. Pin wrench (Fig. 6-2) for bottom bracket adjustable cup. *Note:* Pin diameters differ by make and model of this cup. Buy the one that fits the holes in *your* cup.

5. Torque wrench. Please review the data on torque and use of the torque wrench in Chapter 3.

6. If your bike has a sealed-bearing bottom bracket, you will need a special tool to remove it (A, Fig. 6-3). Use the tool that fits your make and model bottom bracket. If you replace your conventional bottom bracket with this type of bottom bracket cartridge, be sure to buy one that fits your bottom bracket shell and has the same length axle as your old one.

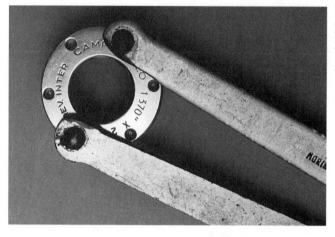

FIG. 6-2: A typical pin wrench to remove or adjust a bottom bracket adjustable cup.

FIG. 6-3: A sealed-bearing cartridge bottom bracket set like this can replace your loose ball bearing conventional bottom bracket.

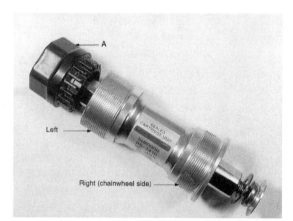

7. A set of 8-, 9-, 10-, 11-, and 12-mm wrenches
8. A set of 11–12-, 13–14-, 15–16-, and 17–18-mm thin open-end wrenches.
9. A tube of grease.
10. A 13-, 14-, or 15-mm socket, for an in./lbs. torque wrench if hubs have axle bolts instead of a quick-release.

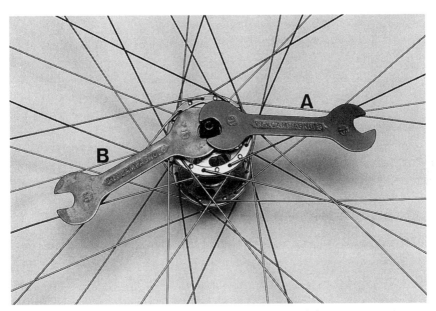

FIG. 6-4: Use two thin cone wrenches when working on hub bearings.

TABLE 6-1: BOLT AND NUT TIGHTENING TORQUE SPECIFICATIONS

(All Torques Are in in./lbs.)

Crank-to-bottom-bracket axle bolt	305–391
Bottom bracket lockring	600–900
Bottom bracket fixed cup (right-hand, chainwheel side)	600–900
Clipless pedal, cleat fixing bolt	44–52
Clipless pedal, axle to crank	305
Standard pedal, axle to crank	305
Standard pedal, toe clip fixing bolt	22
Standard pedal, cone adjustment lockring	70–130
Closing of quick-release lever	79–104
Nuts on solid axles (bolt-on axles)	300–320
Sealed-bearing cartridge bottom bracket set, both left and right sides	435–608
Clipless pedal cleat to shoe (mounting bolt)	44

How to Keep Hubs Rolling Smoothly, Longer

Hub maintenance steps:

1. Remove the wheel from the bicycle.
2. If the wheel is held by axle bolts, remove them, or remove the quick-release mechanism. Hold the quick-release adjusting nut while you turn the quick-release lever counterclockwise until the adjusting nut comes all the way off the skewer threads. (Please see Chapter 2 for information on the proper and safe use of a quick-release wheel retention device.) Grasp the quick-release lever and pull the skewer out of the hollow axle. Catch the little springs so you don't lose them, but remember that the narrow end of these springs faces toward the hub when you replace them. Put the springs and the adjusting nut back on the skewer for safekeeping.
3. From here on out, you can simply lay the wheel on the bench and remove the bearings.
4. Hold the adjustable cone with one cone wrench (B in Fig. 6-4) and turn the locknut counterclockwise with the other cone wrench (A in Fig. 6-4). Remove the locknut and the spacing washer.
5. With the cone wrench, turn the adjustable cone a few turns counterclockwise. You should now be able to unscrew it by hand. Remove it from the axle.
6. Lay a rag out on the workbench next to the wheel. Hold the axle end facing you with one hand and loosen the vise just enough to remove the wheel. Still holding the axle securely in the hub, carefully lay the wheel on the rag.
7. Lift the wheel off the rag enough so you can pull the axle out. You should still have an adjustable cone, washer, and locknut on one end of the hub axle. Leave them on the axle. Be ready to catch loose ball bearings as they fall out of the hub.
8. With a screwdriver, carefully pry off the dustcaps, one on each end of the hub (9 in Fig. 6-5). Remove any bearings still in the hub.
9. Roll the loose balls around in a cup of kerosene to remove old grease and dirt. Carefully spread them out on the rag and dry off the kerosene.
10. Clean both hub cups, the adjustable cones, the dustcaps, and the axle.
11. Examine the hub cups and the adjustable cones (Fig. 6-6) for signs of galling and brinelling. Brinelling is a term denoting wear of ball bearing races, as defined by the Brinell scale of metal hardness (*American Machinist's Handbook*, McGraw-Hill, pp. 27–46). The grooves worn in the adjustable cone in Fig. 6-6 are an example of such wear. Re-

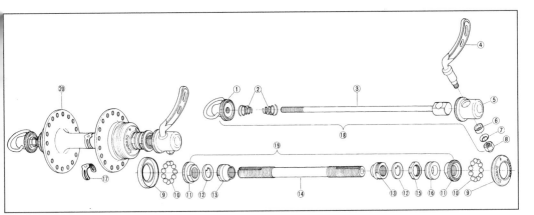

FIG. 6-5: Exploded view of a typical rear wheel hub with ball bearings: 1 is the quick-release locknut; 2 are the quick-release springs; 3 is the quick-release skewer; 4 is the quick-release lever (note cam bulge); 5, 6, 7, and 8 are the lever body, washers, and locknut; 9 is the dustcap; 10 shows the bearings; 11 is the locknut; 12 is a washer; 13 is the adjustable cone; 14 is the hub axle; 15 is the freewheel side locknut; 16 is a spacer; 17 is an oil hole cover for the hub body. But don't use oil on hub bearings unless you are a racer who wants the lowest possible wheel rolling resistance. *Courtesy Shimano American Corporation.*

place such worn cones. If the hub cup(s) are worn, it's time for a new hub, because the cups can't be replaced—they are integral with the hub body.

12. Examine the loose ball bearings themselves for wear. If you've had the bike for three or four years, I recommend you replace them. Take a sample ball bearing to your bike shop to make sure you get the right size. Buy a couple of extra balls in case you drop one on the floor and lose it forever.

13. Hold the other adjustable cone with the cone wrench and remove the remaining locknut, washer, and adjustable cone.

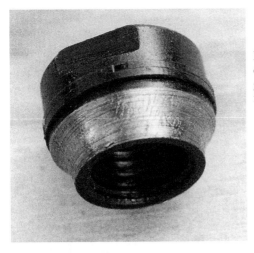

FIG. 6-6: This hub cone shows considerable wear. Note the grooves worn in the bearing surface. It's time to replace this one!

14. Check the axle alignment. Roll the axle on a smooth, flat surface, such as an old piece of plate glass. Replace it if it's bent. Take the axle to your bike shop for an exact replacement. Note: This is a good time to replace a quick-release hollow axle with a stronger, more reliable solid axle. Hollow axles have been known to bend from road impact when the bike is loaded or ridden on rough-terrain trails. Good solid axles can withstand a lot of punishment. A quick-release hub may be stylish and beautiful, but I prefer the reliability of a bolt-solid axle, especially when I am far from a bike shop. Be sure to buy a high-quality solid-steel axle. Ask your bike shop for the cro-moly or titanium solid axles made by Wheels Manufacturing, or contact that firm by phone, 1-303-447-1969, or by FAX, 1-303-447-2676. Inexpensive bikes do come with bolt-on hub axles, but those axles, though solid, may not be as strong as a quick-release hollow axle that comes on a more costly bike. Wheels with bolted-on hubs are also less likely to be stolen. Their bolts are unlikely to be accidentally opened, whereas a quick-release lever can be accidentally opened by, for example, contact with a tree branch, or by having been tampered with while your bike is parked, in which case a wheel may fall out of the dropouts on a bump.

15. Cover the loose balls in grease. Layer grease in both hub cups and on the adjustable cones.

16. Insert loose balls in the freewheel side of the hub. Cover them with grease so they won't fall out when you replace the axle.

17. Carefully replace the dustcap in the freewheel side of the hub.

18. If you have followed the instructions so far, the cone, washer, and locknut should still be in their original position on the freewheel end of the hub. Insert the other end of the axle into the freewheel side of the hub.

19. Hold the axle in place while you turn the wheel over so the freewheel side is now resting on your workbench and the other end of the hub and axle now points up.

20. Place the remaining ball bearings in the hub cup. It's easier to handle bearings if you first roll them around in grease. Put more grease over the bearings.

21. Replace the remaining dustcap.

22. Thread the adjustable cone by hand as far as possible. Hold the adjustable cone with a hub wrench to keep it from turning while you tighten the locknut with another hub wrench. Then look at both ends of the axle. About 1/4 inch of threads should be left where the axle fits into the dropouts. If not, adjust the cones and locknuts as necessary. If you are working on the front wheel, both ends of the axle should

show the same number of threads when you replace the other adjustable cone.

23. Here is the critical step in adjusting not only hub bearings, but all non-sealed bearings in the bottom bracket, headset, and pedals. Twist the axle. If it feels tight (you feel turning resistance), loosen the locknut, hold it with one wrench, and loosen the adjustable cone a half turn with another cone wrench. Then hold the adjustable cone with one wrench and tighten the locknut with the other wrench. Repeat as necessary. Move the axle up and down and in and out to make sure hub cones are not so loose that there is "play" between the axle, bearings, and cones. Readjust the hub cone as necessary. Check and make sure the locknut on the freewheel side of the hub is tight.

24. Replace the quick-release in the hollow hub axle. Be sure the small side of the little springs faces toward the hub. Adjust and tighten the quick-release as described in Chapter 2.

25. Adjust the quick-release lever (see Chapter 2). Again, let me repeat, *it is absolutely necessary that you understand how to adjust and safely tighten the quick-release cam action mechanism. If you do not do it properly the wheel could pop out of the fork when you hit a bump, and you could be hurt.* Turn the release lever to the closed position. Or, if you have a solid axle, thread on the bolts and tighten them to 300 to 320 in./lbs. of torque.

26. Give the wheel a mild spin. Watch as the wheel stops. As it slows it should come to rest with the tire valve at the six-o'clock position. If the wheel seems to resist coming to a stop slowly and instead stops with the tire valve in any other position, readjust hub bearings as described in step 23. Note: When you tighten the axle in the bicycle frame dropouts, hub adjustable cones will tighten up due to thread play.

Sealed-Bearing Hubs

Lubrication of cartridge and sealed-bearing hubs is simple:

1. Follow steps 1 and 2 above (remove the wheel, quick-release, or axle bolts).
2. *Carefully* pry off the fragile seal with a thin-bladed knife (Fig. 6-7). The bearings can now be seen.
3. With your fingers, force grease into the bearing cartridges. Be generous.
4. Replace the seal. Remember, the seal is fairly fragile. If bent it won't seal well. Press it back evenly all around the edges. Eventually cartridge

FIG. 6-7: This is what a sealed hub bearing looks like with its seal removed. The white arrow shows the seal, at right.

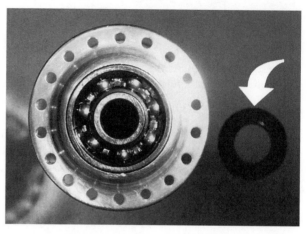

bearings wear out and will need replacement. This requires special tools and is a bicycle shop job. Replacement of the axle and bearings on a sealed-bearing hub is a shop job, but if you regrease these bearings twice a year you won't have to worry about this procedure for some time—years, probably. If you replace your hubs, I recommend the sealed-bearing hubs made by NukeProof. They are very strong and very light, though not inexpensive. See your bike shop for details.

BOTTOM BRACKET MAINTENANCE

The bottom bracket (Fig. 6-8) consists of the axle, A; axle bolts (crank fixing bolts), D; adjustable cup, C; lockring, E; axle bolt washers, G; ball bearings in a retainer, F; and a fixed cup, B, that goes on the right side of the bottom

FIG. 6-8: These are the parts of a typical bottom bracket set. A is the axle (spindle). The AA end is longer, for the chainwheel crank. B is the fixed cup; C is the adjustable cup; D are the crank fixing bolts; F are the bearings in a retainer; G are the washers for bolts D; and E is the lockring.

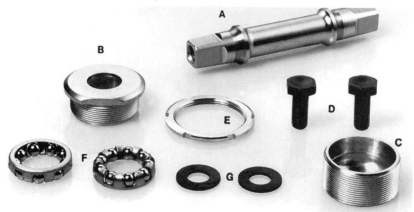

bracket shell. The A side of the axle takes the left crank, the AA side is longer so the crank and chainwheels will clear the chain stay. In fact, if you wish to change from a double to a triple chainwheel set, you can buy a longer axle that offers the wider triple chainwheel set clearance from the chain stay. But make sure that the third chainwheel and the new axle are compatible with your old chainwheels and the bottom bracket axle. The crank arm bolts (D in Fig. 6-8), when tightened, create a press fit between the bottom bracket axle and the crank arms, so the taper of each must match exactly. If the degree of taper is not matched, you may not be able to press-fit the crank arm all the way onto the axle. In that case the crank arm may work loose and come off the axle, or it may move enough on the squared, tapered shank of the steel axle to ruin the softer aluminum cranks.

Let's start with the ball bearing bottom bracket. I will cover sealed-bearing cartridge types later in this chapter.

Disassembly

1. Remove both cranks. See instructions in Chapter 5 on crank arm removal.
2. Remove the lockring counterclockwise with the special wrench, as shown in Fig. 6-1.
3. Remove the adjustable cup counterclockwise with the pin wrench (Fig. 6-2).
4. Remove the outer set of bearings, the axle, the inner set of bearings, and any plastic seal (Fig. 6-9). The bearings in older bikes may be loose instead of in a retainer, so be ready to catch them. Push the axle out the right side of the bottom bracket (the chainwheel side).
5. Clean dirt and old grease from cups, bearings, and axle with kerosene.
6. If your bike is relatively new and hasn't had much use, chances are that all you will need to do, after cleaning the bearings, cups, and axle, is to repack the bearings with grease and replace them. If the balls are in a retainer, you could replace the retainer with a new set of loose balls. This will give you 11 instead of 9 balls per bearing set, so the bottom bracket spindle will run more smoothly. The additional balls will add to both bearing and cup life. Most modern bottom brackets use $1/4$-inch balls, but take your old ones to the bike shop to make sure you get the same size replacements.
7. Inspect the cup bearing surfaces for wear. Fig. 6-10 shows a good cup at left and a worn one at right. Replace any cups that look worn. If you wish to install a sealed-bearing bottom bracket, the fixed cup (right side of the bottom bracket) will have to be removed. My advice is to save

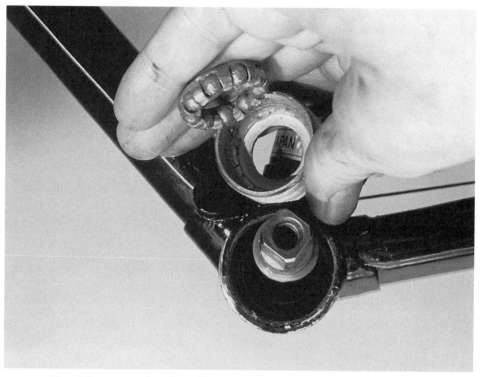

FIG. 6-9: Remove the adjustable cup, bearings, and axle to clean and regrease.

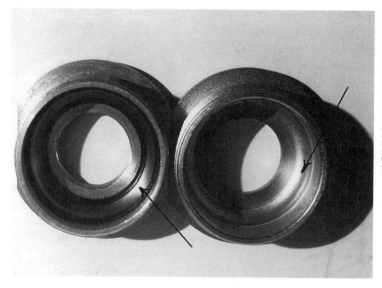

FIG. 6-10: Inspect the adjustable cup for wear. The cup at left is in good shape but the one at the right is worn and should be replaced. Also replace the fixed cup and all the bearings.

yourself the cost of a special wrench that fits it and let the bike shop remove it. Or ask the bike shop to install a sealed bottom bracket cartridge, such as the one in Fig. 6-3. The special tool needed to install the sealed cartridge unit is shown at the left of Fig. 6-3.

Reassembly

Now that you have cleaned your ball-and-cup-type bottom bracket and replaced any worn parts, you are ready to grease and put it back together. Here are the steps for reassembly:

1. Roll the loose balls in grease until they are thoroughly covered.
2. Put a layer of grease on both cups.
3. Put the loose balls (or the retainer with its balls) in the cups. The grease will hold them in place.
4. Insert the spindle (aka axle) into the bottom bracket. Make sure the longer spindle end goes in first, because that's the spindle side for the chainwheels. If your bottom bracket did not come with an internal plastic protective cover, it's a good idea to install one (available from your bike shop) to keep away abrasives and water that get into frame tubes and work down into the bottom bracket shell.
5. Thread the adjustable cup clockwise into the bottom bracket shell and turn it by hand as far as possible. Use the pin wrench to continue turning it until it's snug. Back the cup off a half turn.
6. Thread the lockring onto the adjustable cup by hand. Hold the adjustable cup with the pin wrench so it can't turn and tighten the lockring firmly with the lockring wrench.
7. Check bearing adjustment for tightness. Twirl the spindle with your thumb and a finger. It should rotate smoothly. If it feels rough or is hard to turn, loosen the lockring and turn the adjustable cup counterclockwise about a quarter turn and tighten the lockring. Check the adjustment and repeat this step as necessary. Hold the spindle with your fingers and push it up and down. If it feels loose, loosen the lockring, turn the adjustable cup clockwise a quarter turn, and retighten the lockring. Repeat these adjustments as necessary. See step 9 below for additional check.
8. Install both cranks. *Do not lubricate the spindle flats, where the cranks fit!* The crank-to-spindle is a *drive* fit. Tighten the crank binder bolts to 305 to 391 in./lbs. Replace the dustcaps in the cranks.
9. Again check the bearing adjustment for looseness. Place one crank at the 12-o'clock position. Move both cranks sharply from side to side,

toward and away from you. If you feel looseness, turn the lockring counterclockwise until it's loose and turn the adjustable cup clockwise about a quarter turn. Hold the adjustable cup with the pin wrench and tighten the lockring. Check this adjustment and repeat this step as necessary. The cranks should rotate smoothly and stop gradually.

10. Retighten the bottom bracket crank fixing bolts to 305 to 391 in./lbs. every 50 miles for the first 200 miles. This is important. As I said, the crank-to-spindle attachment is a drive (press) fit. The fixing bolt forces the crank onto the spindle flats. The crank is aluminum (except for bargain-basement cranksets, which are steel); the spindle is steel. Just a few miles of pedaling can destroy a crank if the fit is loose. Then you will be faced with spending upward of $125 for a crankset of equal quality (less labor).

Replacing the Bottom Bracket Unit

If the adjustable cup bearing surface is worn, pitted, or grooved, it should, of course, be replaced. Replace the fixed cup also because it too may be worn. Be sure you buy an exact replacement bottom bracket set that matches the dimensions of your cranks (use your old cranks). Here's how to install a new ball bearing bottom bracket:

1. Remove cranks and adjustable cup and its lockring as described above.
2. As noted earlier, have a bike shop remove the fixed cup. This is a tough job requiring a special tool and know-how. However, if you insist, know that the fixed cup has 36-mm flats for a special wrench, such as the 36-mm wrench, available from your bike shop.
3. Replace the new bottom bracket assembly. See instructions above.

Sealed-Bearing Bottom Bracket Maintenance

There are two types of sealed-bearing bottom brackets. Both types use electric-motor-type cartridge bearings. In one type the bearings are not removable. If they wear out, it takes special tools, such as a machine shop arbor press, to remove and replace them. Fisher, Klein, and some European makes such as Alex Singer come with these bearings. They will last many years if you remove the circlip and seals and press grease into the bearings at least yearly as detailed below. Regrease more often if you ride a lot, especially over sand or through water.

To lubricate these bearings:

1. Remove the cranks. See crank removal instructions above.
2. Remove the circlip (split washer) if there is one (Fig. 6-11).
3. Pry out the neoprene seal with a thin-bladed knife (be careful not to damage the seal).
4. Stuff in grease with your fingers and replace the seal, circlip, and cranks.

Some cartridge-type bottom bracket sets can't be relubricated, but maintenance is nil, so I would install one if you are taking a long trip on your bike. Just be sure, as noted above, that the angles of the flats on the axle match your existing crank flats. Check this with the bike shop before you buy. These units will last a long time and are easy to remove and replace. To install a new cartridge, follow these steps:

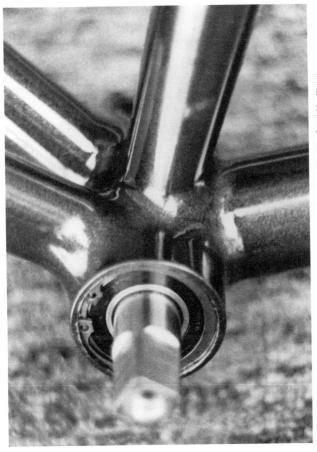

FIG. 6-11: Remove the circlip from this sealed bottom bracket bearing. Then, with a thin-bladed knife, carefully pry off the seal. Press in new grease. Bearing replacement is usually a shop job, however.

1. Remove both cranks as noted above.
2. Remove the old bottom bracket set (bearings, axle, fixed and adjustable cups, and the adjustable cup lockring).
3. Note that the cartridge is labeled with left and right arrows (Fig. 6-3). The right side of the cartridge is the chainwheel/crank side, that is, the right side of the bicycle (the tool is shown on the left side). Insert the cartridge into the right side of the bottom bracket and with the black tool labeled A in Fig. 6-3, tighten the right side threaded section of the cartridge counterclockwise to 435 to 608 in./lbs. Use a 38-mm or adjustable wrench on this tool.
4. Thread the remaining adapter clockwise into the left side of the bottom bracket and tighten it to 435 to 608 in./lbs. with the same tool.
5. Install the cranks. Tighten their bolts to 305 to 391 in./lbs.

PEDAL MAINTENANCE

The pedals on your bike sit closer to the ground than any other part of your bike except the tires, so they take heavy wear from dust, dirt, and water. Their tiny ball bearings are subjected to pressures of 50 pounds in moderate pedaling, 170 pounds when racing, and 350 pounds by strong riders straining uphill. So pedals require periodic cleaning and lubrication, especially after hard riding over trails and through water. Here's how to maintain your ball-bearing-type pedals (for cartridge-type bearings see separate instructions later in this section):

Tools you will need:

1. A set of 8-, 10-, 11-, and 15-mm wrenches.
2. Special wrenches for your pedal if they don't take the tools above. See your bike shop.

Maintenance is pretty straightforward. It simply involves getting access to the bearings, removing, cleaning, and replacing them. Here's how:

1. Remove both pedals. Most pedal axle flats take a 15-mm wrench. A few makes use a 6-mm Allen wrench on the inside end of the axle. I don't want to get you bogged down with right- and left-hand thread instructions. Just remember this: *Pedals always thread on in the direction of crank rotation as you pedal and, of course, thread off in the opposite crank rotation.* If you keep this in mind you can't go wrong. Also remember that most pedals have R and L stamped on the wrench flats. Review pedal parts as shown in Fig. 6-12.
2. Remove the dustcap (Fig. 6-13). Simply reach in and pry (rotate) it counterclockwise with a screwdriver.

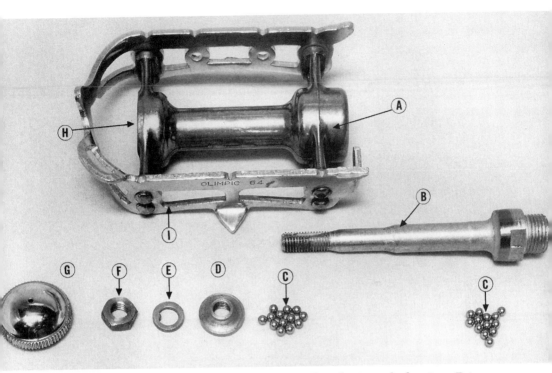

FIG. 6-12: Parts of a pedal: A is the axle end; B is the axle; C are the bearings; D is the adjustable cone; E is the washer between the cone and the locknut, F; G is the dustcap; H is the cone end of the pedal body; and I is the pedal platform.

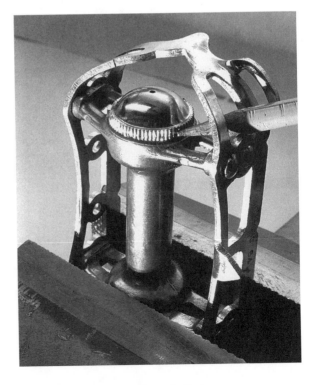

FIG. 6-13: Pry off the dustcap to reach the locknut.

3. With a 9-, 10-, or 11-mm wrench, turn the axle locknut counterclockwise and remove it and the washer under it (Fig. 6-14).
4. Remove the pedal from the axle vise and lay the pedal on a rag on the workbench, ready to catch the small loose ball bearings.
5. Turn the adjustable cone (Fig. 6-15) counterclockwise and remove it. Use your fingers or a screwdriver to rotate the cone.
6. Pull the axle out of the pedal body. Remove all the bearings.
7. Clean the bearings, cones, and axle bearing faces.
8. Put a generous layer of grease on both cups in the pedal body.
9. Replace the balls in both pedal body cups.
10. Insert the axle in the pedal body. Be careful not to knock balls out of the cups as the axle goes in.
11. Thread on the adjustable cone and tighten.
12. Replace the washer and thread on the locknut.
13. Tighten the locknut while you hold the adjustable cup to keep it from turning.

FIG. 6-14: Remove the locknut.

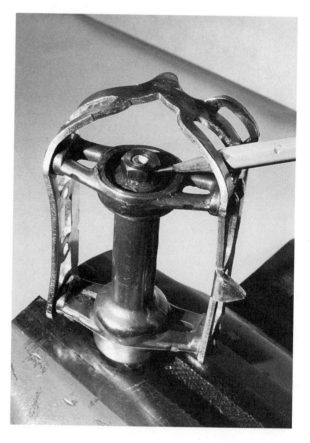

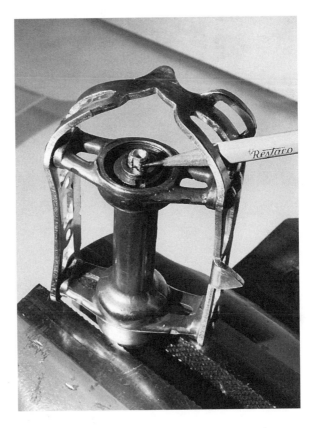

FIG. 6-15: Remove the washer and the adjustable cone under it.

14. Twist the axle between thumb and forefinger. If it feels tight, loosen the locknut; back the adjustable cup off a quarter turn and retighten the locknut as in step 13 above. Now push the axle in and out and from side to side. If you feel play, loosen the locknut, tighten the adjustable cup a quarter turn, and retighten the locknut. Repeat these steps until the axle turns smoothly, without binding or looseness.

15. Replace the pedals on the cranks.

Cartridge-Type Pedals

These pedals use standard industrial cartridge bearings, available from a bearing supply house or from a small electrical motor repair shop (in case your bike shop doesn't stock them). However, it takes special tools to remove and replace these bearings. As Fig. 6-16 shows, it is very difficult and often not possible to regrease these bearings. If the pedal bearings wear out it will probably be less expensive to replace the pedal than to have the bearings replaced.

FIG. 6-16: Cutaway of a sealed bearing pedal.

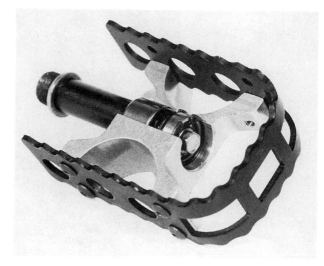

Clipless Pedals

There are many makes and types of clipless pedals on the market today. Their design changes so often that it will simply not be possible to discuss each and every model in this book. I can offer a few suggestions, however, beyond the basic one of having maintenance done by a bike shop.

First, as I said in Chapter 2, clipless pedals, cleats, and their shoes must all be compatible. Otherwise your foot could suddenly and unexpectedly come off the pedal and you could lose control. So if you buy Shimano clipless pedals, for example, attach Shimano cleats to Shimano shoes. For instructions on clipless pedal maintenance use your owner's manual, or if you purchased the pedals separately, use the pedal manual that came with the set. If you can get at the bearings to regrease or replace them, that's great, but it may be difficult to do. Time offers a tool kit just for their pedals, which contains:

1. A needle bearing extractor.
2. A spring fitting tool.
3. A circlip extractor.
4. An axle press.
5. A needle bearing press.
6. A manual.

Shimano clipless pedals are probably the easiest to maintain. Here's how:

1. Remove the pedal from the crank by turning the axle flats with a 15-mm wrench *opposite* the direction of crank rotation.

2. Remove the lock bolt with a special tool (Figs. 6-17 and Fig. 6-18) available at your bike shop or from the Third Hand mail order tool house (see hub instructions above).

Fɪɢ. 6-17: Remove the lockbolt on this clipless pedal with the 7- and 10-mm wrenches shown. Note: Applies only to Shimano clipless pedal. Other models and makes may require special tools. *Courtesy Shimano American Corporation.*

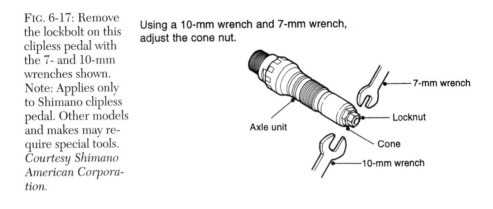

Using a 10-mm wrench and 7-mm wrench, adjust the cone nut.

7-mm wrench

Locknut

Axle unit

Cone

10-mm wrench

3. Remove the axle unit. At this point you could simply replace the entire axle unit, or,
4. Remove the locknut and the cone underneath it, and the bearings.
5. Clean and regrease the bearings, replace them and the cone and locknut.
6. Install the axle unit into the pedal body and replace the pedal into the crank arm.
    (*Note:* When you replace *any* pedal in a crank, do it carefully. Do not force-thread, otherwise you may start the pedal axle cross-threaded. If you should accidentally strip the softer aluminum crank threads, have the bike shop use a tap to straighten them.)
7. Install the cleats in the shoes (if not installed) with a 4-mm Allen wrench and tighten them initially to about 22 in./lbs.

Fɪɢ. 6-18: Remove the entire axle unit from the clipless pedal. Applies only to Shimano clipless pedal. See text for other makes. *Courtesy Shimano American Corporation.*

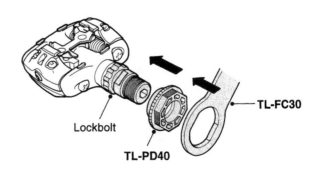

Lockbolt

TL-FC30

TL-PD40

8. Adjust the cleat position to suit your feet. The cleat can be adjusted 20 mm front to rear and 5 mm left to right.

9. When the cleat is positioned correctly for you, tighten the mounting bolts to 44 in./lbs.

10. Adjust the spring tension on the pedal so tension is even at each end of each pedal. As you adjust this tension, look under the pedal to where the tension bolt is visible as you turn it. Do not turn this bolt beyond where shown in Fig. 6-19. Reduce pedal tension if you ride where you might have to get your feet out of the pedals quickly, as on a rough trail or in the city.

Fig. 6-19: Look underneath a Shimano clipless pedal to make sure you do not turn the tension bolt too far. *Courtesy Shimano American Corporation.*

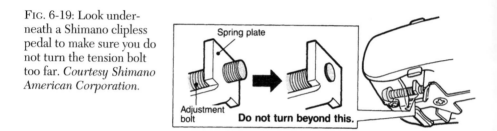

Note: A pedal equipped with strap and toe clip allows you to pull up with one foot while you exert downward pressure with the other foot, and increases pedaling efficiency by about 30 percent. But remember to loosen pedal straps when you might need to remove your foot from the pedal suddenly, as in city traffic. An alternative to strap and toe clip is a platform you can install. It may not be quite as effective as locking your foot onto the pedals with the strap, or a clipless pedal, but it is a lot better than no strap or toe clip at all. Both types of pedal restraints also keep your foot from sliding forward off the pedal when pedaling hard.

THINGS FALL APART

Nothing lasts forever. Even bottom bracket axles can break off under the stomping stress of a strong cyclist. It's called "metal fatigue." Steel gets tired after long years of hard work, so closely inspect all working parts of your bike for signs of metal fatigue, which foretell imminent failure. Look for cracks, crazed lines, and cracked paint on tubing, especially after you have had an encounter with an unyielding object, such as a rock or tree.

Now let's look at the wheels that keep you going and the tires around them in the next chapter.

CHAPTER SEVEN

TIRE SELECTION AND CARE, WHEEL BUILDING AND ALIGNMENT

CARE AND SELECTION OF TIRES

On a bike your connection to the road or trail is your tires and wheels. Here's how to keep them rolling, starting with tire and tube repair.

How to Fix a Flat Tire

When (not if) your tire and tube are punctured and the air hisses out, you will need to know how to patch the tube and possibly the tire well enough to at least get home or to the nearest bike shop. Ideally you should have a spare tube along with you so you can patch the leaky tube later on. Either way, here's how to get your wheel rolling again.

Tools and equipment you will need:

1. Patch kit and tire lever. If you don't have a tire lever, remove the quick-release unit from the hub and use its lever in an emergency.
2. Duct tape to cover tire slits (replace the tire when you can).
3. A tire pump (there's more on pumps later in this chapter).

Steps to patch a tube:

1. Remove the wheel.
2. Release remaining air from the tube by holding down the valve core. Use a twig or pencil on a Schraeder valve or unscrew its core. Or unscrew a Presta valve core and hold it down (Fig. 7-1).

FIG. 7-1: On a Presta valve, unscrew the knurled top and press it down to remove air from the tube before removing the tire from the rim.

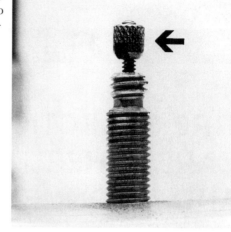

3. Squeeze both sides of the tire all the way around to break the bond between the tire bead and the rim.
4. Remove the tire from the rim, starting on the side opposite the valve (Fig. 7-2). If the tire is really stubborn use two tire levers, one to hold the tire off the rim and the other to separate the tire bead from the rim. Once you get about 10 inches of the bead off, you should be able to remove the rest of the bead with one lever or with your fingers.

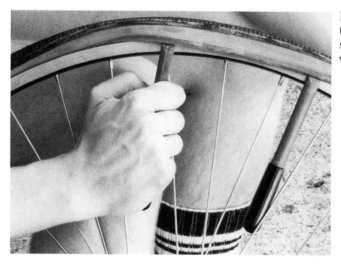

FIG. 7-2: Pry the tire off the rim, starting on the rim side 180 degrees from the valve.

5. Remove the tube from the tire.
6. Pump air into the tube so you can find the leak.
7. Use one of these ways to find the leak:

a. Dunk the tube in water. Watch for the source of air bubbles. If water isn't available, try listening for the hiss of escaping air or put the tube next to your cheek to feel escaping air.
b. Circle leak(s) with chalk, a pen, or anything that will leave a mark on the tube (Fig. 7-3).

FIG. 7-3: Circle the puncture.

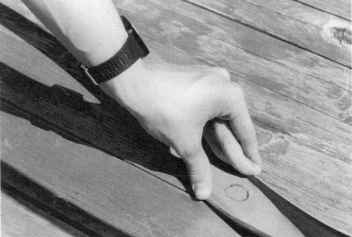

8. Roughen the area around the puncture with the sandpaper that came with your patch kit (Fig. 7-4). Don't use a metal scraper, it can weaken the tube.
9. Put a few drops of patch rubber cement around the puncture area. Spread it out with the nozzle of the glue tube and wait a minute until it gets tacky.
10. Peel the backing paper off a patch. Put the patch on the puncture and press it down firmly with your fingers.

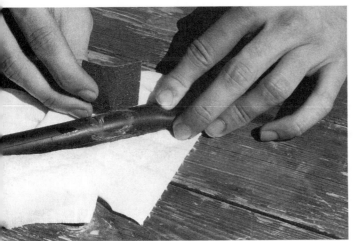

FIG. 7-4: Roughen the area around the puncture with the sandpaper that comes with your patch kit. Never use a metal rasp. Drip patch cement over the puncture, wait till it gets tacky, then apply a patch.

11. Pump up the tube and check it again for punctures and leaks as above. Moisten the top of the valve to make sure the valve core is seated. If you see bubbles, tighten the valve core. If the valve still leaks on a Schraeder valve, buy a new valve core from your bike shop or a service station. Presta valve cores aren't replaceable.

12. Thoroughly inspect the inside tire casing, sidewalls, and tread for whatever caused the puncture. Remove all foreign embedments. If you find a slit in the tire casing, roughen the cut area on the inside of the tire with sandpaper. Cover that area with patch cement. When the cement dries, cover the cut with a canvas patch from your patch kit or with a piece of duct tape, otherwise the slit can puncture the tube. Replace a slit tire as soon as possible.

13. Remove the rim strip and look at where the ends of the spokes poke up. Snip off any spoke ends that protrude past the spoke nipple. Replace the rim strip with a new, thicker, tougher one (see your bike shop).

14. If you have a major cut in the tube and no spare tube, put multiple patches over the slit, then apply duct tape around the patches. If you're lucky, you may have a slow leak and can make it home.

15. Check your patch kit every so often to make sure an opened tube of rubber cement hasn't dried out. Keep a couple of extra patch kits in your bike bag.

To reassemble the tire and tube:

1. Lay the tire on a flat surface and put the tube in it.
2. If the tire has a directional tread, as shown by an arrow on the sidewall, make sure the arrow points in the direction of wheel rotation.
3. Place the tire and tube over the rim and push the valve stem through the rim hole (Fig. 7-5).
4. Place one side of the tire on the rim, fitting the tire in both directions from the valve (Fig. 7-6). Continue until one side is fitted completely in the rim. Make sure the tube is in the tire and does not protrude out over the side of the wheel rim as you replace the tire.
5. Turn the wheel over and finish fitting the tire in the rim, again forcing both sides of the tire away from the valve stem (Fig. 7-7). Finish fitting the tire on the rim. You should be able to work by hand. If you have trouble, use the tire lever but be careful not to squeeze and puncture the tube between the tire lever and the rim.
6. Make sure the tire sits evenly in the rim, especially at the valve area. Push the valve down into the tire about an inch, then squeeze the tire

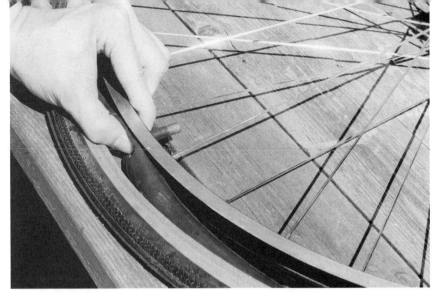

FIG. 7-5: Press the valve into the rim valve hole.

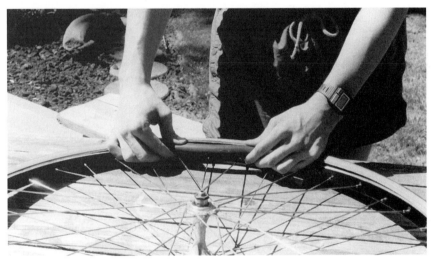

FIG. 7-6: Finish putting the tube into the tire.

FIG. 7-7: Insert the other side of the tire bead onto the rim.

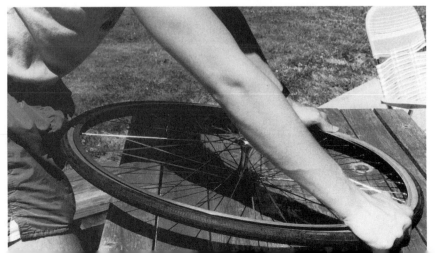

walls until the tire is seated in the rim. Otherwise the tire wall will protrude and cause a blowout.

7. Pump the tire up. If you have Presta valves, remember these are fragile and easily broken if you don't hold the pump steady as you use the plunger (Fig. 7-8). Remove the pump from a Presta valve with a sharp downward blow from the side of your hand (Fig. 7-9). Don't try to wiggle it off—that's a good way to bend and break the valve stem. When fully inflated, thread on a Presta valve retainer nut (Fig. 7-10) and replace the valve cap on either type of valve stem.

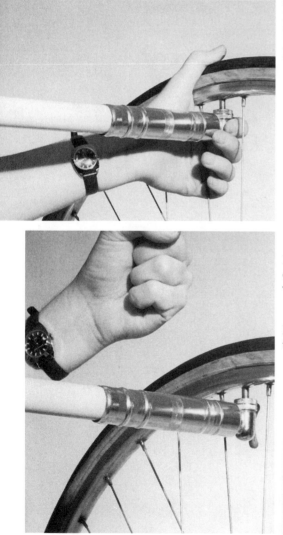

Fig. 7-8: Hold the pump as shown here, particularly on a Presta valve, which can be snapped in half if you wiggle the pump as you inflate the tube.

Fig. 7-9: Remove the pump with a sharp downward blow as shown. Again, do not wiggle the pump to remove it.

Fig. 7-10: On a Presta valve, screw down the valve nut (arrow).

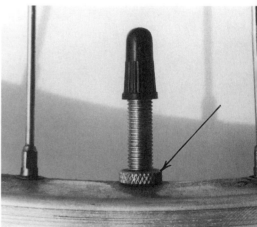

8. Inspect the tire sidewalls to make sure the bead is evenly seated all the way around in the wheel rim. If not, deflate, reseat, and pump the tire up.

9. If you get a flat on a trip and to your dismay find that your pump will only fit a Schraeder valve, but you have Presta valve tubes, use a Presta valve adapter, available from any bike shop. Screw the adapter onto the Schraeder valve and use the pump.

How to Avoid a Flat Tire

You can avoid many flat tires. Start by improving the odds against a puncture:

1. *Reduce impact on your tires* and the chance of a blowout as you come to an obstruction, such as a pothole. Pull back on the handlebars as the front wheel comes to a tire-threatening obstacle. Move forward on the saddle as the rear wheel does the same.

2. *Protect your tubes from punctures by street debris, sharp rocks, and thorns (to name a few puncture sources).* Be aware that the farther apart the knobs on mountain bike tires are, the more prone they are to puncture when used on a hard surface. This is because the tire casing between the knobs is quite thin, so do not be misled by the macho big fat knobs. I learned this the hard way, back when mountain bikes first hit the market. I was circling restlessly around on a rough gravel trail head, waiting for friends to show up, and within a few minutes I had two punctures.

3. *If you ride on very rough roads and trails or where there are thorns, as in cactus country, install a heavy-duty plastic tire liner,* such as Mr. Tuffy, available from your bike shop, between the tire and the tube. This liner comes in sizes to fit most tires. In areas where barbed thorns can cause many flats, such as the Southwest, use thicker thorn-resistant tubes. You could also switch to a semisolid tire as described later in this chapter. These tires have no inner tube so they are immune to punctures. Or use a sealant such as Finish Line's. I can also recommend puncture-resistant Kevlar tubes, although they do cost more.

4. *Before each ride remove anything stuck in your tires,* such as glass shards, nails, thorns, and small stones in the tread.

5. *Replace worn tires and those with weather-cracked sidewalls.* The cost of new tires is a small price to pay to avoid accident-causing tire failure.

6. *Avoid overheating tires.* Alternate braking between front and rear wheels on long downhill runs to avoid heat buildup that could cause

a blowout. When a tube blows out the tire wiggles around on the rim, often to the point where you can lose steering control, particularly if the blowout occurs on the front wheel. In fact, I once had two blowouts so close together that I thought only one tire had blown. Fortunately the road was flat and I was going fairly slowly, about eight miles per hour. The blowouts occurred on a very hot day in California, while I was cycling over a black tar road. The heat from the sun and the very hot pavement heated the air in the tires. When air heats it expands. Keep hot weather blowouts in mind on hot summer days when riding over black asphalt paving. I also recall minding a group's bikes outside a grocery store in rural Vermont when suddenly I heard tires exploding all around me. We had parked our bikes where the sun hit the tires. I counted, as I recall, at least six such explosions within a few seconds.

7. *Match a new tire to your rim width.* Road and mountain bike clincher tires are held on to the wheel rim by the air pressure inside the tube (Fig. 7-11). Mountain bike tire and rim widths vary from 2.25 inches to 1.50 inches. Bead widths of these tires can vary even within the same sizes. Wheel rim widths are more or less standardized to .669, .834, and .992 inches. The rim at the left in Fig. 7-11 shows a narrow mountain bike rim for tires sizes 26 × 1.50 inches up to 26 × 1.75 inches; the tire at the right is for tires 26 × 1.90 inches up to 2.25 inches. If you put a wide tire on a narrow rim, or vice versa, you risk

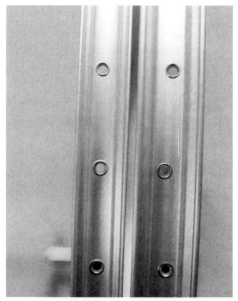

FIG. 7-11: Match the tire width to the width of the rim. The narrower rim at left takes a mountain bike tire width from 1.50 to 1.75 inches. The wider rim at the right is for mountain bike tires from 1.90 to 2.25 inches wide. But check with your bike shop to make sure the tire and rim match, because new rim designs and sizes are coming on the market.

a bead popout and a blowout. To make sure your new tire fits your old wheel, bring the bike, or your wheel, to the bike shop when you buy a new tire. When replacing tubes, also match the size of the tube to the size of the tire. Latex tubes provide the best puncture resistance, and are well worth the $15 or so they cost.

8. *Keep tires inflated to the correct pressure.* For trail and other off-road rides, keep at least 35 psi in the tire. For road use increase the pressure to 50–75 psi, depending on the make of tire. Tire sidewalls usually give safe pressure ranges. An underinflated tire can bottom out and puncture, an overinflated tire can pop the tire off the rim. Vary these pressures to match your weight. For example, an off-road tire may be fine at 35 psi for a 120-pound rider going over loose soil. But a heavier rider may find 40 to 45 psi gives better traction and steering control. For road bike tires, follow the tire recommendation that should be printed on the tire casing. Most road bike tires specify 80 to 100 psi. Be sure to check tire pressure before every ride, or every day on a bike trip. Use an air gauge to be sure you have the correct air pressure.

9. *Scan the road ahead.* Watch for anything on the road immediately in front of your bike that could cause a puncture. Be ready to take evasive action.

10. *Always carry a tire pump.* They come in different lengths to fit specific frame sizes. Take your bike to the shop to make sure the pump fits your bike. Better yet, if you are buying a new bike, buy a pump, patch kit, and tire levers at the same time, along with a couple of spare tubes. You can also buy a minipump that fits in your pannier.

11. *Of course always carry a patch kit and tire levers.* Bring a roll of duct tape (ask your hardware store clerk). Use it to patch slits and large holes in the tire that could cut the tube and make another puncture. The duct tape can get you home, where you can replace the tire. Spare tubes keeps you on the move. Patch the punctured tube later, around the campfire. On a trip, carry a couple of fold-up-type knobby tires, or fold-up-type road tires for your road bike. Stow them in your bike bag or strap them on your carrier or under your seat. If you destroy a tire on a razor-sharp rock or a piece of glass, the spare tire will keep you going.

Match the Tire Tread to the Terrain

Please see Figs. 7-12 to 7-17 for a wide variety of tread designs for road and off-road use on your mountain bicycle. See Fig. 7-18 for typical road bike tire tread patterns and types.

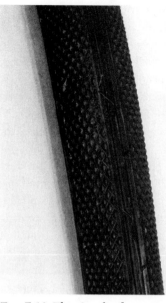

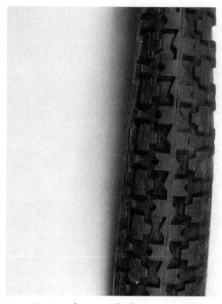

FIG. 7-12: This Overland mountain bike tire by Michelin is great for smooth surfaces on- or off-road.

FIG. 7-13: The tread design on this Michelin Integral tire has a relatively smooth center for paved roads along with knobs for trail rides.

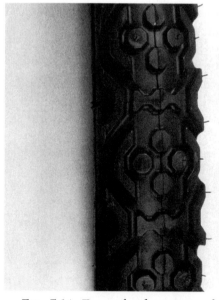

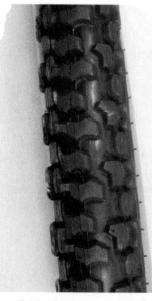

FIG. 7-14: For trail riding on tough, mean, rock-strewn terrain, this Michelin Volcano has thick, closely spaced knobs that offer good adhesion.

FIG. 7-15: Here's a mountain bike tire, the Michelin Chamonix, that grips the trail even in wet conditions.

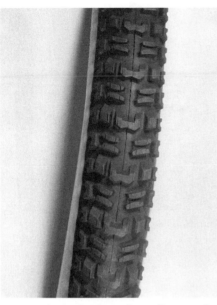

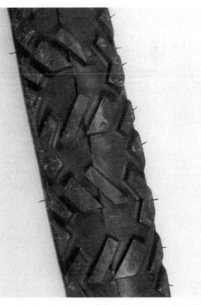

FIG. 7-16: The Transalp LK from Michelin has reinforced sidewalls and resistance to the cuts and bruises of the trail.

FIG. 7-17: Designed for the rear wheel where traction is needed, this Exper Traction lets you move ahead on muddy trails.

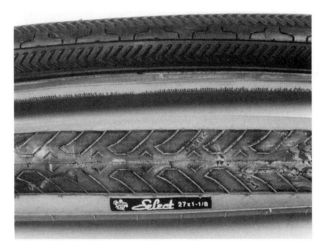

FIG. 7-18: Two tires for your road bike. The tire at the top has side bars for cornering on wet roads. The tire at the bottom will provide smooth riding on paved terrain.

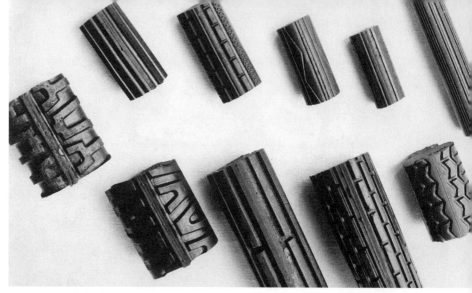

FIG. 7-19: For the busy bike commuter with no time to fix flats, these tubeless tires are immune to punctures. They ride over glass- and tack-strewn roads while you get to work on time.

Solid Tires

I can recommend solid or semipneumatic tires (Fig. 7-19), when you have to ride over poorly swept city streets, can't stop to fix a flat on your way to work, or simply want the utmost in rolling reliability. These tires are not quite as comfortable as pneumatic tires with tubes, but if properly installed they will get you there without ever going flat, blowing out, or popping off the rim. Bike messengers and policemen on bicycles should find these tires a help when there is no time to stop and patch a tube. Select narrower, less aggressive treads for road riding, fatter, more knobby tires for off-road or rough city streets. If your bike shop does not carry these tires, call Green Tyre at 1-800-8973, by FAX at 1-201-952-0185, or write to them at 364 Parsippany Rd., Suite 9-B, Parsippany, NJ 07054.

I use a solid tire on my bike exerciser, where the rear wheel rolls on a drum. When I used pneumatic road tires the heat buildup from the friction contact between tire and drum caused the tread to peel off the tire carcass after a few rides. The solid tire has been rolling on my exerciser drum for over two years and is going strong.

HOW TO KEEP YOUR WHEELS RUNNING TRUE

Your bicycle wheels won't stay true forever—not even wheels built by professionals. Too often I have found misaligned wheels with obvious side-to-side wobble on brand-new bicycles, although to be fair to bike manufacturers and bicycle shops, almost always on inexpensive bikes sold in department or discount chain stores (see Chapter 1). For this reason I will cover wheel alignment first, then get into wheel building from scratch, starting with a handful of spokes, spoke nipples, and a rim.

Wheels become untrue when the spokes stretch. When the spokes stretch they can do so unevenly, so spokes on one side of the rim can be looser than spokes on the other side. A wheel can also become untrue from an impact, such as bumping a curb.

Untrue wheels can cause an accident, loss of control, and injury to you because they:

1. Reduce braking ability (see Chapter 3). As the wheel wobbles from side to side, the brake shoe farthest from the rim can have less stopping power. This is particularly true when the brake shoes are too far from the rim to begin with (Chapter 3).
2. Cause shimmy. Unevenly tensioned spokes contribute to wheel wobble, a major cause of front-wheel shimmy (see Chapter 2).
3. Increase tension on the quick-release skewer that can weaken or snap it, as when you bend a paper clip rapidly to break it. When the skewer snaps, the wheel is free to fall out of the dropouts on an impact or rub on the inside of the fork blades or chain stays.
4. Increase tension on the spokes to the point where a spoke can snap.
5. Reduce the life of hub bearings, cups, and cones.

Check your wheels for alignment this way:

Put your bike on a bike stand, hang it from the ceiling, or lift it up and spin the front wheel. Do the same with the rear wheel. Watch each wheel rim as it passes a brake shoe. If the wheel moves closer to, then farther from the rim, it is untrue and should be realigned.

There are two degrees of wheel truing. The first is the simple type you will probably have to do two or three times a year until you have removed spoke stretch and put each spoke under the same or nearly the same tension. The second and more difficult and time-consuming type of wheel truing is when you have built a completely new wheel from scratch, with new spokes in a new rim. In this chapter I will show you how to do the casual kind of wheel truing first, because that's the kind you'll do most often. Then I'll get into wheel building and after that show you how to true a newly built wheel so it stays truer longer. But let me emphasize, first, that wheel truing does take patience and experience. If you do not feel comfortable at this task, take your wheels to a bike shop. You should, however, at least know the basics of wheel truing so you can bring your wheels back into alignment if you are far from a bike shop.

Tools you will need:

1. A spoke wrench to fit your spoke nipples (Fig. 7-20).
2. A simple truing fixture (stand) (Fig. 21).
3. A bike work stand (optional).

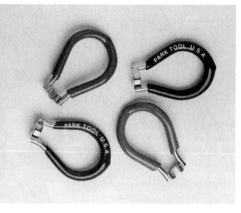

FIG. 7-20: Use the spoke nipple wrench that fits your spoke nipples to true a wheel. *Courtesy Park Tools.*

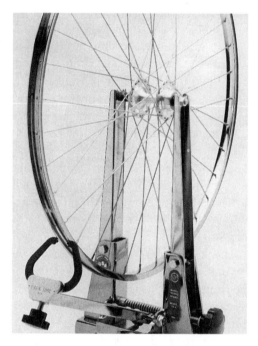

FIG. 7-21: You need a wheel-truing tool to true up your wheels. *Courtesy Park Tools.*

Using your bike as a truing fixture:

1. Put your bike in a work stand, hang it from the ceiling, or turn it upside down.
2. Remove both wheels. Remove the tires, tubes, and rim strips.
3. Look at the rim. If it is badly dented, stop here. The rim should be replaced. If you wish to build (lace up) a new wheel yourself, please refer to the section below on wheel building. You can, of course, use the old hub. But I advise new spokes. Look at the spokes, particularly where they come out of the hub. If you see cracks or if the spokes have been cut by the chain (rear wheel), replace them. Do not cut the spoke. Simply unscrew the nipple, pull out the bad spoke(s), and install new

ones. Be sure to insert the spoke head in the rim as shown in Fig. 7-22. On a rear hub, you will have to remove the freewheel, as shown in Chapter 5. Turn the spoke nipples on any new spokes to bring the wheel approximately back in line, then follow the procedure below to finish truing the wheel.

4. Replace both wheels, sans tubes, rim strips, and tires. Make sure the rear wheel is as far back in the dropouts as possible and that the front wheel is as far up in the fork dropouts as possible.

5. Spin the wheel slowly. Find a place where each side of the rim is the same distance from the seat stays or fork blades (Fig. 7-23). Mark that spot with crayon, on each side of the rim.

6. Find the spot(s) you marked in step 5. You need to true the wheel to them.

7. Spin the wheel. If the rim moves to the right, tighten the spoke nipple on the left side of the rim clockwise a half turn, to pull the rim to the left. Fig. 7-24 shows how the rim moves left or right as you adjust spoke tension. If the rim moves to the right, tighten a nipple

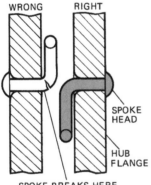

WRONG   RIGHT

SPOKE
HEAD

HUB
FLANGE

SPOKE BREAKS HERE
AT SHARP TURN ANGLE

FIG. 7-22: Insert spokes so the flat undersection of the other spoke head is flush with the flat of the hub flange and the spoke follows the stress-relieving curved part of the hub flange, as shown at the right in this illustration.

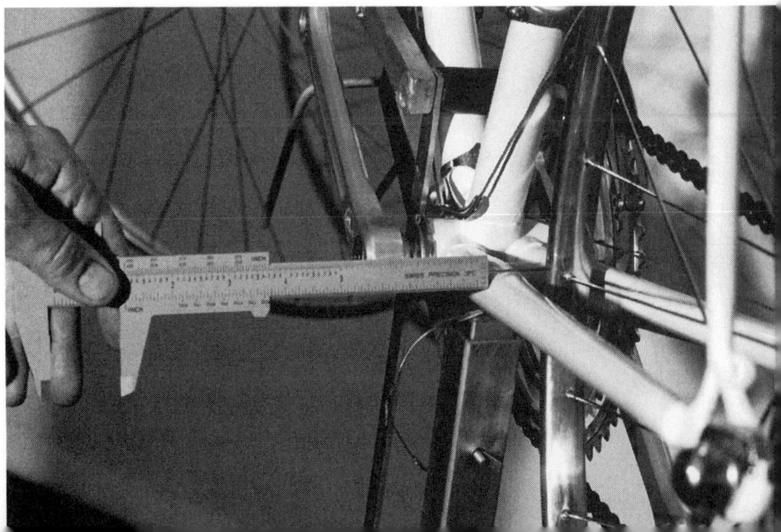

FIG. 7-23: For existing wheels on a bike with sidepull brakes, use a ruler on each side of the rim flats to align the wheel.

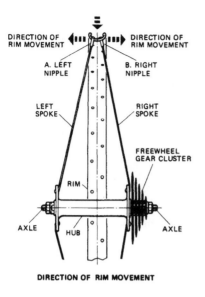

DIRECTION OF RIM MOVEMENT

A. LEFT NIPPLE

B. RIGHT NIPPLE

LEFT SPOKE

RIGHT SPOKE

FREEWHEEL GEAR CLUSTER

RIM

AXLE

AXLE

HUB

DIRECTION OF RIM MOVEMENT

FIG. 7-24: Tightening a spoke nipple pulls the rim to the side of the rim the spoke is on. Loosening a spoke nipple moves the rim away from the side of the rim the spoke nipple is on.

on the left side. If you want to move the rim to the left, but the nipple on that side is already so tight the spoke wrench slips, loosen the nipple on the right side clockwise a half turn. You may have to adjust spoke tension on two or even three spokes if the rim is way out line.

If you use a truing fixture (these steps are for existing wheels; for truing instructions for newly built wheels, see below):

1. Remove both wheels, tires, tubes, and rim strips and the freewheel (see Chapter 5).
2. Put a wheel in the truing fixture.
3. Adjust the truing fixture indicators as you spin the wheel slowly until you find a spot on the rim where the indicators are the same distance from each side of the rim. Mark this spot on both sides of the rim with a crayon.

Follow this truing procedure whether you use your bike or a truing fixture:

1. Put a drop of light oil, such as WD-40, on the top of the spoke nipples in the rim. Wipe off excess oil so it won't damage the rim strip or tube when you replace them.
2. Check the spokes, especially on the freewheel side, where they curve up from the hub, and replace any that are bent, twisted, or cut.
3. Pluck each spoke, starting at the tire valve. Tighten loose spokes by turning the nipple clockwise until the spoke is roughly at the same tension as the rest of the spokes. If the nipple keeps turning but the spoke won't tighten, the nipple is stripped. Replace that spoke and

nipple and tighten it until it's about at the same tension as the rest of the spokes.

4. Study Fig. 7-24. Note that tightening a left spoke nipple (clockwise) pulls the rim to the left, and tightening a right spoke nipple pulls the rim to the right. Loosening a left-side spoke moves the rim to the right, loosening a right-side spoke nipple moves the rim to the left. The "right" and "left" sides of a rim are arbitrary. If you're working on the side of the wheel that's on the left side for you, then that's the left side.

5. Make sure the truing indicators (on the bike or in the truing fixture) touch the side of the rim you marked with the crayon. That mark is where the rim is true laterally from side to side and that's your starting point.

6. Rotate the rim until one side moves as far away as possible from the truing indicator. Mark that spot with the crayon.

7. Tighten a nipple 1/4 turn on a spoke that will pull the rim toward the indicator. If the rim is too far to the left, tighten a right-side nipple.

8. Make rough truing adjustments, 1/4 nipple turn at a time, until the rim is almost true.

9. Make final touch-up truing adjustments 1/8 nipple turn at a time until the rim is true from side to side.

10. If you can't true the rim by tightening a spoke, loosen a spoke on the opposite side 1/4 turn. For example, if the rim is too far to the right, and you can't tighten a left-side spoke to pull it back, loosen a right-side spoke 1/4 to 1/8 turn.

11. With side-to-side (lateral) untrueness removed, now check for concentric (roundness) trueness. With the truing guide, note the average concentric trueness and mark any place the rim moves up or down from that average.

12. Correct concentric untrueness by tightening adjacent left-side right-side spoke nipples 1/8 turn at the high place, or loosening one right- and left-side nipple 1/8 turn at the low place. *Use two adjacent spokes to pull the rim up or move it down. That way you keep the wheel laterally true while you correct concentric untrueness.* Repeat this step until you have removed all high and low spots and the rim is concentric.

13. Check the rim once more for side-to-side trueness and if necessary true it up as shown above.

14. When the rim is true, make sure spoke nipples do not protrude above the nipple inside the rim, where they can pierce the tube and cause a flat. File down or snip off protruding spoke ends.

15. Prestretch each spoke. Squeeze a pair of spokes by hand. This is an important step when you build a new wheel, with new spokes. Do this during the wheel-building process.

16. Turn each spoke another 1/8 turn to remove spoke stretch. If you build a lot of wheels, it pays to use a good spoke tensionometer, such as the Wheelsmith (Fig. 7-25) or the Hozan (Fig. 7-26). Instructions with either unit are easy to follow, and they are available from your bike shop or from the Third Hand (see their catalog in the Bibliography). These units help to strengthen wheels by tightening spokes to the same tension, eliminating wheel wobble and later misalignment if loose spokes stretch.

17. Check the wheel for lateral and concentric trueness and true it again if necessary. Again squeeze pairs of spokes together to relieve tension, recheck trueness, and true up as above.

18. If necessary, readjust brake shoe clearance as shown in Chapter 3.

19. Replace the rim strip, tube, and tire.

20. Put the wheels back in the bike.

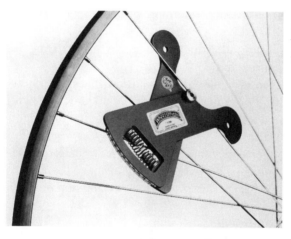

FIG. 7-25: Use a spoke tensionometer like this Wheelsmith unit to tighten spokes evenly.

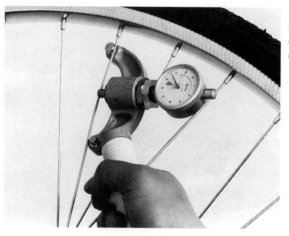

FIG. 7-26: This Hozan spoke tensionometer has a dial indicator to speed even spoke tensioning.

How to Build a Wheel

If you have dented a rim beyond repair, want to upgrade your hubs, want to add your own components to a new frame, or want an extra set of wheels for your ATB—one set for the trail, one for the road—you have a choice of having a professional wheel builder build (lace) the wheels or doing it yourself. You save about $22 in labor cost when you build and true one wheel yourself, but it takes three to six hours if you're not used to it. With practice you should be able to cut this time to an hour.

Bike shops charge about $45, including the spokes, to build and true a wheel. This does not include the cost of a new hub, of course, or a new rim. Every bicycle enthusiast should build his or her own wheels at least once to understand what it takes to create wheels that will see you through hell and high water. You'll appreciate your newfound skill if you ever get stuck in the boonies and have to replace busted spokes or if you live where bike shops are scarce. If you tour in third-world countries, wheel-building ability is a *must*.

Tools you will need:

1. Wheel truing fixture (Fig. 7-21).
2. Accurate straight ruler (Fig. 7-23).
3. Spoke nipple wrench (Fig. 7-20).
4. Push-type screwdriver (an ordinary screwdriver will do, but it's slower).
5. "Dishing" tool (Fig. 7-27) for centering a front wheel and dishing a rear wheel (more on dishing later). You could make such a tool out of a straight piece of two-by-four with offset blocks at each end. Use a 10-inch bolt with two nuts and lockwasher for the center indicator. The homemade version is cumbersome, though. A Park dishing tool can be used on any size wheel.

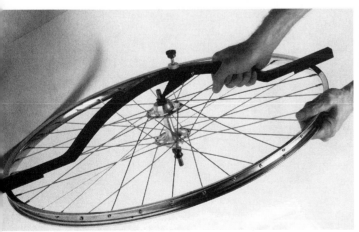

FIG. 7-27: You need a dishing tool like this Park unit to true newly built wheels so the rim is evenly located between hub axle locknuts.

Spoke Length

If you use your old hub, or a duplicate, and the same rim or a duplicate, take your spoke to the bike shop for a new set of the same length. If you use a different hub or rim, or decide to lace up your wheels with spokes crossed three instead of crossed four (see below), or change to a hub and rim drilled for 32 spokes instead of 36, ask your bike shop for the correct length spoke for the new combination. There are too many possible variations of these factors. Do it the easy way, ask your bike shop mechanic, who will consult a spoke chart and select the spokes you need.

Spokes come in three gauges, 14, 15, and 15 double-butted. The lower the gauge, the thicker and stronger the spoke. For example, a 14-gauge spoke is 2 mm thick, a 15-gauge spoke is 1.56 mm thick, so the 14-gauge spoke is about 22 percent thicker. Fifteen-gauge double-butted spokes are 14-gauge thickness for about 50 mm (two inches) at the spoke head end, the part that goes into the hub. Use 14-gauge spokes if you want a strong, durable wheel, 15-gauge double-butted spokes for some sacrifice in strength to save a few ounces in weight, and 15 straight-gauge spokes for lightness at the expense of strength. I prefer 14-gauge double-butted DT spokes, which should be available from your bike shop.

Four-Cross Versus Three-Cross Lacing

You can lace your wheels with spokes crossed three, as in Fig. 7-28, where spoke A crosses over spokes B and C and under spoke D, or crossed four, as in Fig. 7-29, where spoke A crosses over spokes B, C, and D and under E. You get a stiffer wheel with three-cross spoking. The stiffer wheel more ef-

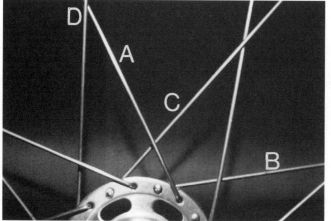

FIG. 7-28: This wheel has spokes crossed in threes. Spoke A goes over spokes B and C and under spoke D.

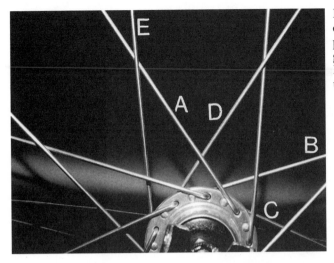

FIG. 7-29: A four-crossed spoking pattern. Spoke A goes over spokes B, C, and D and under spoke E.

ficiently translates muscle power to go power. But the stiffer wheel also sends more road shock back into the frame, which can be fatiguing on a long ride.

Four-cross spoking requires longer spokes, which soak up road shock better than the stiff three-cross pattern. Use three-cross for racing and four-cross for casual and long-distance riding and touring.

Steps in Building Four-Cross Wheels

1. Select the correct spoke length as noted above.
2. Note that *rim* holes are staggered so that every other hole is closer to one side of the rim than the one preceding it or the one following it (Fig. 7-30).

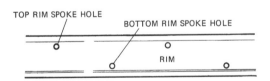

FIG. 7-30: Every other spoke hole in a rim is on the opposite side from the rim hole preceding it, as shown here.

3. Note that hub flange holes are offset with respect to the spoke holes in the facing flange (Fig. 7-31).

    (*Note:* Some hubs have one side of every other hole chamfered so the spoke bends gradually, instead of at a sharp angle [Fig. 7-22]. Insert spokes in the hub as noted in step 6 below, so the spoke bend follows the curve of the chamfer. If you don't, the spoke bends sharply and can break where it angles up out of the hub. Most modern hubs have a slight chamfer on both sides of all holes.)

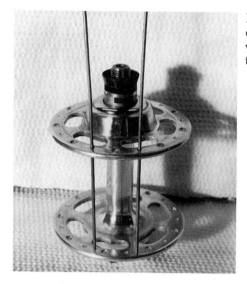

Fig. 7-31: Note that spoke holes in one side of a hub flange are offset with respect to the spoke holes in the facing flange.

4. Poke a spoke through the rim hole to make sure it's big enough to accept the spoke, but not so big the spoke can bounce around in the hole under the stress of road shock and break. For example, some hubs are drilled for 15-gauge spokes and are too small for 14-gauge spokes, and some hubs drilled for 14-gauge spokes are too large for 15-gauge spokes. Exchange hubs rather than drill out holes that are too small, or use 14-gauge spokes instead of 15-gauge spokes if the holes are too big. If you drill out rim spoke holes you probably won't get them at the right angle.

5. Drill a half-inch hole in your workbench or in a 12-inch square of 2-inch planking to hold the hub while you lace up the wheel. Remove the quick-release skewer or the axle nuts.

6. Put a spoke down every other hole in both flanges, so the spoke heads face upward (Fig. 7-32).

7. Sweep the spokes up, turn the hub over, and insert spokes as in step 6. The hub should look like Fig. 7-33, so every other spoke hole has a spoke head facing up.

8. Sweep both sets of spokes up and put the hub in the hole in your workbench or block of wood (see step 5).

9. Lay the rim over the hub on the workbench.

10. Locate the valve hole in the rim (Fig. 7-34). Look at the first hole to the *right* of the valve hole. If it's a *top* rim hole, take any spoke in the *top* flange of the hub that has its spoke head facing *up*, and insert it in this rim hole and thread on a nipple four turns. If the first hole to the *right* of the valve hole is a *bottom* hole, insert this spoke into the first hole to the *left* of the valve hole.

11. Count off four empty rim spoke holes to the *right*, not counting the valve hole. This should be a top rim hole. Take the next spoke with its spoke head facing up in the top hub flange and put it into this fourth rim hole.

12. Put every spoke with its head facing up in the top hub flange; insert into every fourth top rim hole, working to your right. You should now have eight spokes in the rim, each with a nipple threaded on four turns. There should be three empty rim holes between spokes (Fig. 7-35).

FIG. 7-32: Insert spokes with spoke heads on the flange as shown.

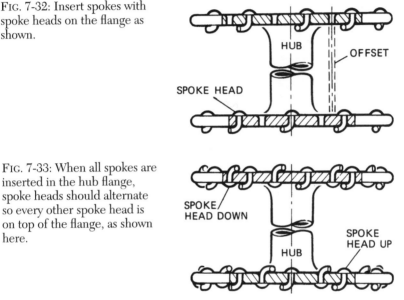

FIG. 7-33: When all spokes are inserted in the hub flange, spoke heads should alternate so every other spoke head is on top of the flange, as shown here.

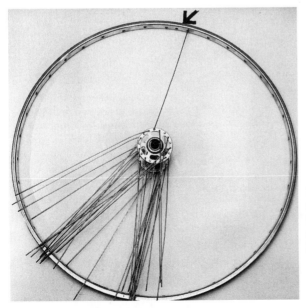

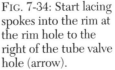

FIG. 7-34: Start lacing spokes into the rim at the rim hole to the right of the tube valve hole (arrow).

13. Hold the hub so it can't turn and *twist* the rim to the right so the spokes are at an acute angle, just grazing the outside of their adjacent empty *hub* spoke holes. If a spoke crosses over the *rim valve hole*, twist the rim to the *left* instead of to the right.

14. Take any *head-down spoke* (a spoke with its head under the hub flange) in the top hub flange (Fig. 7-33), and, going in the *opposite* di-

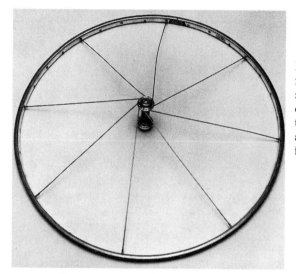

FIG. 7-35: First sequence in wheel lacing should show spokes with three empty rim spoke holes between spokes, and spokes at an angle to the rim flange as shown.

rection from the first nine spokes, cross it *over* three and *under* the fourth spoke. For example, in Fig. 7-36, spoke A goes to the left and crosses *over* spokes B, C, D, and *under* spoke E. Continue this spoke-lacing pattern until the wheel looks like Fig. 7-36 and Fig. 7-37, with one empty spoke hole between each pair of spokes and with each

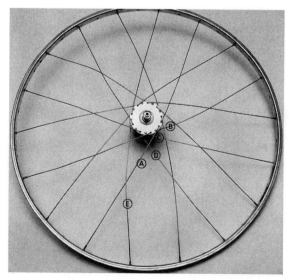

FIG. 7-36: Spokes are in sets of two in this step of wheel building. Note that spokes are crossed in a sequence of four, so, for example, spoke A goes over spokes B, C, and D and under spoke E.

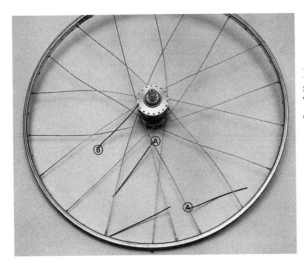

Fig. 7-37: Beginning spoke crossing pattern. The first set is in a group of three. See text.

spoke going in an alternate left-right direction, with nipples threaded on four turns.

15. This is the most critical step in wheel lacing. Turn the wheel and hub over. Sweep all but one of the unlaced spokes out of the way. Refer to Fig. 7-31 and note that the top and bottom hub flange spoke holes are offset, so that if you poke a spoke straight down in a top flange hole it stops midway between two of the bottom flange spoke holes. Now look closely at Fig. 7-38. Find spoke A and note that its spoke head, facing up in the top hub flange, is just to the right of spoke head B and is centered midway between spokes B and C in the bottom hub flange.

16. Put any spoke with its head up on the top hub flange into the position shown by spoke A in Fig. 7-38, starting in a top hub hole. Note that this spoke goes to the right.

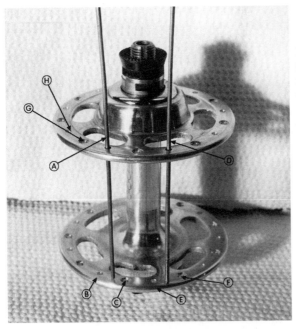

Fig. 7-38: Spoke holes in one side of a rim flange are offset from spoke holes in the other side of the flange. Spoke A, for example, falls between spoke holes B and C. Spoke D falls between spoke holes E and F.

17. Put all the remaining head-up hub flange spokes in the rest of the top rim holes (every other empty spoke hole), working to the right. Spokes should now be in groups of three (Fig. 7-39).

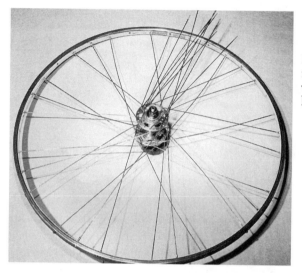

FIG. 7-39: Spokes are now in groups of three, with one empty spoke hole between trios.

18. Pull any hub top flange head-down spoke to as sharp an angle to the *left* as possible, so it's almost touching a head-up spoke in the top hub flange, and put it in the only bottom rim hole it will reach. If it sticks out more than half an inch from the rim spoke hole, move the spoke to the next left bottom rim hole. If it won't go that far, go back one bottom rim hole to the right.

19. Continue lacing the remaining head-down spokes to the left, crossing *over* three spokes and *under the fourth spoke*. When you are finished, the spokes should be in groups of four and look like Fig. 7-40.

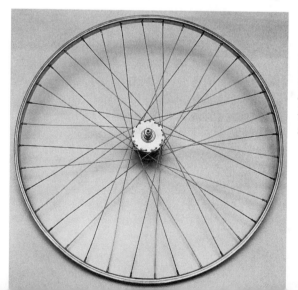

FIG. 7-40: Here's what a finished four-crossed built wheel looks like. The wheel has not been trued up, and spoke tension is as yet uneven.

20. Tighten each spoke two turns at a time, then one turn at a time, then a half turn at a time until spokes are about evenly tensioned and the wheel looks almost straight. It won't be, but you will correct and true up the wheel as noted earlier in this chapter, except for the rear wheel, which will need to be dished.

Three-Cross Wheel Building

For a stiffer wheel, build one with spokes crossed three instead of four. Lacing three-cross is essentially the same as for a four-cross wheel, with these exceptions:

1. Place the first nine spokes into every other hole in the top of the hub flange (see step 7).
2. A crucial step. Put another nine spokes into the bottom hub flange, spoke head up, as you would when lacing four-cross, *but* offset the first spoke in the lower hub flange one hole to the right of the spoke above it in the upper flange.
3. Put one spoke from the upper hub flange through the first spoke hole to the right of the valve stem hole in the rim. This should be a hole on the side of the rim facing upward, toward you. Thread a nipple on this spoke a few turns. Skip the next three holes to the right of the one into which you just inserted a spoke.
4. Take the next spoke to the right of the first one on the upper hub flange and put that spoke into the fourth rim hole, which should also be on the upper side of the rim, facing you.
5. Continue this spoking pattern to the right until all the spokes from the upper hub flange are laced into the rim. Make sure the spokes are evenly placed and are only in the holes on the upper side of the rim.
6. Twist the hub so the spokes make an acute angle to the rim. Spokes should nearly touch the holes adjacent to them in the hub flange.
7. Find the first spoke you laced, the one to the right of the rim valve hole. Now look down at the lower hub flange. Take the unlaced spoke offset directly to the right of the first spoke you laced and put it into the rim hole next to the first spoke and thread a nipple a few turns on it.
8. Skip the next three holes. Put the next spoke to the right into the fourth rim hole. Continue this pattern all the way around the rim until all nine spokes from the lower hub flange are laced into a rim hole, which should be on the *lower* side of the rim, the side farthest away from you.

9. Continue this lacing pattern. Make sure you cross over the first two spokes to the right and under the third one. Every spoke from the upper hub flange should be laced into a rim spoke hole on the upper side of the rim.

10. Place the last set of spokes from the lower hub flange into the remaining rim holes (lower side), passing over two spokes and under the third one.

How to True a Newly Built Front Wheel

It's easier to true a freshly laced front wheel because it doesn't have to be dished like a rear wheel. I'll explain the dishing process in the section below on truing a rear wheel. Follow these steps in truing a front wheel:

1. You will need the spoke nipple wrench (Fig. 7-20) and a centering (dishing) tool (Fig. 7-27).

2. The hub and rim measurements used below in the sample truing process are examples only. They may not apply to the hubs and rims you use. However, follow the measuring process shown here on your own hubs and rims and consider the measurements given as illustrative only.

3. Measure the width of the rim. In Fig. 7-41 it's 23 mm or about one inch.

4. Measure the space between hub locknuts. In Fig. 7-42 it's 100 mm or about 4 inches.

5. Subtract the rim width, one inch, from the width between the axle locknuts, four inches. You get three inches.

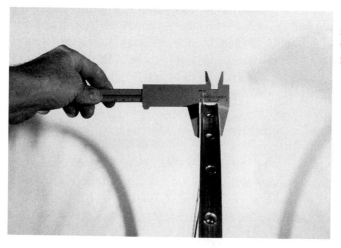

FIG. 7-41: First step in truing is to measure the rim width.

FIG. 7-42: Next step in truing a front wheel is to measure the distance from lock-nut to locknut, as shown. The idea is to center the rim between the hub flanges and the hub locknuts. See text.

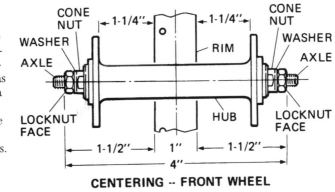

CENTERING -- FRONT WHEEL

6. Divide the figure obtained in step 5, 3 inches, by 2, which equals 1.5 inches, which is the distance each side of the rim should be from each hub axle locknut *in this example* (Fig. 7-42) *when the rim is trued.* Again, these measurements apply to one make of hub—make your own measurements on the hub/rim combination you are using.

7. Lay the centering tool (Fig. 7-27) on a flat surface and adjust the center "feeler" so it is 1.5 inches from the flats. This is a sample measurement for this example only. Be sure you use the measurements of your own hub and rim if they differ from this example.

8. Put the centering tool on the laced-up rim (Fig. 7-27) with one of the tool's flat ends on the flat side of the rim just over the valve hole and the other side (of course) on the opposite side of the rim, as shown in Fig. 7-27. Now tighten (adjust) the spoke nipples, until the centering (dishing) tool flats lie evenly where both flat surfaces of this tool touch the rim.

9. Turn the wheel over and repeat step 8 above. Now the rim will be laterally aligned at these two locations. Mark these locations with chalk.

10. Put the wheel in the wheel truing stand. Turn the wheel until the chalk marks on each side of the rim are aligned with the feeler arms of the alignment tool (Fig. 7-43). This is your starting point.

11. Finish truing the wheel as shown earlier in this chapter. Remove the wheel from the truing fixture and check side-to-side adjustment with the centering gauge a few times to make sure the rim is centered between the hub flanges and axle locknut.

12. Look closely at Fig. 7-43, where the adjustment feelers rub on the rim. You will notice that the feelers rub on both the sides of the rim and the top of the rim. As you adjust spoke nipples in the truing process, be sure to align the rim to be true both side to side (laterally) and around (concentrically). Be patient. Truing a rim accurately takes

FIG. 7-43: Install the wheel in the wheel truer so chalk marks (see text) are being touched by the truer arms.

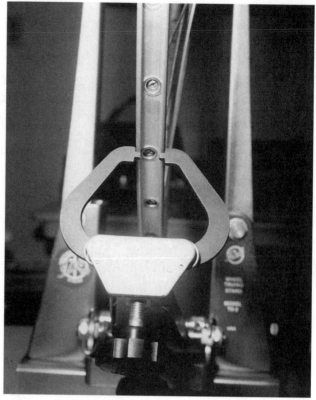

time. When you are finished, use the spoke tensionometer to make sure the spokes are equally tensioned, or close to it. On a rear wheel, because it has to be dished or pulled to one side so the spokes clear the freewheel, spoke tension should be even, but less, on the freewheel side than on the left side of the rim.

How to True a Newly Built Rear Wheel

You trued up the front wheel so the rim was centered between the axle locknuts. Do the same with the rear wheel, but dish it so the rim is centered between the locknuts (Fig. 7-44). Dishing will be automatic as you follow steps 1 through 12 above. Just make the measurements of the rim as you did for the front wheel, make the same computations as you made for the front wheel, and set your wheel-dishing tool accordingly. Dishing puts the rim closer to the right hub flange than to the left hub flange (Figs. 7-44 and 7-45).

Spokes will stretch so the wheel will eventually have to be retrued. Reduce the number of times you have to retrue wheels by prestretching a newly built wheel, as shown in Fig. 7-46.

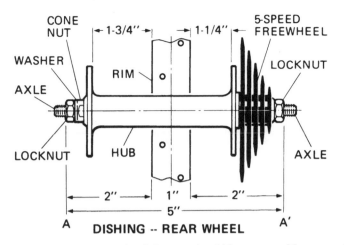

FIG. 7-44: When truing a rear wheel the rim should be centered between the hub locknuts, so the rim will be closer to the freewheel side.

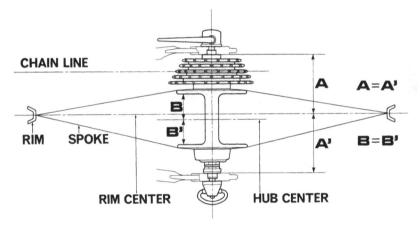

FIG. 7-45: Another view of centering the rear wheel rim between the axle locknuts.

FIG. 7-46: After truing the wheel, exert pressure on the spokes as shown here to pre-stretch them. Check trueness again and retrue as necessary.

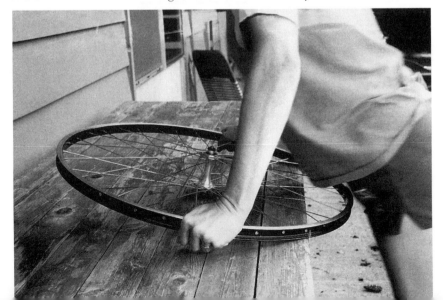

Radial-Wheel Building

I have put radial-wheel spoking last because it is an unusual way to lace wheels, and it applies only to the front wheel. Think of a wagon wheel and you will see what I mean by radial spoking. Do not attempt to lace a rear wheel this way, because the torque applied to the wheel as you pedal will pull that wheel rapidly out of alignment. Follow the spoking pattern shown in Fig. 7-47. Follow truing instructions above for truing a radially spoked wheel.

FIG. 7-47: A radially spoked front wheel. Note that spokes are not crossed.

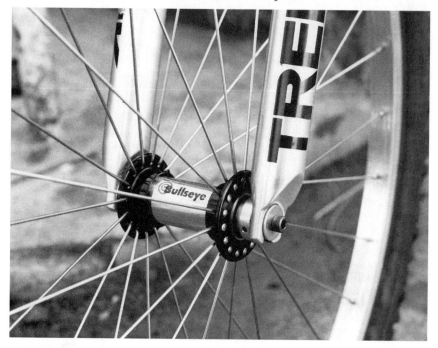

Now that you know how to keep your wheels rolling, Chapter 8 shows you how to do so comfortably.

Chapter Eight

HEADSETS, SUSPENSION SYSTEMS, SADDLES, AND STEMS

In this chapter we will review the care and adjustment of your headset, which consists of the mechanical parts that make steering easier, safer, and more accurate. I will also review the various types of suspension forks and saddles. Let's start with the headset. The headset bearings, cups, and cones are located inside the head tube (see Fig. 1-2).

Headset Maintenance

The headset (Fig. 8-1) takes a terrific beating, especially on rough roads. The lower set of balls is under thrust stress, the upper set is under radial stress. Thrust stress is force applied toward or away from an object, like the reactive force on the springs of a car on a rough road or when you strike a nail with a hammer. Radial stress is force spread outward, like the ripples a pebble makes when it's dropped in a pond. Road shock tends to flatten bearings. The bottom set takes most of the beating. Road shock will also wear grooves in the headset cups and cones. Fig. 8-1 shows these parts: locknut (A), spacer washer (B), adjustable cup (C), top cone (D, a press fit into the top of the fork steerer tube), bottom cup (E, a press fit into the bottom of the frame steerer tube), bottom cone (G, a press fit into the bottom of the fork steerer). F and H are bearings in a retainer. Fig. 8-2 shows the location of the headset parts on a bike frame and fork.

Loose headsets can cause wheel shimmy, loss of control, and an accident. Please see Chapter 2 and the text below under "More About Wheel Shimmy" for a review of the hazards of this condition, which are very real.

Check headset adjustment every few months if you ride a lot. Straddle the

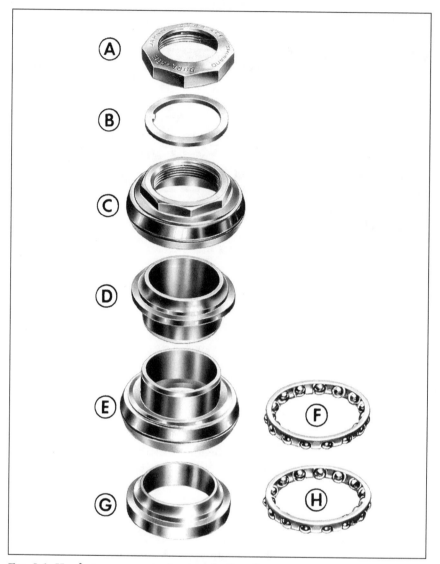

FIG. 8-1: Headset components. See text for list of parts.

bike, squeeze the front brake lever hard, rock the bike back and forth (Fig. 1-13), and watch the headset locknut as you do so. If you feel looseness, if the locknut moves in any direction, or if it's so loose you can turn it by hand, readjust the headset bearings to prevent hazardous wheel shimmy, as shown below. Readjust headset bearings if necessary, also shown below.

Disassemble, clean, and, readjust the headset every four to six months and install new bearings every year. Here's how to do it.

Tools you will need:

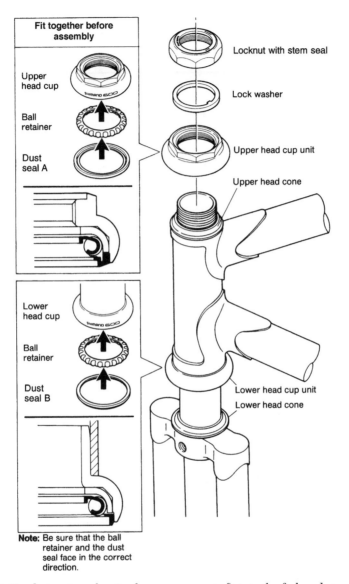

Fit together before
assembly

Upper
head cup

Ball
retainer

Dust
seal A

SHIMANO 600

Locknut with stem seal

Lock washer

Upper head cup unit

Upper head cone

Lower
head cup

Ball
retainer

Dust
seal B

SHIMANO 600

Lower head cup unit
Lower head cone

Note: Be sure that the ball
retainer and the dust
seal face in the correct
direction.

FIG. 8-2: Headset system showing how components fit into the fork and steerer
tube of the bike frame. *Courtesy Shimano American Corporation.*

1. A pair of headset wrenches that fit Campagnolo, SunTour, and older
   Shimano headset locknuts and adjustable cups. The new larger headsets take a 36-mm wrench, the older ones, 32 mm. Shimano has special headset wrenches (Fig. 8-3), but standard 32-mm wrenches will
   also fit their newer headsets as well as other makes with this size headset locknut.

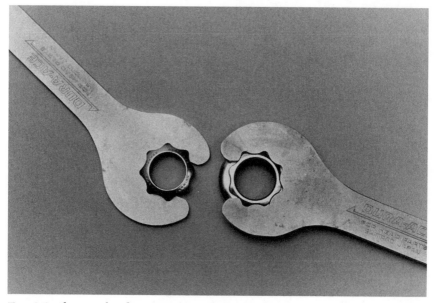

FIG. 8-3: Shimano headset wrenches. However, you can also use 32-mm headset wrenches. *Courtesy Shimano American Corporation.*

2. An Allen wrench or an open-end wrench to fit your stem binder bolt.

Headset Disassembly

1. Remove the front wheel.
2. For a mountain bike, mark the stem where it comes out of the lock-nut, so you can replace it at the same height. This is important, because if you change the stem height, you will have to readjust the front brake shoe-to-rim clearance, as I noted in Chapter 3.
3. Loosen the stem binder bolt with an Allen wrench or open-end wrench (Fig. 8-4), but do not remove it all the way. The expansion bolt has a nut that expands against an angle cut in the nut (see Chapter 1). As it's tightened, it wedges the stem tightly inside the fork steering tube. The stem bolt must be tapped down to break the wedge lock. Tap this bolt down with a hammer over a block of wood (see Chapter 1). One tap should break it loose.
4. Remove the handlebars and stem (Fig. 8-5). Drape them over the top tube, out of the way.
5. Remove the locknut. Hold the adjustable cup with one wrench while you loosen the locknut with another wrench (Fig. 8-6). Remove the washer under the locknut. If you have an inexpensive bike, the adjustable cup may have a knurled edge instead of wrench flats. In my

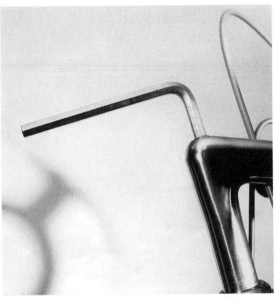

FIG. 8-4: Loosen the stem binder bolt to remove the stem.

FIG. 8-5: Remove the stem and handlebars with brake and shift cables attached, and drape the handlebars over the top tube so you can remove the headset.

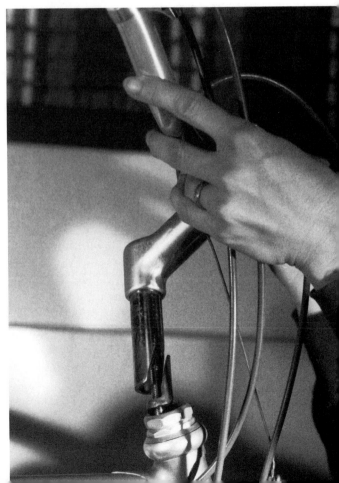

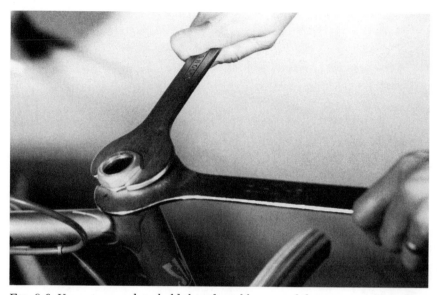

FIG. 8-6: Use one wrench to hold the adjustable cone while removing the locknut with the other.

opinion a knurled cup is a design defect because you have no convenient way to hold it in place while you tighten the locknut, other than by pliers. If you don't hold the adjustable cup while you tighten the locknut, the cup can wind up too loose and cause front-wheel shimmy and an accident. If the cup is too tight, headset bearings will wear faster and eventually the cup bearing surface will be grooved to the point where its adjustment will become loose and again, wheel shimmy could occur. If you do have such a knurled cup, use a locking-type pliers to hold it firmly in place as you tighten the locknut.

6. Loosen the adjustable cup until you can turn it by hand. Hold the fork of the bike with one hand while you remove the adjustable cup (Fig. 8-7). Carefully remove the fork. Catch loose bearings if they're not in a retainer. Or put a rag on the workbench, put the bike on it, and catch loose balls as you withdraw the fork.

7. If the headset has a dust seal (Fig. 8-2), remove it so you can remove the ball bearings.

8. Remove the bearings. Clean off old grease. If the bearings are in a retainer, check retainer and bearing wear. If the bearings easily fall out of the retainer, it's time to replace them, as noted below. Actually, I recommend replacing headset bearings every time you disassemble the headset. New bearings are not expensive, and they help reduce

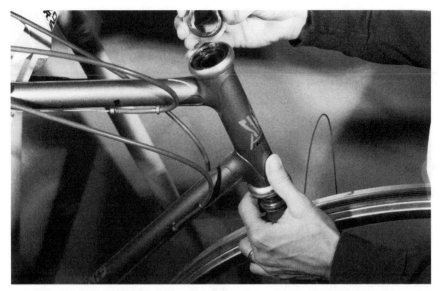

FIG. 8-7: Hold the fork with one hand while you remove the adjustable cup and top set of bearings. Carefully pull the fork out. Be ready to catch any loose bearings that may fall out of a worn retainer. In some cases, balls may be loose and not in their retainer.

the likelihood of wheel shimmy and make it easier to adjust the headset bearings as you reassemble them.

9. Clean old grease out of the adjustable cup, the top and bottom cones, and cup.

10. Examine cups and cones for grooves, rust, or wear. If you see grooves or dents in the cups or cones, take your bike to the bike shop and have them replaced. Don't do this yourself. This job requires special tools and skills. Have your bike shop check the seats where the cones and cups fit to make sure the factory has accurately machined them. If not, have them remachined so that the cups and cones seat accurately. This permits the bearings to absorb road shock evenly and wear uniformly. Uneven bearing wear can loosen the headset and cause wheel shimmy.

Headset Reassembly

1. Forget the retainer. Just buy enough of the same size balls that came out of your bike so you can replace the number of balls in the retainer plus two or three more. As you can see in Fig. 8-8, you can get more balls, at least two more, in the same space. More balls means greater headset life and improved protection against bearing wear.

2. Reassemble the headset. Grease the bearings, cups, and cones. Replace any seals. *Note:* If you leave the bearings in the retainer, be sure

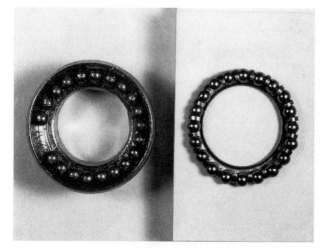

FIG. 8-8: Replace headset balls when you take the headset apart. At left, the same number of bearings taken from a retainer. Note there is still room for two more bearings. At right, the extra two bearings are on a headset cone. The balls are tiny, the beating they take is big, and their cost is small. Use loose bearings and you get two extra balls to absorb road shock. Buy extra balls to replace those you lose.

you replace the retainer correctly. The curvature of the retainer must be matched to the curvature of the cone, as shown in Fig. 8-2.

3. Place the bottom set of bearings in the bottom cup with enough grease to hold them in place.
4. Put a lot of grease in the adjustable cup. Fill the cup with the ball bearings.
5. Replace the fork. Be careful not to knock any balls off the bottom cup. Hold the fork in place while you thread on the adjustable cup by hand, as far as possible.
6. Tighten the adjustable cup with a wrench until it is snug, then back it off 1/4 turn.
7. Install the washer over the adjustable cup.
8. Thread on the locknut. Hold the adjustable cup with one wrench and tighten the locknut with the other wrench.
9. Replace the handlebars. The stem should be at the height marked earlier. Remember, if you don't replace the stem at the original height, you will have to readjust brake shoe clearance, for which please see Chapter 3. Also, and this is very important, at least 2 1/2 inches of the stem *must be inside the steering tube!*
10. Tighten the expander bolt to 174 to 260 in./lbs.
11. Replace the front wheel.
12. Check the headset adjustable cup setting:
   a. Check for looseness. Mount the bike. Hold the front brake lever tightly closed. Rock the bike back and forth (see Chapter 1). If the fork feels loose, hold the adjustable cup with one wrench and turn the locknut counterclockwise one turn. Turn the adjustable cup

clockwise 1/4 turn, hold it with the wrench, and tighten the lock-nut. Repeat until the fork has no free play.

b. Check the headset for tightness. Lift the front wheel off the ground and turn the handlebars in both directions. Tilt the bike so the handlebars move freely by gravity, without binding or tightness. If the handlebars stick or bind, hold the adjustable cup with a wrench, loosen the locknut, then loosen the adjustable cup 1/4 turn and hold it with a wrench while you tighten the locknut. Repeat until the fork turns freely.

More About Wheel Shimmy

I've mentioned the dangers of wheel shimmy several times so far in this book. Once started, shimmy is difficult or impossible to stop. You can easily lose control and take a spill. Loose headsets are a prime cause of wheel shimmy accidents. Headsets work loose more often in all-terrain bicycles than in other bike types, because trail shock ultimately flattens the headset just a fraction of a thousandth of an inch. The flattening effect comes sooner if the headset is loose. It always creeps up on you gradually, unnoticeably. Sometimes, the headset locknut and adjustable cup work loose as bearings wear down. Sometimes, the adjustable cup is loose to begin with, right out of the bike factory. Then, one day, at speed, down a rough, steep hill, the front wheel assumes a quick left-right-left life of its own.

A new headset, the AheadSet, introduced by DiaCompe, Inc., is designed, according to the manufacturer, to maintain the headset bearings at the original tightening adjustment. Of course when the bearings wear down this adjustment will change so that the headset will become looser. Which is a good reason to give your bike the push-pull test at least annually, as described in Chapter 1 and shown in Fig. 1-13. But at least the AheadSet, in my opinion, is very unlikely to loosen up on you until the bearings, or the bearing races, or both wear. A word of caution, though. The AheadSet is designed for threadless steering tubes. So if you are installing a suspension fork on your existing bike, order a fork with an unthreaded steering tube with the same diameter as your existing or old fork steerer tube. Have the bike shop install the AheadSet, because it involves remachining of the bike's steerer tube for a precise fit of the lower bearing cup, and of the fork crown for precise fit of the fork crown race. However, if you are good with tools and have all the proper equipment, just follow the installation instructions that come with the AheadSet. Of course, once it is installed, you can easily remove the Ahead-Set, pretty much as you would any other type of headset, and proceed to clean, regrease, and reinstall the headset and its bearings.

Suspension Forks, Bikes, Saddles, and Seat Posts

At my last count there were some 25 manufacturers of suspension forks of various designs, just a few of which are shown in Fig. 8-9, at prices ranging from $150 to $750, less installation. There were also at least 12 manufacturers of bicycles with full suspension, at prices ranging from $1,200 to $4,000. A full-suspension bicycle has an articulated frame (Fig. 8-10) with suspension front and rear.

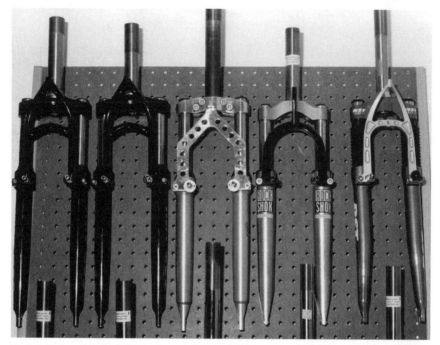

FIG. 8-9: Just a few of the makes and types of suspension forks now on the market.

You can of course try out a full-suspension mountain bike (full-suspension road bikes are only on the horizon at this writing), because it is fully assembled and ready to go. But you probably won't be able to borrow such a bicycle long enough for a real tryout on a variety of off-road trails, hills, and sharp turns. So what I suggest is that you ask friends or members of your local bicycle club for their experience with suspension forks or full-suspension bicycles. If you are good with tools and have experience with bicycle maintenance, you can install a suspension fork yourself. But this is a complex process, even involving remachining of your existing bike's steerer tube, so I recommend you have your bike shop make this installation. Suspension forks are quite complicated in themselves. If they are not correctly installed

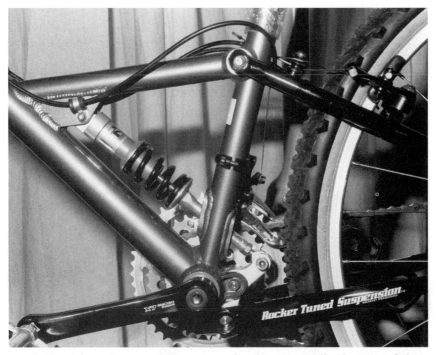

FIG. 8-10: A bike with rear suspension. Note that the rear triangle (the seat and chain stays) can pivot up and down.

and adjusted you could be in for a spill and injury. In fact, the manuals that come with suspension forks are quite explicit with this warning. One of the pioneers of suspension forks warns, on the first page of its installation instructions: *"It is extremely important that your . . . fork is installed correctly by a qualified technician with proper tools. Improperly installed forks are extremely dangerous and can result in severe injuries."* So I am not even going to attempt to describe how to install suspension forks on your old bike. I do urge you to have the bike shop do this. Or, better yet, buy a new bike that comes with such a fork. On the other hand, a correctly installed suspension fork can add a lot of comfort, control, and safety to off-road riding and even to riding on mildly bumpy paved roads. I wish I had had a suspension fork on my last trip over the cobbled roads of Belgian cities. You could also install, on your mountain or road bicycle, an Allsop suspension saddle, which gives excellent bump control over the rear wheel, and an Allsop or Girvin suspension stem, which absorbs bumps from the front wheel, or a Hydra-Post suspension seat post (Fig. 8-11). Installation of the suspension saddle is fairly easy if you know how mechanical things go together. The manufacturer of this saddle has excellent installation instructions and can even loan you a videotape that shows how to install this unit. Installation of the suspension

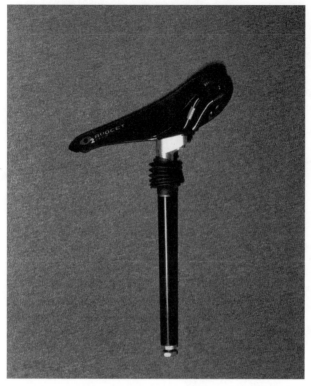

FIG. 8-11: A Hydra-Post seat post, which adds a form of rear-suspension comfort to your saddle.

stem is also quite easy, but you need to adjust the brakes (Chapter 3) and front and rear derailleurs (Chapter 5) to do so.

Here is what to look for if you contemplate adding a suspension stem to your current road or mountain bike, or are thinking of buying a full-suspension bicycle.

Types of Suspension Forks

The four types of suspension forks (at this writing) are:

1. Air/oil using a combination of air pressure and oil, which is forced through valves, such as Rock Shox.
2. Elastomer, which uses a type of rubber called a "bumper" that absorbs road shock.
3. Elastomer, with coiled spring.
4. A fork with a heavy coil spring. Early high-quality suspension forks used springs only. You will see inexpensive bicycles that have a spring in plain view on the fork, which as far as I am concerned is a blatant attempt to

impress a potential buyer that here is a suspension bike at very low price. In actuality this fork shows the spring for purely cosmetic purposes. If you push down on the handlebars you will find that there is no compression at all. Some models of these bikes do have springs that can be compressed, but they cannot be adjusted and can, in my opinion, be dangerous on some types of terrain.

Variations of the above are many and their number is growing. My advice is to try riding a bike equipped with suspension on a variety of surfaces, uphill, downhill, the flats. See how it fits your riding style. Ask yourself these questions:

1. Does the fork twist sideways when it hits a bump (torsional stiffness)? Do the brakes rub on the rim under road shock and does this affect braking power?
2. Does the fork have links, and do these wear and negatively affect torsional stiffness?
3. On a suspension stem, does your riding position change as the stem moves up and down, and is this change fatiguing?
4. Can the suspension fork be adjusted for various terrains? Quickly? Without special tools?
5. Does the suspension fork bottom out easily? Does the fork stay compressed and not bounce back quickly and easily?
6. Does the bike bounce up and down and so affect handling and steering on very rough terrain?
7. Does the suspension fork handle small bumps well but not big bumps, or vice versa?
8. Does the suspension fork work for the kind of riding you do, or can it be adjusted so it will?
9. Does the suspension fork let you handle bumps with comfort and corner well on a high-speed downhill run?
10. When you climb uphill standing on the pedals, does the front wheel bounce up and down as you pedal and use up your energy? Is the suspension so soft that it absorbs your energy?
11. When it gets cold outside, does the suspension fork ride harder and absorb bumps less well?
12. If you adjust the fork for small bumps, do you have to readjust it for big ones, and vice versa?
13. Does the suspension fork you like have a history of seals that leak air and oil? Is maintenance high and costly for these forks?
14. Is the ride so bouncy that you have trouble with steering on uphill runs and when cornering at speed?

15. Does the suspension fork change frame geometry to the point where wheels do not track? Does the frame feel so springy that it seems made of rubber?

16. Does the fork dive downward as you brake hard and reduce the stable handling characteristics you are used to?

17. When the fork is installed on an older bike or one with a frame not designed for a suspension fork, does handling become so stable that steering becomes very sluggish?

18. When the fork is fully compressed, does the fork crown rub on the tire? This is a potentially dangerous situation and can lead to an accident.

19. Last, but by no means least, can you understand the owner's manual?

Handlebar Accessories

I have covered handlebar height adjustment and stem lengths for reach and rise on mountain bikes and stem length and fall for road bikes in Chapter 1. But there are a few other items concerning handlebars that I will mention here.

Use bar ends such as the Onzas in Fig. 8-12 to give you a firm grip when you power up steep hills or go all out on the flats. They fasten on the ends of your handlebars and give you a couple more places to grip, which can relieve pressure on your hands.

For distance racing on your road bike, install either handlebars like the ones in Fig. 8-13 or an add-on version so you can lean far forward, resting your torso on the elbow pads and gripping the top of the bars. These bars increase aerodynamic efficiency by letting you get your back down almost par-

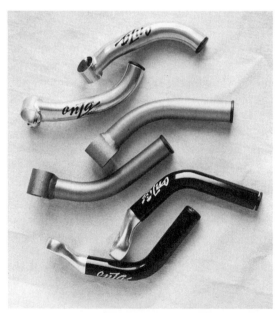

FIG. 8-12: Use these bar ends on your mountain bike for hill climbs.

allel to the top tube. One warning, though. It's all too easy to see only the first 10 feet or so in front of your handlebars. So I don't recommend them for casual road cycling, especially where the traffic can get heavy. One solution for forward vision with aerobars is to install a Windcheeta (Figs. 8-14

FIG. 8-13: Install this type of handlebar on your road bike, or put an add-on version onto your existing handle-bars, for comfort when you race in an aerody-namic position or just for elbow and arm rest on long rides.

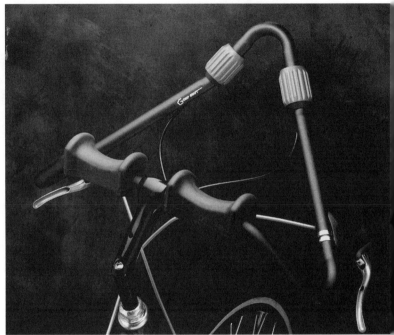

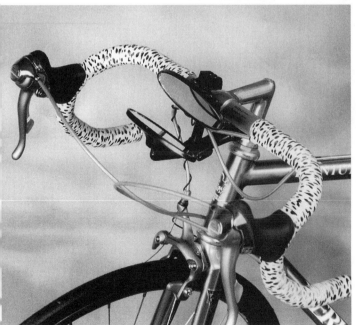

FIG. 8-14: Mount a forward viewing mirror on your stem when you in-stall the handlebars shown in FIG. 8-13, so you can see the road ahead when you crouch over the handlebars to reduce wind pres-sure in a race. *Courtesy Wind-cheeta, Inc.*

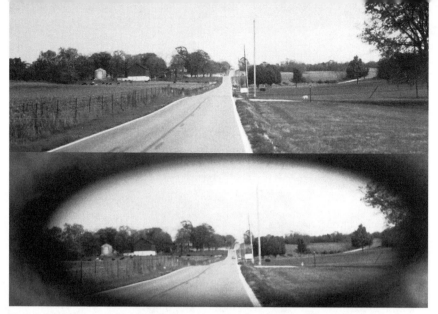

FIG. 8-15: The view ahead with the stem mirror. *Courtesy Windcheeta, Inc.*

and 8-15) on your stem, which costs about $40. If your bike shop does not carry one, write or call Windcheeta, Inc., for a source: 187 Bellbrook Ave., Xenia, OH 45385, 1-800-691-0011, or 513-376-4150.

If your handlebars are too close, too far away, too high, or too low, consider installing a stem that has the "rise" and the length to fit your arm and torso. See Chapter 1 for more details. If you get sore hands on a long ride, try one of the many soft, cushiony grips you can buy in your local bike shop (Fig. 8-16).

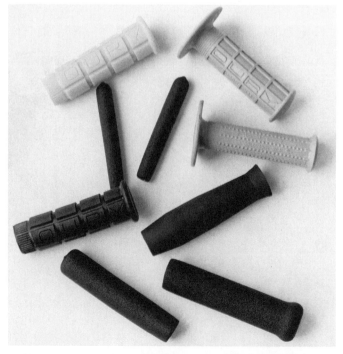

FIG. 8-16: Comfortable bar grips ease pressure on the palm of your hands.

Saddle Suggestions

Personally I prefer leather saddles. I have been riding on them for more years than I care to think about. There are other saddles, in other materials and different configurations, and if one of them is comfortable, great! But I have found that the contour-shaping and comfort aspects of a leather saddle are more important than the weight saving in a lighter plastic type with titanium frame. I use a Brooks Pro leather saddle, which, over the years, has shaped itself to fit my nether extremities, as you can see by the saddle at the top of Fig. 8-17. Obviously there is more of me on one side of that saddle than on the other. The Brooks spring-loaded leather saddle in Fig. 8-18 brings sighs of comfort from my friends who ride on it. Sure it's heavy, but if comfort is more important to you than squeezing that last extra millisecond out of a race, you have made a good decision. But you do have to give a leather sad-

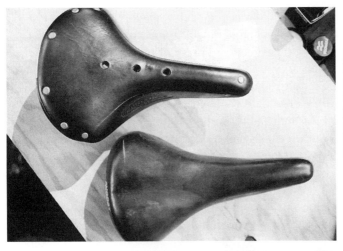

Fig. 8-17: A leather saddle shapes itself to the contours of your derriere, as you can see by the saddle at the top.

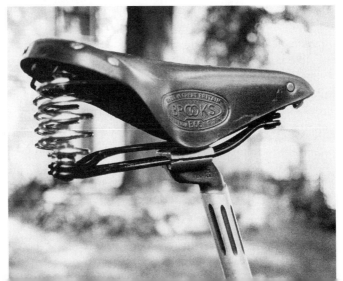

Fig. 8-18: This leather saddle has springs that absorb road shock.

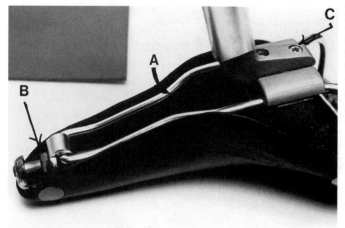

FIG. 8-19: Leather saddles stretch. Remove the stretch by turning nut B until the saddle is taut once again.

dle lots of TLC, such as keeping it supple with a saddle dressing and taking out stretch by turning nut B in Fig. 8-19.

Most mountain bikes these days come with a quick-release saddle clamp, like the quick-release on a wheel hub but, of course, a lot shorter. See Chapter 2 for information on the use and adjustment of a quick-release mechanism. This release permits you to adjust seat height to suit your riding style and the terrain. You can also install one on your road bike, to facilitate change of saddle height, which can ease the pain of saddle sores. Review the instructions on the adjustment and use of the quick-release mechanism in Chapter 2. If the saddle moves when you apply rotational pressure to it, the quick-release clamp is too loose. A quick-release on your seat post also lets you remove the saddle when you park your bike, so the saddle won't be stolen.

An excellent solution to saddle comfort is offered by WRS SportsMed. Fig. 8-20 shows a selection of their gel-filled saddles. Going clockwise, at the lower left is a road bike saddle, above that is a wide saddle that women like, the next one over is a touring saddle, and at the lower right is a super-lightweight gel saddle with titanium rails that weighs only 7.2 ounces. Your bike shop can get these saddles for you, or call WRS at 1-800-299-3366 for the name of a bike dealer near you who does carry this line. WRS also makes a gel-filled saddle cover that fits over your existing saddle. There is also a saddle designed for women, by a woman, Georgena Terry. This saddle has a specially shaped nose to, as Ms. Terry says, "promote airflow, which leading gynecologists say helps prevent yeast growth." If your bike shop does not carry this saddle, call Terry Precision Cycles for Women at 1-800-289-8379 or write to this firm at 1704 Wayneport Rd., Macedon, NY 14502.

One of the problems you might face during a mountain bike ride is the need to readjust saddle position for optimum steering and handling. The need is there, but the problem is that it's a bother to stop, get off the bike,

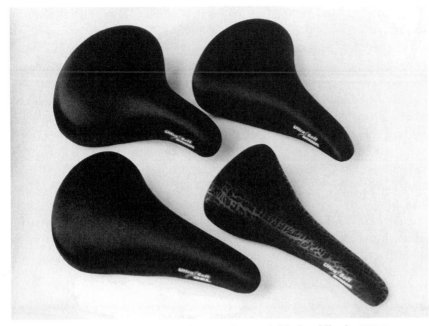

FIG. 8-20: Saddle solutions for comfort are these gel-filled saddles by WRS SportsMed (see text).

FIG. 8-21: Change saddle position up, down, fore, or aft with this Power Post for optimum powering and steering control of your mountain bike.

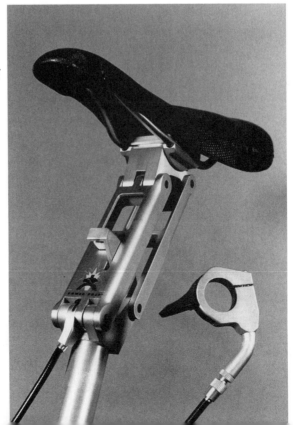

and readjust saddle height. More than that, you should also adjust saddle fore and aft position, but that's even more of a hassle because it requires loosening the saddle clamp bolt (not just the seat-tube clamp on the seat post), shoving the saddle fore or aft, and retightening the bolt. I doubt that anyone ever does this, considering the work and the time involved. Up to now one had to compensate by moving one's body back or forward, not the ideal solution. Now, though, there's a new product just on the market that lets you readjust the saddle position in all these positions, up, down, fore or aft. It's called the Power Post (Fig. 8-21). Saddle repositioning this way is fast, quick, and accurate. See your bike shop or contact Centerline Sports, 370 S. Crenshaw Blvd., Suite E202J, Torrance, CA 90503, phone 1-800-900-POST, or FAX 1-310-787-7096.

Chapter 9, coming up next, tells you all about the accessories that make bicycling fun to ride cross-country or commute to work, and to pedal in foreign countries. Also in Chapter 9, you'll find tips on bike clothing for all seasons.

CHAPTER NINE

ACCESSORIES THAT ADD PLEASURE, SAFETY, AND SECURITY TO CYCLING

Here is a quick overview of bicycle-related products that can make your bicycle trip more enjoyable and safer and add security and peace of mind, whether you ride to the corner grocery or embark on an overland safari on the road or trail. Let's start with security.

Locks

Your bicycle, especially if it is costly, is a prime target for thieves these days. A good bike is very saleable and almost untraceable, even if you registered it with your local police or sheriff. So never leave your bike unlocked. I've had two attempts, both unsuccessful, by thieves lusting after my beautiful Klein road bike. One try was at a campground on the Sacramento River north of Berkeley. I woke up at around 2:00 A.M. to odd noises outside my tent. The sound of the zipper on the tent fly alerted the would-be thieves, so all I saw was a pair of jean-clad buttocks disappearing. My fishing tackle box had disappeared with them, but my bike, U-locked to a picnic table anchored in cement, was intact. I am sure I would have lost that bike had I not locked it. Another try was at a grocery store, when I noticed scratches on the keyway on the lock from someone trying to pick it. All locks are pickable, of course, but mine was more difficult to open without a key than most. So I love U-locks (Fig. 9-1). If your bicycle is stolen, remember that your homeowner's insurance will pay for it. But of course your trip will come to a halt if your bicycle is swiped. So lock that bike up, always and forever! Older U-locks can be snapped by inserting an iron bar or even a two-by-four between the U-arms and twisting. Newer locks are stronger, beefier, and more resistant

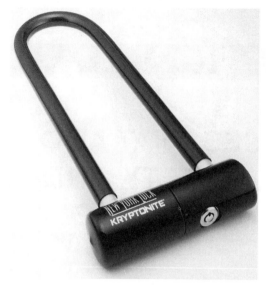

FIG. 9-1: This Kryptonite U-lock is reinforced to resist twist breakage of the shank and is one of a line of such locks, which fit any size bike and security situation. The shank is hardened steel to resist cutting and the lock is pick-resistant. This lock is available from your bike shop.

to such breakage. The Kryptonite lock in Fig. 9-1 is a new version with 5/8 hardened steel, which, according to Kryptonite, will withstand a pulling force of over 8,000 pounds of hydraulic force. The cylinder is of hardened steel and is "pick and drill resistant." The lock mechanism tests at up to 7.5 pounds of pull force, according to the manufacturer. If you lose your key but have registered your lock with Kryptonite, they will provide a new key within 24 hours from receipt of order. Locks are available from your bike shop. Another modern U-lock that also resists being broken by a twisting force is the Bad Bones lock, which incorporates sliding bars. Use this lock by inserting the metal bars so there is no room for a twist bar to be inserted in the arms. The Bad Bones lock is from Integrated Cycle Systems, Inc., 101 Townsend St., No. 333, San Francisco, CA 94107.

A quick-release on your expensive wheels and on your saddle clamp is as quick for crooks as it is for you. So if you are going to be away from your bike, say in a grocery store or in a tent, take the saddle and the front wheel in with you. Then lock the bike with the U-lock through the frame and the rear wheel to an immovable object, such as a support post of a chain-link fence, or a parking meter if you are sure your locked bike can't be lifted up and over it.

Panniers (Saddlebags)

Yup, another French-derived word, like derailleurs. The bike industry calls them panniers, cowboys call them saddlebags. I've been calling them panniers so long I'll just stick with that name. Anyhow, a good set of panniers is vital to an enjoyable trip, however long or short. You need something reliable in which to carry spare tubes and tires, parts, tools, wet gear if it rains, and camping gear for overnight rides. Here is what to look for in a set of panniers:

1. *Size:* Panniers come in cubic-inch sizes of around 600 (Fig. 9-2); 1,100 (Fig. 9-3); 1,615 (Fig. 9-4); 2,500 (Fig. 9-5); and 3,050 (not shown).
2. *Detachability:* Easy fastening to the carrier (aka rack) and easy detachability. The Mountain Minded pannier (Fig. 9-6) is a good example of a 2,300-cu.in. pannier that, once the disc/cam buckle is fastened to the carrier, can be quickly detached and reinstalled without a lot of hassle. Great idea when you need to remove the pannier and contents for security, or for day rides without it. This is one pannier set that stays put on the roughest terrain. What you don't want to happen is unexpected detachment, which could cause an accident, or loss of the pannier and contents if a vehicle runs over it. Outside straps to hold a

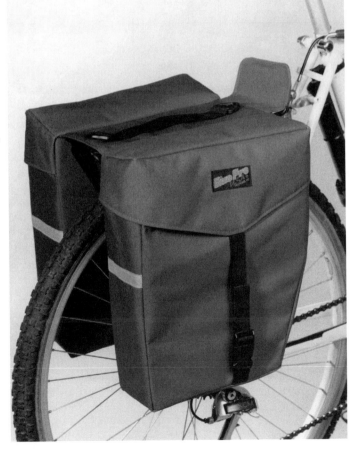

FIG. 9-2: This Bike Pro DayTripper pannier is a single-compartment bag of about 600 cu.in., which is quickly detachable and ideal for grocery shopping or for day trips.

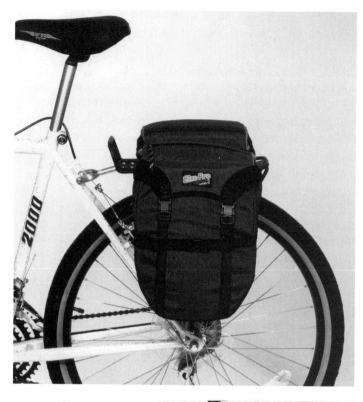

FIG. 9-3: A 1,100-cu.in. pannier from Bike Pro, the Canyon.

FIG. 9-4: A 1,615-cu.ft. pannier, the Ascent, is great for longer trips.

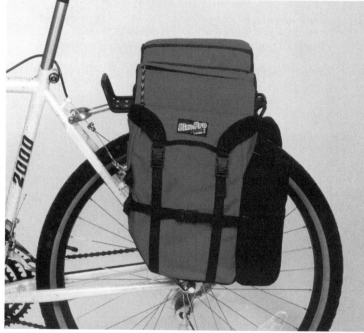

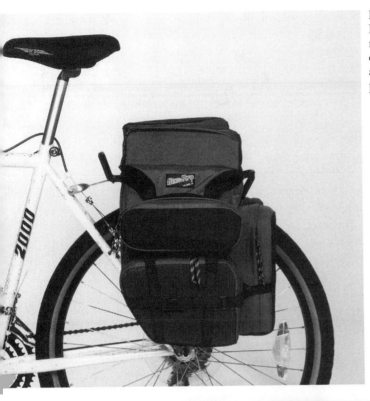

FIG. 9-5: Bike Pro's Summit model has 2,500 cu.in. of space and a detachable fanny pack.

FIG. 9-6: The Meridian pannier from Mountain Minded is an extremely well-made set featuring quick detachability along with a removable fanny pack.

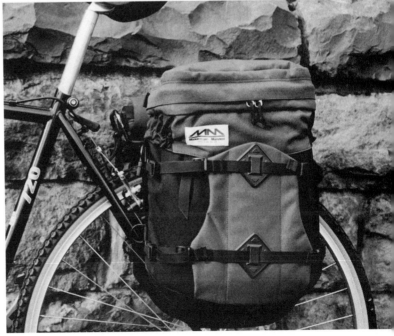

loaded pannier in place so contents don't move are also important (Fig. 9-6). Another good feature of the MM pannier in Fig. 9-6 is the upper section, which is detachable, so you can take your wallet, maps, keys, and so forth with you without taking along the entire pannier. That's a good idea when you just want to run into a store to buy food (but have a friend watch your locked bike or keep an eye on it yourself from the store).

3. *Commuting ease:* The garment pannier made by EccoSport is a combination pannier and garment bag in which you can carry your suit, shirt, tie, and shoes to work or on an airplane (Fig. 9-7). Cycle Smith also has combination pannier/briefcase (Fig. 9-8) and a set of 1,100 or so cu.in. panniers with an over-the-shoulder tote strap.

4. *Convenience:* You need panniers with many pockets of different sizes. When you need a specific tool, the salt shaker, or matches, you want to be able to find them quickly without having to rummage around inside two big pockets.

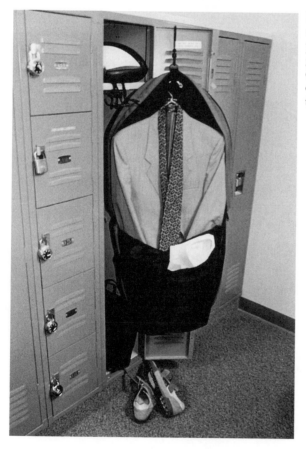

FIG. 9-7: For bicycle commuters, here's a pannier that doubles as a garment bag, from EccoSport, in which you can carry your suit, shirt, tie, and shoes to work.

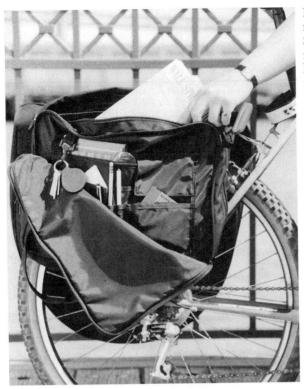

FIG. 9-8: Also for commuters, use this Cycle Smith briefcase/pannier to carry your homework between office and home.

5. *Protection from the elements:* No pannier is submersible, but some, such as the MM line, have optional covers that keep out the rain. Rain-soaked clothes are a tad dispiriting on a bike trip. *Note:* You could wrap clothes in plastic garbage bags. Carry a couple of heavy-duty bags to keep your sleeping bag dry. You never know when or how hard the rain will fall.

6. *Construction:* Try opening and closing the zippers on the panniers you like. If the zippers catch and bind on loose threads or the pannier fabric, that's a sign of shoddy construction as well as a source of frustration. The better panniers do not have zipper bind—where the zippers get caught on loose threads. Look for quality heavy-duty snap fasteners, strong fabrics, such as 1,000-denier Cordura, lined inside with rip-stop nylon. Good panniers cost around $195 for 2,300 cu.in. a pair.

Sidetrak, Inc. in Seattle makes a line of very convenient pouches that can be fastened to the seat post or top tube, or double as a fanny pack tool holder. You can carry a rear light in the one mounted on your seat post. If space in your home workshop is limited, consider Sidetrak's ToolRap Pro, which displays all your tools and can be wall-mounted. Other pouches I have found convenient include Sidetrak's ToolRaps. Reach Sidetrak at 1221 Harbor Ave. SW, Suite 104, Seattle, WA 98116, phone 1-206-575-0335.

Tools and Spare Parts

A breakdown or a flat far from a bike shop can be a disaster. Which is why you should carry at least the minimum number of tools needed to get you going again, and those spare parts that you can replace on the road or trail. Carry this equipment in your pannier:

Tools:

1. Allen and open-end wrenches in 5-, 6-, 8-, 9-, and 10-mm sizes.
2. Spoke wrench (see Chapter 7).
3. Small standard and Phillips head screwdrivers.
4. Small adjustable wrench to fit nuts no other tools you brought will fit.
5. Needlenose pliers.
6. Chain rivet tool (see Chapter 4).
7. Headset wrenches (see Chapter 8) to fit your headset (32 or 36 mm).
8. Two hub wrenches to fit your hub locknuts and adjustable cones.
9. Tire levers to pry tire off rim, such as the Sidetrak kit in Fig. 9-9.

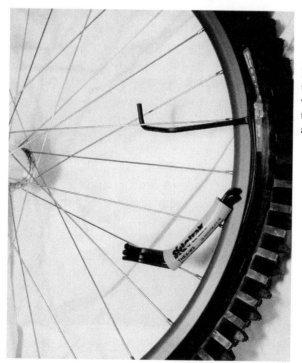

FIG. 9-9: A combination tire lever and Allen wrench is a handy addition to your set of take-along tools.

10. Patch kit to repair tube punctures.
11. Duct tape (to mend a rip in the tire wall as an emergency repair, or to patch a tear in a tent, to name a few uses for this versatile tape).
12. Pouch to carry these tools.
13. Tire pump.

Spare parts and equipment:

1. Two or three spokes for each wheel (same length as existing spokes) and spoke nipples.
2. Rear derailleur cable (can be trimmed for front derailleur).
3. Rear brake cable (can be trimmed for front brake).
4. Crossover cable for cantilever brake (if you have this type of brake).
5. Five or six lengths of chain links to fit your chain, or an entire chain if you are on an extended trip.
6. Pair of brake shoes (you probably won't need them, but I like the comfort of having them—they don't weigh much or take up much room).
7. Small container of chain oil.
8. Tube of grease.

Other equipment:

1. Front and rear racks to carry your panniers. Use a "low-rider" carrier over your front wheel for better balance. I like the Blackburn racks (Figs. 9-10 and 9-11) for adjustability and strength, available in your bike store. Be sure to check tightness of mounting bolts (35 to 50

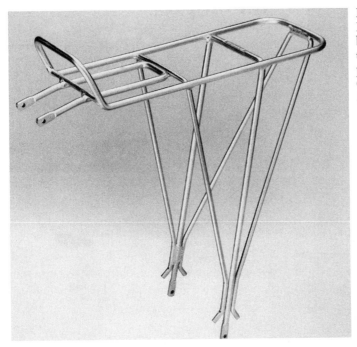

Fɪɢ. 9-10: Rear Blackburn carrier to hold your panniers. *Courtesy Bell Sports, Inc.*

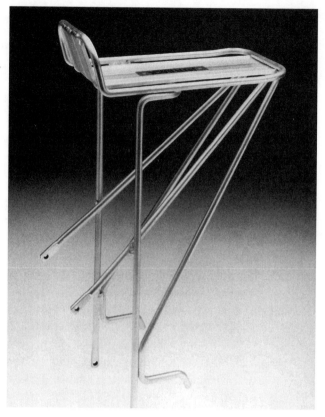

FIG. 9-11: Blackburn low-rider front carrier keeps the load low for safe bike handling. *Courtesy Bell Sports, Inc.*

in./lbs.) before each trip (Fig. 9-12). Your bike should have brazed-on mountings on the seat stays and dropout ears for the rear carrier as well as for the front carrier. If not, use carriers that can be clamped onto these fittings, but on a trip check their tightness daily to avoid a spill should the clamps loosen and let the carrier slide down onto the tire. Be sure that the carrier clears all brake cables, both tires, and fenders. One lament: At this writing, at least, forget touring on a full-suspension bike. There is no way you can mount carriers on that type of bike. Nor can you mount a carrier or a fender on a suspension fork. However, you can install a handlebar bag such as the Cannondale model that clips onto a fitting mounted on the handlebars. This is handy for removing and taking into a store, restaurant, motel, or tent at night. Buy the bar bag that has a map holder, very handy for road trips and tours.

2. A bicycle computer (Fig. 9-13) with a digital readout that gives speed, mileage, and pedal cadence. Be sure to fasten electrical wires so they don't tangle in the spokes. Carry a spare battery for the computer.

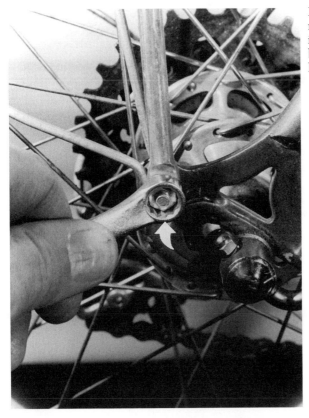

FIG. 9-12: Check tightness of carrier mounting bolts often and before every tour with loaded panniers.

FIG. 9-13: Use a bicycle computer to tell you how fast you pedal and how far you have traveled.

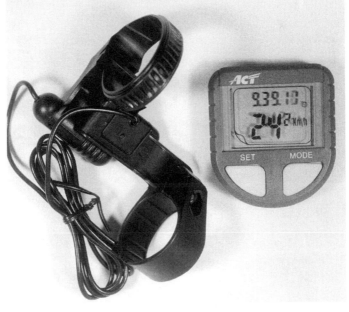

3. A first-aid kit in a handy pouch (Figs. 9-14 and 9-15). The kit in Fig. 9-14 is from Outdoor Research, 1000 1st Ave. So., Seattle, WA 98134, phone 1-800-421-2421. The three kits in Fig. 9-15 were designed by Dr. Eric A. Weiss, assistant professor of emergency medicine at Stanford University Medical Center and chairman of the editorial board of the Wilderness Medical Society Letter. These kits are available directly from Chinook Medical Gear, Inc., 2805 Wilderness Place, Suite 700, Boulder, CO 80301, phone 1-800-766-1365.

4. A water purifier kit. Necessary for travel in Mexico, China, or anyplace sterility of the water supply is questionable. The best models remove *Giardia,* pathogenic bacteria, flukes, tapeworms, cysts, larger protozoa and fallout, herbicides, pesticides, other chemicals, asbestos, and foul odors.

5. Small flashlight and extra batteries for it.

6. Mosquito lotion (a must, in my opinion).

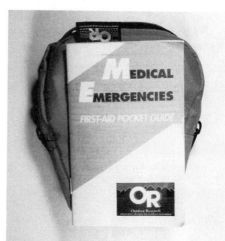

FIG. 9-14: This first-aid kit comes in a Velcro canvas package that can be attached to your bicycle. It also comes with a compact 60-page first-aid manual from Outdoor Research, Seattle.

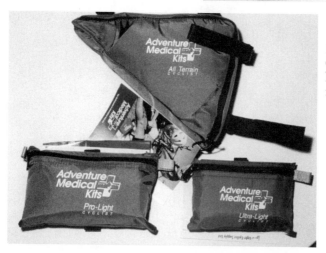

FIG. 9-15: These Chinook first-aid kits are frame-mountable.

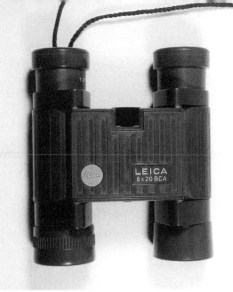

FIG. 9-16: Use precision Leica binoculars to enjoy the pleasures of outdoor life on a bike tour. This pair of minibinoculars has 8 × 20 power and weighs only 7.98 ounces.

7. Minibinoculars. The Leica compact binoculars in Fig. 9-16 are 8 × 20, have the excellent precision optical quality expected from Leica, weigh only 7.98 ounces, and have a field of view of 380 ft. at 3,280 ft. Diopter compensation is plus/minus 3.5, short-range focus is 3.5 ft. Brunton compact binoculars are 8 × 24, have fine optical design, weigh about 8 ounces, and are armored and waterproof. With either pair you can enjoy the scenery, and watch birds and other humans. Reach Leica at 156 Ludlow Ave., Northvale, NJ 07647, phone 1-201-767-7500, FAX 1-201-767-8666; reach Brunton at 620 E. Monroe, Riverton, WY 82501, phone 1-800-443-4870. For a fine pair of powerful 10 × 42 binoculars I can also recommend Bausch & Lomb's Trophy model, which is also armored, waterproof, and fogproof (Fig. 9-17). Reach Bausch & Lomb at 9200 Cody, Overland Park, KS 66214, phone 1-800-433-3537, FAX 1-913-752-3550.

FIG. 9-17: View distant vistas up close with this pair of Bausch & Lomb 10 × 42 waterproof binoculars.

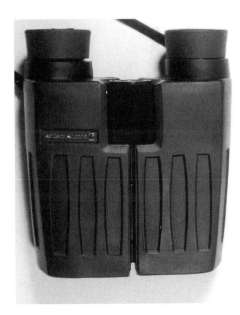

8. A handlebar-mounted inclinometer that gives you the percent grade and degree grade of a hill (up and downhill). An optional but fun unit from Sidetrak, Seattle.

9. Compass, the kind used for orienteering on remote mountain trails (Fig. 9-18), such as a Silva or the excellent compasses from Brunton, at 620 E. Monroe, Riverton, WYO 82501, phone 1-800-443-4870. Brunton also has a videotape titled *The ABC's of Compass and Map,* which teaches you or small groups the essentials of land navigation using map and compass. Topics included in this tape are understanding magnetism; the earth's magnetic field and magnetic declination; the importance of a compass in the field; taking a bearing; types of maps; reading maps and scales; visual and poor-weather navigation; and using a map and compass together. The complete package includes a 25-minute video, a basic map compass, an instruction book, and a USGS topo map symbol guide.

10. A signaling mirror (Fig. 9-18) that can bounce a solar ray for miles, such as off an airplane overhead or toward a person far away. This mirror is on the inside of the altimeter cover flap in Fig. 9-18. If you get lost, or incapacitated, or your bike does, and you need help, this mirror can alert someone who may see its bright glare and respond to your need for assistance. Available in sporting goods outlets.

11. An altimeter, so you can follow map contour lines, which give altitude, a great help to mark your position accurately. If you know approximately where you are and have an altimeter to tell which contour line you're on, you're halfway to orienteering yourself accurately. I use a Swiss-made Thommen 15,000-ft. altimeter (Fig. 9-18) and find it highly accurate, light, easy to read and, at around $160, a comforting instrument to have in the wild. For off-road trail rides into the wilderness, you really should know orienteering, how to find your way with contour map and compass. I urge you to take courses in this subject. Your local sporting goods outfitter should know who offers them. Or read and study books on this subject, such as:

Bjorn Kjellstrom, *Map & Compass,* 215 pages. Orienteerists say this book is their bible. Once you read it you'll agree. It covers map symbols and what they mean, how to travel by map alone, by compass alone, or with both together, how to find bearings, and sketching maps and wilderness travel. Charles Scribner's Sons, Inc., New York.

Hans Bengtsson and George Atkinson, *Orienteering for Sport and Pleasure,* 224 pages. Emphasizes orienteering as a sport unto itself. The Stephen Greene Press, Brattleboro, VT.

June Fleming, *Staying Found,* 159 pages. A practical guide to the use of map and compass. Vintage Books, New York.

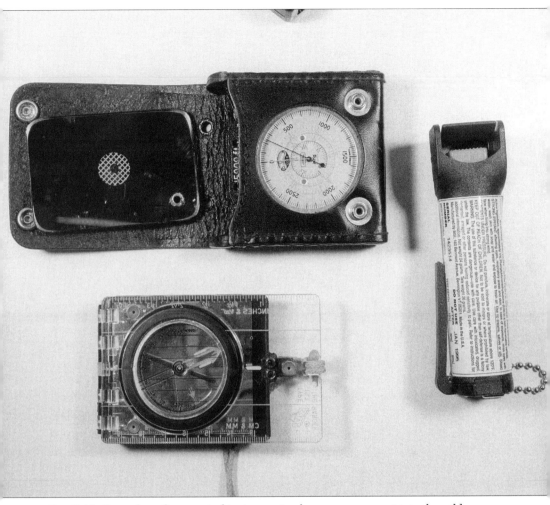

FIG. 9-18: Carry these four survival instruments when you go way out into the wilds on a trail ride. At the top, a Thommen altimeter. On the altimeter case lip, a separate precision solar signaling mirror, which can reach a plane high in the sky. Bottom center, a Silva compass for orienteering work. At right, a Mace/pepper spray to protect you against four- and two-footed animals.

Harold Gatty, *Finding Your Way on Land or Sea,* 272 pages. This book is subtitled "Reading Nature's Maps." Teaches you to use Mother Nature herself to find your way, without the use of maps or compass. Stephen Greene Press, Brattleboro, VT.

W. S. Kals, *Land Navigation,* 230 pages. This is the Sierra Club's guide to the map and compass. Also covers use of the altimeter as an aid to finding your way on the land. Sierra Club Books, San Francisco, CA.

These books are available from sporting goods outfitters.

12. Mace/pepper combination spray (Fig. 9-18) for obnoxious wild animals and humans.

13. One or two water bottles and bottle cages to hold them.

14. An extra-large water container (Fig. 9-19). If your bike does not have water bottle cages you'll need them. If the frame has no brazed-on fittings for water bottle cages install at least one clamp-on bottle cage. Two bottles and cages are advisable for long trips.

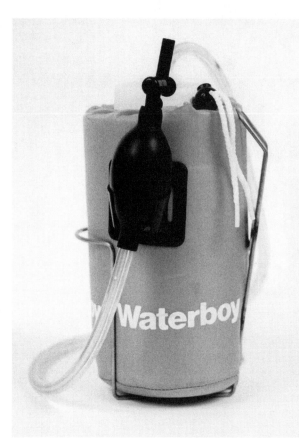

FIG. 9-19: You need water and lots of it when riding on a hot day. This oversize liquid container comes with its own frame-mountable carrier, an insulated wrap, and a pump so you can reach down for a drink.

15. Tire chains, if your route may take you over ice- or snow-laden roads or trails. You will have traction on the rear wheel and steering control on the front wheel. Your bike shop should have them or be able to order them for you. Practice installing them.

16. Small radio (Fig. 9-20) so you can pick up weather reports and news. I like the Grundig Yacht Boy 205 model because it is a bit bigger than wallet size, yet has an excellent tuner and nine shortwave channels

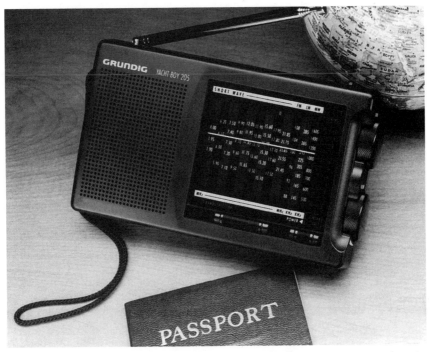

FIG. 9-20: This great little radio, which comes in a sturdy carrying case, is about as big as two (God forbid) packs of cigarettes. It has 9 shortwave channels and one channel each for AM, FM, and longwave. *Courtesy Grundig.*

plus FM, longwave, and AM, so you can use this little gem of a radio throughout the world. It has an earphone outlet and telescopic antenna, and comes in a sturdy leatherette pouch. It weighs only 16 ounces with its two AA batteries, costs only $79.95 (suggested retail) and is available through electronic and radio outlets. Call 1-800-872-2228 for more information and technical support (if you want the Radio Moscow frequency, for example).

Camping Equipment

Here is one place where economy does not pay. Cheap tents can leak and cheap sleeping bags are uncomfortable and may not be warm enough on a chilly evening, especially at high altitudes. Look for a tent made of breathable fabric, such as GoreTex, and one with handy pockets inside for storing small stuff such as personal gear, flashlight, and a book. The tent should be quickly erectable, and sturdy when up, which may not be true of cheap tents. Here is the camping gear I have used on long, overnight trips, where I stayed mostly at campgrounds.

1. Tent for two. The extra space is handy even if you travel alone. On a cross-country bike camping trip you'll see as many makes, sizes, and designs of tents as there are cyclists to tote them. Good tents have common characteristics, which you should look for in the one you select. First, any cyclist's tent should have a small vestibule, so you can store panniers and other gear *outside* the tent living area but protected from the elements and light-fingered thieves. The tent should be made of fabric that breathes. I once had a tent that didn't breathe. Moisture from our bodies and breath would collect on the cold inner surfaces of this tent at night. By morning a slap on the tent sides would send drops of moisture down on us. We usually rinsed the inside of this tent in a bucket to wash out this moisture. The one time we didn't, and packed it away wet from body moisture because we were in a hurry to get started, the tent became unusable the next night. What happened was that the moisture went sour, and it smelled as though 10 people had spent the entire night barfing on its walls. We took the tent to a launderette and machine-washed it. No use. That odor was now a part of the tent. We wound up throwing this tent away and buying one that breathed, just so we could get a night's sleep. So get a tent made of a breathable fabric, such as GoreTex. Moss Starlet tent (Fig. 9-21) is a good example of the kind of tent I am describing. This tent weighs six pounds (but that's only three pounds apiece for two people), has a floor

FIG. 9-21: This Moss Starlet tent sleeps two comfortably and has a rain cover, inside nets to stow personal stuff, and a covered lobby (not shown) that keeps panniers and other gear out of the weather.

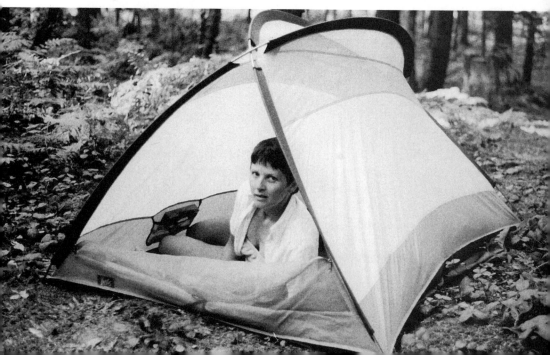

area of 29 sq.ft., and with the vestibule (not shown in Fig. 9-21) has a total of 37.5 sq.ft. This tent and its rods fit into a tote sack you can carry on the back of your bike. It also comes with a rain cover and has a double-thick floor that comes up to six inches on the inside of the tent. In a hard rain you'll appreciate this floor, because it will keep water out. (Which reminds me to urge you *not* to dig a trench around your tent to funnel away rainwater. Camp authorities take a very dim view of this practice and usually forbid it, and it does not help the local ecology.) Without the rain cover, the top of the Moss tent is open to the night sky, which can be pretty romantic while avoiding the crowded feeling of a small tent. Available from your sporting goods store or contact Moss Tents, P.O. Box 577, Camden, ME 04843, phone 1-800-859-5322.

2. Sleeping bag(s). Down-filled sleeping bags are lighter than synthetic-filled bags at the same temperature rating, will compress and take up less space in a smaller tote bag. But if a down bag gets wet, it clings to you so sleeping is impossible, takes forever to dry, and is soggy and heavy. Man-made insulating fibers are quicker to dry, in my opinion, and you can even get some sleep in a wet one once your body warms the bag. You can buy "mummy" bags, which configure to a point at the toes. I find this design constrictive, especially when I turn over at night. For comfort I prefer the rectangular sleeping bag, such as the Therm-A-Rest bag in Fig. 9-22. If you have a friend along, this bag can be truly

FIG. 9-22: If you travel alone, this rectangular Therm-A-Rest sleeping bag will keep you warm down to 20 degrees, and with its self-inflatable mattress under it, comfortable on uneven soil. The bag is shown with an optional insert for sleeping two, a good idea that saves having to carry two sleeping bags if you travel with a friend. *Courtesy Cascade Designs, Inc.*

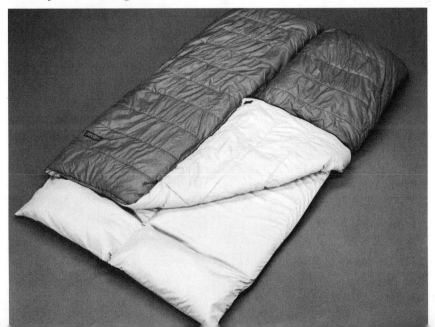

friendly, because it is expandable to sleep two. Use it with a self-inflating mattress that weighs but 10 ounces. For more info or a nearby dealer call Therm-A-Rest at 1-800-531-9531. In the summer at moderate altitude, say a maximum of 3,000 feet, a sleeping bag rated for 20 to 40 degrees Fahrenheit should keep you warm at night, especially if you are in a tent. Please see Table 11-5 for more information about the relationship between thermometer temperature and the wind-chill factor. A sleeping bag rated at 20 degrees Fahrenheit, for example, may when outdoors, in the wind be exposed to a temperature of minus 10 degrees, so select the sleeping bag that will protect you at the lowest temperature you can expect. That's a decision only you can make because only you know where you camp. If in doubt, check with the local U.S. weather people for the temperature and wind speeds where you will camp.

3. Small cookstove. I like the MSR dual fuel stove (Fig. 9-23) because it burns white gas or kerosene. I use white gas because it leaves less carbon residue inside the stove, so the stove requires cleaning less often. This stove will burn on the high setting for about 2 hours or on the simmer setting for 12 hours and uses about 20 ounces of fuel to do so. So on a trip away from a fuel source, expect 20 ounces of fuel to last about

FIG. 9-23: This MSR stove burns white gas and kerosene.

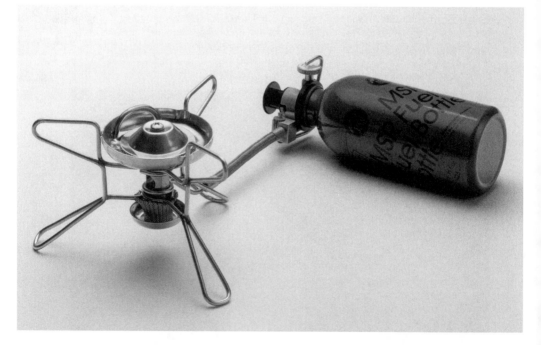

a week for one person. But be on the safe side and carry 40 ounces, 20 in the fuel tank, another 20 in a separate fuel can. You can buy compact propane stoves, which are easier to use because they don't need priming and fire up to full blast at the touch of a match flame (carry waterproof matches or ordinary matches in a waterproof container for any stove). The Coleman Peak 1 stove uses a 16.4-ounce disposable propane cylinder that provides 2.75 hours burning time on high, 5.5 hours on low. But you will need to tote empty tanks back for disposal. No big deal, but you should know about it.

4. Dual fuel lantern. You can get by without it, but a small camp lantern such as Coleman's dual fuel model (Fig. 9-24) brings cheer to the camp

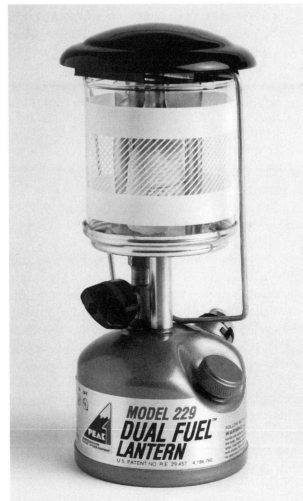

FIG. 9-24: For cheery nights at the campsite this Coleman dual fuel lantern uses the same fuels as the stove in FIG. 9-23.

on dark nights. Don't use it inside the tent, though. Use the same fuel for this lantern as for the stove in Fig. 9-23, but remember burn time is 3.5 hours on high and the lantern uses 8 ounces of fuel in that time.

5. Cooking utensils. Coleman makes a set of nesting stainless-steel pans and a double-walled coffeecup that fits compactly into your panniers.
6. Maintenance kit for your stove.
7. Extra fuel bottle (can fit in a bottle cage).
8. One or two tubes of fire ribbon for starting campfires (so you don't have to carry old newspapers).
9. Sunshower kit. Not every campground will have shower facilities. This kit holds 2.5 gallons of water. You hang it in direct sunlight and in three hours you'll have enough hot water for two short showers.

This seems like a lot of equipment. But each item is small and light. Even with your personal effects, tent, sleeping bag, and a foam plastic ground cloth to go under the sleeping bag, you will still probably keep your total load under 30 pounds. If there are two of you sharing a tent, that reduces your load to one tent, and undoubtedly you will only carry one cook stove and one each of any other items that obviously serve you both. Two can travel a lot lighter than one.

BICYCLE CLOTHING

I am indebted to clothing expert Carol deChelle-Mosteller for providing the following data on clothing, about which I admit ignorance, as I am barely able to sew a button on my shirt. Carol says:

Let's begin with an explanation of clothing (activewear) design. Some cycling activewear on the market today seems to fit the body so closely that it appears to leave just enough room for the bones, muscles, and skin. This skin-tight fit is aerodynamic; garments cling so closely that they add very little wind resistance. Garments are light because fabrics are lightweight (it's not much fun to carry around excess baggage on a bike). Some fabrics are stretchy; they move as the body moves. Better cycling fabrics breathe, in other words, they allow cooling air to flow over the body (breathing equals ventilation). Conversely, in this ventilating process, fabric should allow perspiration to be wicked away either to outer layers of clothing or to the outside air. ("Wicking" means moisture absorption by capillary attraction.) Some types of activewear offer protection for the skin and insulation for the body, with minimal bulk and weight. In other words, cycling activewear is streamlined, utilitarian, and comfortable.

Streamlined utility and comfort are basic to the design of cycling jerseys and shorts (in later paragraphs other specific types of clothing, such as mountain biking and women's clothing, will be discussed). There are variations on a few common themes of design detail for both jerseys and shorts. So, get out just a few sewing terms you might remember from basic survival home economics in high school and let's begin.

Basic Jersey Pattern Design

Usually the jersey front and back panels and the sleeves are designed in one of two ways. One jersey pattern is constructed simply by sewing a single-unit front piece to a single-unit back piece at side and shoulder seams. The second jersey combination is narrowly cut front and back panels and four contoured side panels (two under each arm). As a result there are more seams. Whenever side panels appear in nonactivewear, it means that portion of a garment will allow more flexibility of movement while it more accurately fits proportion and shape. Therefore, in theory, a jersey with side panels should have a more defined fit and allow for unhampered movement. However, the designers of both types of jersey patterns are working with stretchable fabric, which would automatically allow for close fit and body flexion. Choice of side panel detail depends on individual taste or body shape and size.

The sleeve design detail also has two basic pattern options. One option is the set-in (cap) sleeve, which, according to advertising, has been cut to allow for the forward body and arm position of the biker. A set-in sleeve is cut in one flat piece, stitched together at the underarm seam, and the resulting sleeve is sewn into the armhole opening of the jersey. The second sleeve pattern option is cut so that it begins at the neck edge and extends over the shoulder to the midbicep or wrist in one continuous piece. When the sleeve sections are sewn to the front and back of the jersey, the seams lie diagonally from neck side-front to underarm (a raglan sleeve). The raglan sleeve is used most often in jackets. Both types of sleeve, if cut properly, should prevent pulling and binding across the upper back and arms.

Other design details of cycling jerseys are somewhat standard. One standard detail is the added length in the back panel (sometimes called a tail), which is designed to cover the waist-to-hip area. When the body is bent forward, this is an area where gaping easily occurs in an ordinary shirt and shorts combination. At times, the tail or the entire hem is elasticized as added insurance against shirt sneak-up or to prevent flapping in the breeze. Another standard feature of jerseys is a two- or three-section pocket across the lower back. This sectioned pocket is handy for storing things you might need while riding, such as quick snacks and maps or directions. A final standard feature is a stand-up and close-fitting collar with a front zipper that extends into the body of the jersey (some collars taper down to the zipper). Snug fit should prevent wind resistance that other types of collar might cause by catching or flapping in the wind. The zipper is designed to be opened with one hand for ventilation. A casual or an off-road cyclist might choose to wear a cotton or cotton/polyester blend T-shirt with a crew neck. A crew neck lies flat against the neck. One drawback to a crew neck is that it does not protect the neck from chill on cool days. A more detailed description of fabric types, characteristics, and value to cyclists will follow in later paragraphs.

Shorts Design

As jerseys have optional design details, so do cycling shorts. There are two basic shorts designs, which can have various modifications or additions. Shorts are designed to stretch and move with the rider in any riding position without bunching up or binding in the crotch or at the waist. The first type of shorts design is the skin-fitted nylon/spandex model. These shorts are sewn together in a series of panels, which may vary from four panels in one pair of shorts to eight in another pair. Without going into detail, it can probably be assumed that quality of the contoured fit and the amount of mobility the shorts allow is in direct proportion to the number and cut of panels in the shorts. The legs of the shorts are also cut to about midthigh to prevent the inner thigh from brushing constantly against the bike saddle. In time, brushing can cause irritation and chafing of the inner thigh. Grippers have been added to the inside of leg hems of some shorts to prevent any fabric creep while riding. Shorts have an inner back pocket tucked inside a high-rise back waist that protects the lower back. They also have a lower-cut front waist to minimize bunching when the biker leans forward. For additional adjustments at the waist, some shorts have drawstrings inside the waistband.

Another type of shorts design is for casual riders, for riders who are figure-conscious, or for off-road cyclists. These shorts are usually made with a fabric that has a tougher, more resilient (yet soft to the touch) finish. Because of the combination of fibers in the fabric, some of these shorts do have limited stretch. These shorts are generally cut in panels but the cut is fuller, the shorts roomier. The legs also appear to be shorter than the nylon/spandex shorts, and some have a V-slit in the lower side-leg for added ease. Some also have elastic or a drawstring in the waistband.

Crotch Liners

Finally, one of the most important parts of any pair of cycling shorts, as far as comfort and anatomical protection are concerned, is the crotch liner.

Most liners look like a pliable eggshell that has been flattened and has had a broad V inserted at the narrow end. This is called a Y-cut liner. The flattened shape protects the crotch and sit-bone area. The pubis is protected by the V-insert, which cups up and over the nose of the saddle. In some liners, seams are required for construction and could be a source of irritation if they are bulky or poorly placed. Cannondale Corporation (for one) now offers a molded one-piece Ultra-Suede chamois liner that has a second layer of fleece bonded to its underside to provide wicking action and extra cushion. The original and probably still most expensive liner is made of chamois, which is not as washable as the synthetic liners. It is claimed that chamois offers more resistance to saddle chafing. Most often, the chamois liner is one layer thick.

Usually, unlike chamois liners, the synthetic liners are constructed in layers. Each layer is a different type of fabric, and each fabric has a separate purpose. For example, the Descente liner has four layers: 1) the top layer (closest to the crotch) is a chamois mimic (sometimes called Ultra-Suede) to reduce the risk of chafing (it is quick drying and pliable); 2) a layer of fleece to aid in moisture absorption; 3) a layer of polyurethane padding to cushion the road bumps and to help prevent numbness; and, 4) a tricot layer, which, it is claimed, allows the liner to move with the body and not the outer fabric of the shorts, further reducing the chance of irritation. Another liner, which sounds unique, is the Spenco Biosoft gel. This liner is a sandwich of 1) Supersuede synthetic chamois; 2) terrycloth; 3) foam, gel; and 4) tricot. Spenco adds the gel, which, they claim, is "fluid like" and "cushions both vertical and lateral pressure" when the crotch, sit-bones, and muscles meet the saddle.

There certainly are differences in liners. For instance, compare those already mentioned to those used most often in the casual cycling shorts. These liners are generally made of a single layer of polyester fleece. Andiamo makes padded bike briefs that look like men's underwear shorts so you can use them under regular unpadded shorts for biking comfort. The five-layered padding is of polyester stretch fleece bonded to foam and nylon tricot sandwiched between two layers of Coolmax hydrophobic fibers, which speed evaporation.

Fabrics for Cycling Activewear

Construction detail for dynamic fit is only one of the necessities for cycling activewear. Quality fabric is also a necessity. Fabric is a film or sheeting, woven or knitted from fibers of various types, used to manufacture activewear. Activewear fabrics, at a basic level, should mimic our skin's excellent adaptive and protective qualities. For example, one of our skin's many functions is to moderate extremes of body temperature. When our normal core temperature is maintained we are able to perform at an optimal level of focus and energy. When we are active, we perspire, and perspiration gradually evaporates to cool our skin and body core. If perspiration did not evaporate, we'd have heavier bodies, which would slow us down. When our body is chilled our skin tightens and puckers up, which, along with surface hair and a subsurface layer of fat, provides insulation and prevents heat loss. Our skin serves as a protective shield for underlying muscle. It is also soft, lightweight, and flexible enough to allow muscles and bones to move freely. Finally, skin can be washed and dried without shrinking, and, when clean, does not retain odor.

Ideally, fabric should perform as well as or better than our own skin, especially while we are active. Many fiber and fabric manufacturers today are searching for ideal fabrics. It is exciting to read about research and high technology being used to develop efficient fabric for activewear. First of all, new synthetic fabrics are being designed to meet the distinct thermostatic needs (temperature maintenance) of individual athletes. Modern fabrics accomplish this by wicking perspiration from the skin. Excess moisture is held in a sort of suspension in or between fibers of the cloth until it exits through evaporation, which takes very little time. Rapid evaporation prevents saturation, and fabrics remain lightweight. Another advantage of some newer fabrics is toughness and durability. They provide excellent abrasion-resistant surfaces while maintaining good looks. Some fabrics resist or repel water and wind or insulate against cold. Most synthetics wash easily and dry rapidly, without shrinkage or fading. If washed properly, they are nonabrasive and supple, and retain their shape. Odor retention is not the problem it once was.

Some folks believe that synthetic fabrics are best. Others believe in or will use only natural fabrics such as cotton, silk, and wool. One reason for using only natural-fiber fabrics is that some people have allergies to synthetic fibers. In the following paragraphs, qualities of both natural and synthetic fabrics will be reviewed, some briefly. It will be easiest to describe fabrics (from here on referred to as fabric, although this could mean fiber, yarn, or fabric) according to the climatic conditions in which they could be used. *Note:* there are many trademark names for fibers or fabrics that appear to be similar in character and function. One reason for this is that a major design and engineering company (such as Dupont) might develop a new fiber or fabric. Activewear manufacturers, by adaptation or invention, may design a fabric with similar qualities to meet their own specifications and purposes. Therefore, there may be several names for fabrics with similar qualities. Trademark names for some similar fabrics are included in the following paragraphs, which should be helpful to you when you shop and read labels.

Lightweight Fibers/Fabrics: Moderate to Hot Weather

Fabric that is used to construct cycling activewear for moderate to hot weather should have the latest synthetic's advantageous qualities (listed earlier). Most of the fabrics mentioned in this category are used primarily for jerseys, shorts, and some jackets.

Natural fibers such as cotton and silk can be soft and smooth to the touch and give a relaxed, comfortable feeling when worn. Cotton does not require too stringent washing and drying procedures, although it takes longer to dry than synthetics. On the other hand, silk does need special handling when washed or dried. It can retain odor unless washed with gentle detergents made especially for silk and other fine washables. (Try REI's REFRESH.) Both cotton and silk are generally less fade-resistant than synthetic fabrics. Neither fabric has as much wicking capability as synthetics. When they become saturated with moisture fibers swell and block ventilation, creating a soggy jersey. On a day of cool breezes a soggy jersey next to your skin can be extremely chilling. Both fabrics might be used more effectively as a second layer over one of the wick-efficient synthetics.

Synthetics

Of the synthetics specifically targeted for activewear, nylon, polyester, and acrylic are primary. All three are tough and resilient and can be dyed in vivid, fade-resistant colors. You will find these fibers blended, layered, sandwiched around insulating fibers or fabric, laminated to membranes, or coated with film or finish. Sunlight can weaken these fibers. Black absorbs more rays than light colors do, so black or dark garments will not wear as long.

Among the synthetics (knit rather than woven fabric) are Dupont's 100 percent Coolmax, Milliken Mills's WickTec, Descente's X-Bio (a dual-layered fabric of cotton and polyester), Toray's Fieldsensor, and Asahi's Sofilia Sport. Dupont claims to have achieved an ultrafine, soft, light fiber with dynamic wicking and insulating characteristics in its newest development, Microfine (fabric by Milliken Mills). These synthetics and others like them are used in jerseys, tanks, bras, and mesh liners and inserts.

In a class by itself is spandex. Spandex is an elastic fiber. When it is knitted together with other fibers, the result is a stretchy fabric. Activewear made from this fabric will fit closely but not tightly because it adapts to your shape and movement. Body oils and tanning oils and lotions, as well as perspiration, can discolor or yellow spandex. Common trademarks are Dupont's Lycra, BASF's Vivana and Zefsport, and Hoechst-Celanese Corporation's ESP. Spandex/nylon fabrics are used in skin-fitted cycling shorts, bib-shorts, tights, full-body tights, portions of gloves, and T-back tops and bras. Spandura is a heavier, more abrasion-resistant type of spandex that may be used in the side panels of off-road shorts.

Finally, a group of fabrics that are woven (some with a textured finish) rather than knit, are more abrasion- and snag-resistant (tough-wearing), and have a light cottony feel are Dupont's Supplex, ICI Fiber's Tactel, and Allied Signal's Trek. When Dupont's Cordura is added to the fiber mix the resulting fabric is extra-rugged. These fabrics are used most often for casual and off-road shorts and various styles of jackets.

Wind and Rain Gear: Jackets, Ponchos, Tights

Wind and rain gear sold for cycling is either "resistant" or "repellent." To date there is no fabric that is absolutely wind- or waterproof. The term "resistant" means that the garment will shed rain or wind for a short time and then penetration will occur and you'll get wet. The term "repellent" means that the garment is the closest to waterproof that you will be able to purchase (fabric stays dry the longest). Buy only garments with labels that state that they have sealed seams or prepare to seal them yourself with seam sealer. If seams are not sealed, they will leak.

In order to make a garment resistant or repellent manufacturers use finishes or coatings (Burlington's Ultrex, Dupont's Zepel), membranes (MicroPore's Microtex, Akzo's Sympatex), or fabrics specifically woven for this purpose (Allied Signal's Dryline, Toray's Entrant, W. L. Gore's Gore-Tex, Helly-Tech's Tactel). Note: Gore-Tex is a well-known example of a microporous fabric. Its pores are minute and wind and rain cannot pass through although perspiration vapor, from inside, can. Not all of the processes mentioned above allow garments to breathe.

Venting systems are added to some jackets. Mesh fabric, zippers, and strategically placed openings are common to these systems. A mesh insert is sewn across the upper back and shoulders (the yoke). It is covered by a second separate piece of fabric (generally the same fabric that has been used in other parts of the jacket). Vapor dissipates through large holes in the mesh. The outer fabric resists/repels the wind or rain. Vents, with or without mesh, may be part of underarm seams. Sometimes underarm seams are zippered to form vents. You can control the amount of venting by zipping or unzipping the vents and jacket front.

Ponchos are a one-piece rain covering. Make sure yours has elastic thumb loops to prevent fly-up. It should have a contoured hood large enough to fit over a helmet. The hood should have a drawstring or adjustable closure to ensure a close fit, otherwise it could block peripheral vision.

Looser-fit nylon shell pants and cycling tights are also part of the wind/rain gear scene. If you choose the nylon shell variety make sure that the knee area has stretch or pleated panels for flexion. Another must for these pants is an adjustable ankle band, ankle strap, or clamp. These keep the pants leg out of the chainwheel. Side zippers make it easier to get pants on and off. Cycling tights are made of stretch fabric. The nylon/spandex tight is not necessarily rain functional. However, there are some with top-leg panels of wind/rain-resistant or fleece-bonded insulating fabrics. What you wear under any wind/rain gear would depend on weather conditions at the time of your ride.

Boots, also known as booties, to pull on over cycling shoes (in rainy or cold conditions) are available. They either pull on or have zippered backs. Neoprene, a molded (yet stretchy) material that can be sandwiched between layers of nylon, is used as insulating material in boots. It is durable, blocks wind, and (when wet) maintains body warmth. Neoprene is also used in headbands and facemasks.

Weightier Fabrics: Cool to Frigid Weather

If you cycle in cold weather or in areas where temperatures can fluctuate drastically or suddenly, it is wise to be familiar with causes, effects, and preventions of hypothermia.

It is important to wear a hat because a great amount of heat is lost from a bare head. Layering is still the best defense against variable or cold weather. Wearing clothing in layers makes it possible for you to adjust, not only to weather, but to your body's heat and perspiration output. Gloves that are flexible, thin, wind/rain resistant, and warm are a must. Finally, a wind/rain shell is the icing on the cake. This lightweight covering takes the brunt of wind, rain, or snow. It can increase the effective warmth of a wool shirt or sweater or polar fleece jacket without adding much weight.

Following is one system for layering garments. Choose at least three layers and adjust them depending on your body's requirements and the harshness of the climate. The layer closest to the body should be long underwear. Follow this layer with appropriate activewear. A final layer is some form of outerwear, which might incorporate batting as an insulator. An active outdoor person should, in each layer, choose the fabric and garment that gives the most warmth for weight, as well as maximum flexibility and comfort.

Underwear Layer

To be most effective underwear should fit snugly. Silk underwear works only if you perspire lightly. Washable lightweight wool or wool blends are effective if you are not allergic. Even when wet, wool can keep the body warm and dry in wind and rain. (SuperWash wool is Australian merino wool, which is soft, nonabrasive, durable, and washable.) Polypropylene is a synthetic with excellent wicking action. It insulates against wind. It stays warm when wet although it does not stay wet long. Follow washing instructions carefully (REI's REFRESH). Machine drying can cause the fabric to feel abrasive. New technology has eliminated the odd odor previously associated with this fiber. Dupont claims its Thermax (hollow-core fiber) fabric meets and exceeds all of polypropylene's characteristics. Other items that fit in this underwear category and also available in the same fabrics are socks, knit hats, earbands, glove liners, and helmet liners.

Activewear Layer

This group includes all the styles of activewear described earlier. However, jerseys have long sleeves and higher collars and are made from fabrics that insulate, such as Superwash Wool, Dupont's Thermax, W. L. Gore's Thermodry, and Allied Signal's Hydrofil. (Activewear available: Performance's Apex and Terminator winter jerseys.) Winter tights are also available in the above fabrics. Another option is leg and arm warmers, tubular casings that slide over the arm and legs. (Baleno offers both spandex/nylon and fleece in single- or double-knee styles. ShaverSport also has leg and arm warmers.) A fabric used for jerseys that has not been mentioned is synthetic fleece (pile). Synthetic fleece is lightweight and soft. It comes in varying thicknesses known as weights. It resists water and when water is absorbed, dries quickly. The warmth-to-weight ratio is excellent. Some stretch and resist pilling. Neck warmers, earbands, vests, jackets, and jacket liners are also made of pile or fleece. (Names to look for are Dupont's Polarlite and Polartek, Maiden Mills's Polarite and Polarplus.)

Insulating Layer

Synthetic insulation, in the form of batting, is lofty (thick in appearance but lightweight). It is constructed to trap body heat and to prevent its rapid dissipation to colder air. Trapped warm air maintains warmth. Batting is designed to imitate goose down, which (when dry and of good quality) is the best insulator for its weight. Synthetics, however, absorb less water and retain much of their warming capability even when wet. Jackets, parkas, and insulated pants are among the activewear items in this group, as well as other smaller but equally important items, such as balaclavas, gloves, insoles (3M's Thinsulate) for shoes, earbands, and ear coverings that slip onto helmet chin straps. Insulation material represented in this group is also used in sleeping bags. (Trade names: Wiggy's Lamilite, Dupont's Holofil II, Moonstone Mountaineering's Moonlite, Hoechst-Celanese's Novaloft, 3M's Thinsulate.)

Off-Road Wear

For cyclists who use their all-terrain bikes on roads or city paths, the activewear already described is recommended. The activewear needs of an off-road cyclist are somewhat different. The off-roader sits in a more upright position on the bike and terrain is varied and, at times, much more difficult. An upright position places less stress on the back and sleeves of a jersey. On hot days or dry trails, underarm mesh inserts provide rapid evaporation and cooling. Rough terrain calls for tough padded or reinforced shorts or tights. If shorts are worn, thick wool knee socks or neoprene guards protect vulnerable shins and kneepads cover knees. Socks (for any type of cycling) should be chosen carefully. Look for flat toe seams, extra cushioning on top for protection on the upstroke, dual layers that have been designed to protect against friction (which can cause blisters), and added padding for heels. Long-sleeved shirts help protect arms from abrasive foliage. Stretchy shorts or tights are necessary for the muscular expansions and contractions and twisting and turning movements required to climb hills and to maneuver on tricky terrain. Sorry, jeans are too confining— you'll exert more energy and wear out sooner because you are working against stiff fabric.

Excellent lines of clothing for bicycling in all sorts of weather, cold, wet, dry, or hot, are made by Pearl Izumi, Inmotion, Andiamo, Jogalite and WRS SportsMed, Descente, and Jackson & Gibbens. Burley makes fine rain gear.

WRS makes a back support for lower-back problems (Fig. 9-25) and a patellar support for knees (Fig. 9-26). Here's where to find a dealer near you for these fine products:

Pearl Izumi: 2300 Central Ave., Suite G, Boulder, CO 80301, phone 1-303-938-1700, FAX 1-303-938-8181.

Inmotion: 6407 Cecilia Circle, Minneapolis, MN 55439, phone 1-612-829-0144, FAX 1-612-829-7085.

WRS: P.O. Box 21207, Waco, TX 76702-1207, phone 1-800-299-3366, extension 292, FAX 1-817-751-0221.

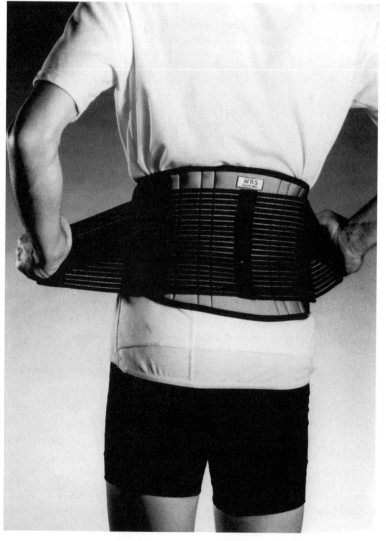

FIG. 9-25: Cycle in comfort even with minor backache with this WRS back support.

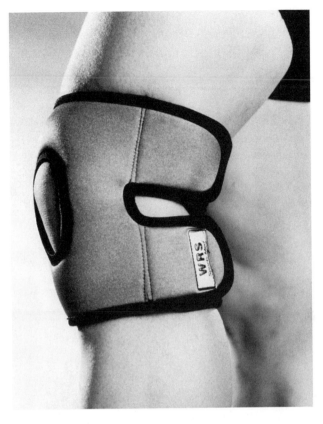

FIG. 9-26: Knee pain from an inflamed patella or strained ligament can be helped with this knee support from WRS

Descente America, Inc.: 109 Inverness Drive East, Englewood, CO 80112, phone 1-800-999-0475, FAX 1-303-790-2149.

Jogalite: Silver Lake, NH 03845, phone 1-800-258-8974, FAX 1-603-367-8098 (also makes reflective vests, great bike lights, bike horn, chemical and electronic animal repellents).

Andiamo: P.O. Box 1657, Sun Valley, ID 83353, phone 1-208-726-1385.

Burley Design Cooperative: 4080 Stewart Rd, Eugene, OR 97402, phone 1-503-687-1644, FAX 1-503-687-0436 (also makes bicycle trailers and tandem bicycles).

Jackson & Gibbens: 70 E. 39th Ave., Eugene, OR 97405, phone 1-800-452-3938, FAX 1-503-345-2459.

Gloves for Off-Road

Gloves for any type of cycling need to pad palms against road and trail shock, have finger openings that fit snugly without binding, and have no bulky seams in the palm. If your ride could be a chilly one, you will need gloves with some sort of insulation, such as wool or synthetic dot-gloves (dot-gloves have little gripper dots on the palm and fingers), glove liners, or Thinsulate lining. In addition to the above characteristics, off-road gloves need to have longer finger lengths for added protection against scrapes, an effective gripping system for control on rough trails, and fabric that provides excellent ventilation. Two examples of available gloves are WRS UltraSoft gel gloves (Fig. 9-27) and the excellent gloves made by Kinco (Fig. 9-28). Reach Kinco at 927 SE Marion, Portland, OR 97202, phone 1-800-547-8410. If you have carpal tunnel syndrome, characterized by pain in the palm of your hands, use the special gloves shown in Fig. 9-29, designed by neurologist A. Robert Spitzer, M.D., of Detroit and made by Saranac. Contact Dr. Spitzer at 3535 W. Thirteen Mile Road, Suite 305, Royal Oak, MI 48073, phone 1-313-551-0615.

FIG. 9-27: Padded bike gloves from WRS (shown over a gel-filled saddle cover) help cut pressure on the palm of your hands.

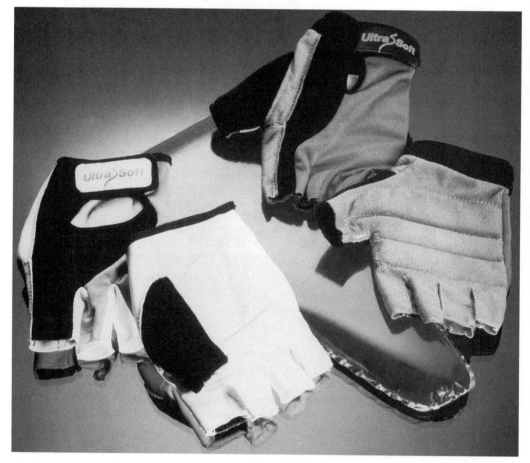

Fig. 9-28: Another pair of well-made bike gloves, by Kinco, also adds comfort to cycling. And if you should fall, gloves can help prevent skin loss.

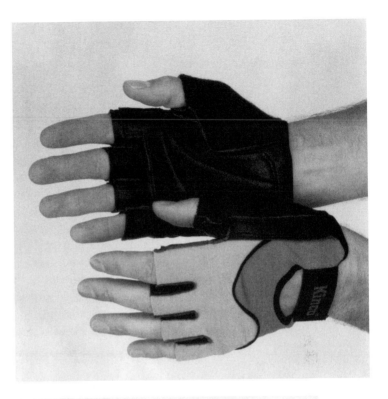

Fig. 9-29: If you have carpal tunnel syndrome, these gloves are designed to keep pressure off the carpal tunnel in the palm of the hand. Made by Saranac, designed by A. Robert Spitzer, M.D. The dotted white highlight line was made by your author and shows the area of pressure relief.

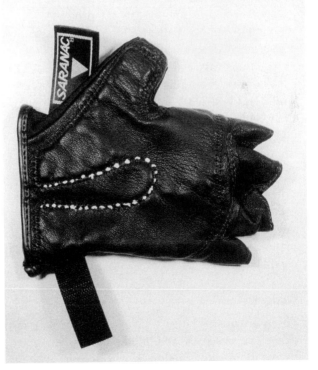

Women's Activewear

Until recently many manufacturers have used "unisex" sizing only. However, women do differ from men in their anatomical structure. Women have longer legs than torso, smaller and higher waists, larger hips, and wider pelvis. Therefore, some companies are now extending their lines to include activewear constructed and sized specifically for women. All of the aforementioned manufacturers now have women's lines. Along with better fit come new items of activewear that directly accommodate female anatomy. One item is T-back (or crop top) bras with or without mesh liners for added support. The T-back allows for support, as well as freedom from mid-shoulder straps, which can slip or bind when the body is in cycling position. It also affords the coolness of a swimsuit-style top (as long as you keep sunscreen applied). Another article designed with cooling quality in mind is the sleeveless tank top, which has the same construction as cycling jerseys with the exception of sleeves. Blackbottom offers a more feminine look in its jersey and culotte combo. Women's activewear lines should improve with age and ingenuity.

Designed for Safety

Safe riding any time of the day (and, if you must, evening) is absolutely necessary. Safety-conscious cyclists can promote safety in their activewear additions and choices. Reflector tape is a safety feature that can be added to activewear. Reflective leg or arm bands and vests can be worn over other garments. Cyclists can choose more visible colors, called "day-glo" or neon. Finally, Hind is offering reflective 3M Scotchlite (300 times brighter than white, visible at 2,000 feet) decorative panels on the side-thighs and rear of their Night-Blade shorts.

Shoes

In hot weather wear low-cut, well-ventilated shoes designed for off-road riding, such as Nike's (Fig. 9-30). These shoes have thick, sturdy soles that protect the tender underside of your feet from the pressure of pedaling on sawtooth-edged pedals. The shoes also have a grip pattern in case you have to put a foot out to stay upright, or walk your bike up a slippery trail. Wear good hiking shoes in colder weather and on rougher terrain.

Gadgets

There are many gadgets for cycling, such as suspenders, watches, cyclometers, seat pads, and helmet covers. Some items, such as sunglasses, have a more vital function. If you buy glasses especially designed for cy-

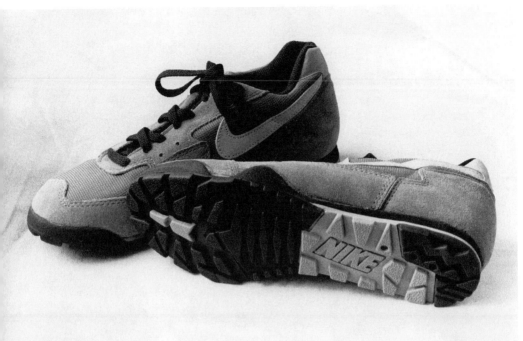

FIG. 9-30: Nike makes excellent shoes for bicycling both on- and off-road.

cling watch for scratch/shatter/fog resistance, good depth perception and upper and peripheral vision in the cycling position, UV ray blockers, and ventilation. Some glasses are designed to use interchangeable lenses for different light conditions. Others have elastic headbands or built-in sweatbands. Most specially designed sunglasses are expensive.

Conclusion

Sunglasses are not the only pricey items for cycling. To complete a functional activewear wardrobe requires some expense. At the least, be an informed buyer, shop, consider, and choose wisely (based on your own needs and pocketbook). You need to 1) talk to other cyclists, 2) read labels, 3) ask questions and continue to ask questions until you are satisfied or totally confused, 4) try on garments (bend, sit, and move in them), 5) check construction details (try zippers for ease of movement, see that layers of cloth are evenly sewn into seams, look for broken seam threads and even hems, stretch the stretchy garments, and listen for thread pops), and 6) think about the safety factors you need. In the end, check your pocketbook and then "pay your money and take your choice."

Bicycle Carriers

If you have a van or a pickup truck equipped with a Class 3 receiver, you can carry two, four, six, or seven bicycles on one of the hitches made by Spearing's Welding (Fig. 9-31). Reach Spearing at 776 Newton Way, Costa Mesa, CA 92627, phone 1-800-554-9956, FAX 1-714-645-0749.

Yakima makes excellent bike racks, sold through bike shops. One model is for the top of your car, another is for a pickup truck (Fig. 9-32). Yakima

FIG. 9-31: Carry up to seven bicycles on this Spearing carrier mounted on a van.

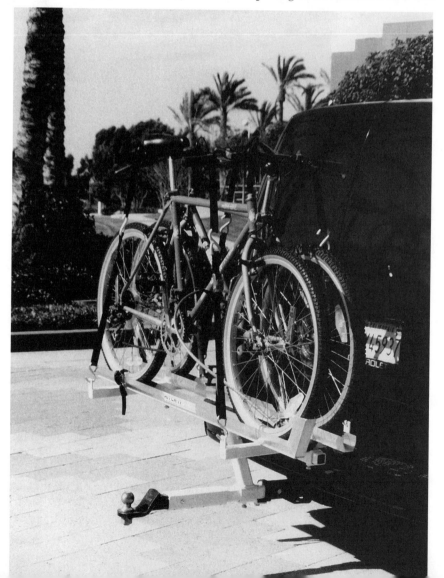

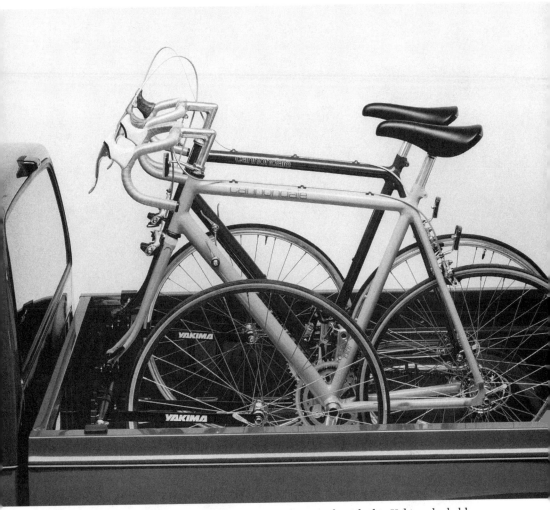

FIG. 9-32: Transport your bicycles in your pickup truck with this Yakima lockable carrier to keep them safely secured.

also makes a Load Alert that mounts on the roof of your car and that activates when you slow to parking speed, to remind you that you have a bike on top so you won't drive into the garage with it. I can testify that the crunch of a good bike being demolished is not the happiest sound I have ever heard.

I also like the bike racks made in Sweden by Thule (Fig. 9-33). For added security the fork can be locked in the carrier and the carrier to the roof of your car. Reach Thule at 42 Silvermine Rd, Seymour, CT 06483, phone 1-800-238-2388, FAX 1-203-888-4252.

If you don't want to lift your bike up onto the roof of your car, use a rear-

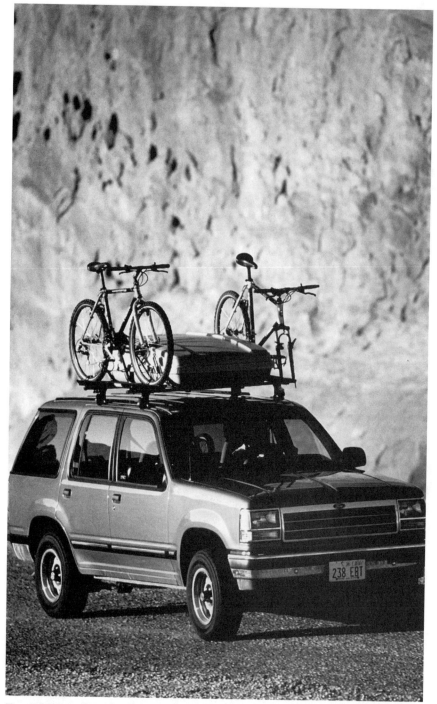

FIG. 9-33: A well-made rooftop bike carrier is this Thule model, which also locks the carrier to the car and the bike to the carrier.

bumper-mounted carrier. Fig. 9-34 shows an excellent carrier of this kind, by Rhode Gear, which holds up to three bikes, attaches in minutes to the bumper and rear trunk, and has restraints designed to hold the bicycle securely onto the padded arms of the carrier.

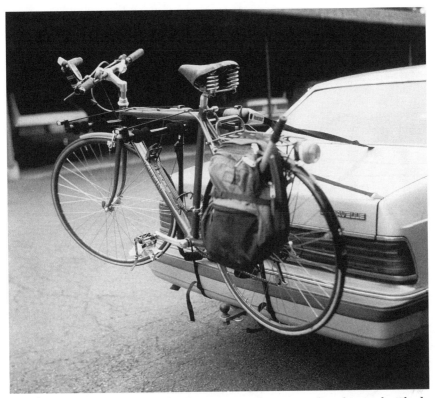

FIG. 9-34: Use a trunk- and rear-bumper-mounted carrier such as this one by Rhode Gear, which holds up to three bikes. This way you won't have to lift bikes up onto the roof of your car.

Ride Assist

A little battery-powered electric motor that weighs only 5.7 pounds (with battery and control circuitry) can help you make that really steep hill. According to the manufacturer, the motor is 0.2 horsepower yet can give you up to three hours intermittent or about 10 to 15 minutes of continuous full-power operation on one battery charge. The power boost is said to be equal to two other cyclists. I would have welcomed this little item on some of the 15 percent grades I hit in the Alps on my loaded bike. It can also help you keep up with stronger riders, ease muscle and heart strain, and keep pulse rates to a safer level on hills. Called the Hammer, the motor assist automatically disengages when the bike speed exceeds 12 miles per hour. Reach Chronos, the maker, at 11408 Sorrento Valley Road, Suite 04, San Diego, CA 92121, phone 1-800-364-8894 or 1-619-455-7345.

Speaking of ride assists, if you pedal in temperatures below 28 degrees Fahrenheit your feet are going to get cold, even to the point of pain. One solution is to use electrically heated shoe inserts (Fig. 9-35) from Chinook Medical Gear. The kit comes with rechargeable batteries and a battery charger. Reach Chinook at 1-800-766-1365.

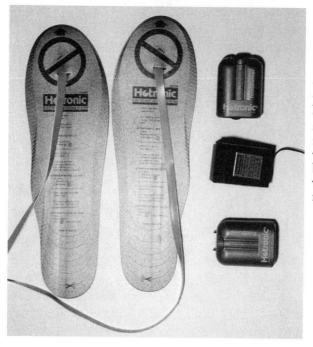

FIG. 9-35: Your feet are probably the most vulnerable part of your body. Use these electrically heated inserts when you commute to work in the winter. Recharge the batteries at work and when you get home, recharge them again.

Now that you are all equipped and know how to keep your bicycle in tiptop safe operation, let's go to bicycle commuting, touring, and camping in the next chapter.

CHAPTER TEN

RIDING YOUR BICYCLE TO WORK AND ON CROSS-COUNTRY TOURS

This chapter explores the benefits to you and to your employer of commuting between home and work on your bicycle. The chapter also gives you tips that make bicycle touring safer, less expensive, and more enjoyable in this country and abroad.

CYCLE COMMUTING

The Advantages of Commuting to Work

If your company does not yet have a policy of encouraging you to bicycle to work, I suggest you show this section of the book to management because it explains why bike commuting is cost effective for your employer.

No matter how you add it up, the payback from commuting 10 miles round-trip, five days a week, will pay for a good bike in a year through savings in fuel, in wear and tear on the car, or in not having to ride a bus or train to work. Your bike doesn't have to pass vehicle inspections (although this is not such a bad idea, given the awful condition of some bikes I've seen on the road) or suffer the slings and arrows of outrageous repair bills. Parking fees are nil, and you'll never have to circle endlessly around the block looking for a parking place. Best of all, you'll benefit in *at least eight* ways.

First, your transportation costs will be zero, or close to it. *Second,* you'll find yourself in radiantly good health after a few months of biking to work.

Third, because your energy level is heightened and can be sustained all day, you can be more effective on the job. You'll eliminate that "wiped-out" feeling that seems to creep up around three in the afternoon. *Fourth,* because your waistline will shrink, you can get back into your prebulge clothing or avoid the expense of new clothes to fit the larger (spell that "fatter") you. *Fifth,* if you want to move up the corporate ladder, take a look at the people on the rungs above you: Today's executives are a slimmer, healthier bunch than those of a generation ago. If you're fighting for promotion, a simple bicycle can be the leverage that can get you there in more ways than one! A *sixth* advantage of commuting on a bike is time. Studies have shown that while you can indeed drive a bit faster than you can bike to work, this time difference is misleading. You still have to get into your car, warm it up in the winter (assuming it starts and you don't have to wait for a jump start from a tow truck), and park the car in a garage. On a bike *you* provide the jump start, warming up as you exercise your body. In the winter you actually have to peel off layers of clothing as you ride, even when the temperature is in the twenties and overcoated, sedentary commuters are shivering while they wait for the bus or train. If you commute by public transportation, try going to work on your bike—you'll get there faster most of the time. I'm excluding New York suburbia here, unless you count the boroughs of Queens and Brooklyn as suburbia to those who live there and work in Manhattan. I am thinking of cities such as Philadelphia, Chicago, Boston, Seattle, and Denver. By the time you walk from the house to public transportation and walk to the office at the other end, you have lost out to the bike. That has been my own experience. I vividly remember the time I was in New York at a hotel in mid-Manhattan. I had to go to the New York Stock Exchange on business. As I contemplated the cab ride I thought, no, I'll ride my bike. Friends with me on the same business jaunt took a cab. I arrived first. I learned that the New York joke "Shall we walk or do we have time to take a cab?" is all too true.

I also found that I could plan my day's activity while biking to work, whereas if I took the train I tended to doze off or read the paper on the way.

A *seventh* benefit of getting from home to work on a bike is sustained energy and rejuvenation of the spirit. You'll find that even though you may feel tired at the end of the day, by the time you get back home you are invigorated, more alive, hungry for good food, and capable of a great love life. You'll have energy to spare for the kids, too. Since you'll be physically healthier, you'll be healthier emotionally as well. At least that's what I found for myself. I became more stress-resistant and got along much better on the job and in interpersonal relationships.

Which brings me to the *eighth* benefit. After you read Chapter 11, on bicycling and health, you can understand why your bike-conditioned body will need less attention from the medical profession. When I first started biking to work, my blood pressure was 130/70. That's pretty good, actually, within the norm for my age at that time. But within six months my blood pressure had dropped to 110/60, which is the norm for persons in their twenties, if they're healthy. Twenty years later my blood pressure is still the same, 110/60. The rare times I see a doctor, the nurse has to take my blood pressure twice, once on each arm, to make sure she has read her instrument correctly. I love it! The eighth benefit, then, is reduced illness as well as money and time saved in medical bills and visits to physicians. For example, I recently took a stress test at the hospital. This involves keeping upright while the attending physician gradually speeds up the treadmill as he monitors my pulse rate and blood pressure. At the highest speed I was a bit winded but not in distress. As the nurse peeled electrodes off my body the doctor, who was a bit overweight, asked what I did for exercise. His reaction to my reply was "I'm going to buy a bike."

Cycle Commuting Is Business Cost Effective!

Used to be that you stood out from the crowd as a kind of weirdo if you biked to work. Not anymore. Check your company to see if it offers incentives for you to bike to work. Many firms across the country are setting up bike parking areas and offering lockers and showers for bicycle-commuting employees. Industry is beginning to realize that two-wheel commuting is cost-effective enough to more than pay for the cost of shelter, secure bike parking, and the amenities I just mentioned.

An investment in these facilities pays high dividends in many ways. For example, healthier employees:

- *Are more productive.* It stands to reason that a wide-awake, healthy person can perform at maximum physical and mental efficiency longer than a couch potato.
- *Are at less risk for health problems,* so health insurance costs paid in full or in part by the company can be lower. Employees will be more alert and less accident-prone. Insurance costs can be lowered along with time lost to on-the-job injury. Absenteeism due to non-work-related illnesses, such as the common cold, will be reduced, as will the cost of floating fill-in workers to take the place of workers home ill.
- *Make for happier customers* because alert employees make fewer mistakes, so the quality of their output will be higher.

- *Eliminate the need for the expensive perks of corporate-sponsored health club memberships, along with the time wasted at them.* I note also that some companies, and municipalities, actually pay employees a percentage of the money saved by using their bike for short trips, instead of a company car. More efficient employees give greater return on fixed labor costs, more bang for the salary buck.

Now let's look again at how much you save by bike commuting, in terms of dollars and cents. First, a few assumptions, which you can change to suit your own circumstances:

- Work days per week, 5; work weeks per year, 48; work days per year, 5 × 48 = 240.
- Mileage, round trip, home to office: 20.
- Miles per year: 20 × 240 = 4,800.
- Miles per gallon, your car: 20.
- Auto fuel consumed per year: 4,800 ÷ 20 = 240 gallons.
- Cost of fuel for your car: $1.20 per gallon.
- Cost of fuel consumed per year: 240 × $1.20 = $288.
- Parking your car downtown: $5.
- Annual cost of parking: 240 × $5 = $1,200.
- Estimated annualized cost of car maintenance and insurance: per mile, $0.23; per year, $0.23 × 4,800 = $1,104 (not including interest on an auto loan, if a loan is outstanding).
- *Yearly total cost of commuting by car 20 miles round-trip: Auto fuel $288 + parking $1,200 + maintenance and insurance $1,104 = $2,592!* Or, if you use public transportation, and you pay $3 a day round trip, that's 240 days × $3 = $720 a year. Still worthwhile savings if you eliminate just public transportation by riding your bike to work! And that's not counting time lost stuck in traffic jams.
- Yearly cost of commuting 20 miles round-trip by road or mountain bicycle: one pair of high-quality tires with Kevlar-reinforced nylon casing, $70; one pair of latex tubes, $30; total, $100.

TABLE 10-1: ENERGY COMPARISONS*
(Calories per Mile)

BICYCLE	WALKING	RAIL	BUS	CAR, SINGLE PASSENGER
35	100	885	920	1,860

* President's Council on Physical Fitness and Sports, *Transportation Energy Data Book*, Oak Ridge National Laboratory, April 1987.

How to Make Bike Commuting Even More Practical

In Chapter 2 you learned about safe cycling on city streets. I would like to add one more observation. The first time you set out for work you may be terrified. Every car may seem to be aiming at you. But within a few days, as you become more confident of your biking reflexes and street sense, you'll get used to the city traffic around you. Believe me, you will get nerves of steel. So don't give up because the first few days are highly stressful. We all go through that. There are usually safe roads for biking downtown, either through parks, on off-road bike trails, or on safe streets. Scout various routes to work in your car first. Your local bicycle club or bicycle shop often has bicycle routes already mapped out. Some cities have full-time bicycle coordinators who can help you plan a safe route to work. The construction of freeways connecting suburbia to the high-density mess downtown is a boon to cyclists, because it takes the traffic off city streets. Just watch out for cabs and buses! In New York, avoid crosstown streets if possible. If there is no safe place to park your bicycle, try to get your company or the municipality to install a compact bike rack such as the one in Fig. 10-1. This rack holds 16 bikes, costs only $249, and is available from Bicycle Bay Parking Systems, P.O. Box 281084, Papillion, NE 68128, phone 1-800-253-2378, FAX 1-402-331-8259. It requires only 4.25 sq.ft. and comes assembled.

FIG. 10-1: This rack holds 16 bicycles, and requires only 4.25 sq.ft. to install.

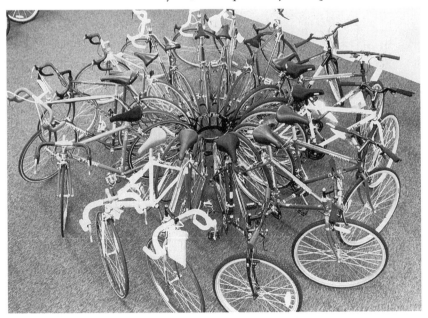

Here are a few tips on what to take along when you commute. First, you can use a garment pannier (Fig. 9-7) to carry fresh clothes to work.

You'll need a couple of spare tubes, because if you get a flat on the way to work, changing the tube is faster than finding the leak and patching it. Practice changing tubes until you can do it in minutes. Bring the tools to do it, along with a tire pump. Or use tubeless semipneumatic (solid) tires so you can't get a flat no matter what you ride over (see Chapter 7).

If you live where the weather is unpredictable, carry rain gear (see Chapter 9) designed for bicycling. I did say you can bike through snow. If you live in the "snow belt" the city usually has the streets plowed before you set off in the morning. I find snow amazingly stable. It's only when there's ice under the snow, or the snow has turned to slush, that the going gets treacherous enough that I can't bike to work. In any case, up to two inches of newly fallen snow should not keep you from riding to work.

I would not ride if the temperature falls much below 20 degrees Fahrenheit, unless you are in good shape. Three or four layers of clothes are advisable in cold weather, because you can peel off layers as you warm up. In cold weather, wear shoes a size larger so you can wear heavy wool socks. Or keep your old shoes and slip a neoprene bootie over them. The bootie is a wet- and cold-weather ankle-high shoe covering, available from your bike shop or from Spokes Wear, P.O. Box 71098, Seattle, WA. Spokes Wear also distributes an excellent wet/cold-weather glove of leather and neoprene. MSR (Mountain Safety Research) makes helmet liners with earmuffs for any helmet, called Helmuffs, that add warmth to your head and ears. Down-filled mittens keep fingers warmer than fingered gloves, but make braking more awkward. Try finger-type down-filled gloves first, along with a wool glove liner. If your fingers still get cold, graduate to the mittens, keeping the liner if necessary. You can order these gloves from the Performance Bicycle Shop catalog (see Bibliography).

If you plan to bike after dark, you *must* use a bright headlight and taillight. Some cities and states require bike lights. Please see Chapter 2 for more information on bike lights. If you ride a lot at night you might also consider a modern high-performance generator-powered bike light (Fig. 10-2). There's no battery to die and leave you without lights. For information on this light see your bike shop or contact International Bike Lights, 4403 N.W. Seneca Ct., P.O. Box 1133, Camas, WA, phone 1-206-601-0979, FAX 1-206-834-6902. You still need a rear light, preferably the blinking kind. I replaced the conventional bulb in my taillight with a quartz halogen bulb. These lights give you good visibility, and more important, tell motorists where and what you are. For chargeable bike light batteries keep a charger at home and one at work. You should get at least two hours out of each charge. Carry a couple of spare bulbs with you. Remember not to touch the

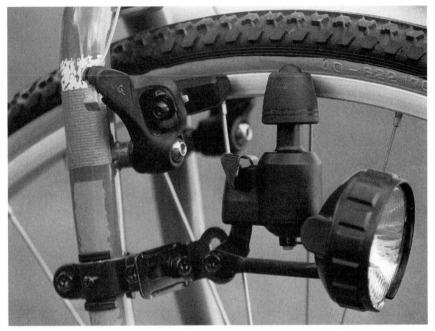

FIG. 10-2: For light without batteries try this generator-powered frame-mounted light.

bulb with your fingers when you replace it. There's something on human skin these bulbs don't like, and they don't last long if they are touched. You can use a rag to install one.

A Word About the Future

When you commute by bike to work you will be immune to rising gasoline prices and fuel shortages. Contacts in the petroleum, natural gas, and coal industries tell me that the world has about a 30-year supply of oil, a 150-year supply of natural gas, and a 250-year supply of coal, at the present rate of consumption of these fuels. This forecast is based on present technology of resource recovery and exploration and known reserves. Of course, when oil begins to be depleted, the other fuels, if converted to gasoline, will cost a bundle and will be depleted much faster. If you're 30 years old now, you are probably going to be glad that you will be a healthy 60-year-old with a good bicycle and bicycling skills, when we run out of nonrenewable liquid fossil fuel, and the cost of its replacement goes sky-high. I like the non-air-polluting aspects of electric vehicles, but I don't see their per-mile cost, at this writing, as less than that of conventional fuel-powered autos.

LONG-DISTANCE TOURING

When you travel through the countryside on a bike, you move at a leisurely pace. You're not stuck in a metal box with the windows shut, air-conditioning on, radio blaring, oblivious to the world around you. On a bike you're keenly aware of the surrounding countryside and the people who live there. The hum of the tires, the feel of fresh air in your face, the music of songbirds in your ears, the tingle of well-being as you pedal down the road—all are your reward for touring by bike rather than by car. You can savor the countryside as you would a fine wine—tastefully and with appreciation. Wave at people working in the fields or walking along the road, and they wave back. Stop when and where you will, break out a loaf of bread, some cheese, and a flask of wine and lunch by the side of the road. Cool your toes in a nearby brook, watch the sky and the endless variations of clouds passing by (and hope they don't portend rain).

Whether you make camp at night, or go deluxe and stay in a motel, it's your choice. Tour alone or with a friend, or take a packaged, planned bike trip with a larger group. There are advantages to each type of bike touring. Let's look at them now.

Going It Alone

When you tour alone, or with just one other person (Fig. 10-3), you are free to plan your own route and go where you wish. You can stop and stay for a day or a week in one campsite, make exploratory trips in different directions and return to the same camp each night. You go as fast or as slowly as you wish. Your schedule is your own.

There are days, and I speak from experience, when you have so much energy you burst out of your sleeping bag, zip open the tent, throw on some clothes, and after the morning necessary, can hardly wait to breakfast and get back on the road. Then there will be days when you just have no energy at all, when you want simply to roll over in the sack and only get up when the sun is blasting down on you. On those days it's fun just to laze around the campsite, read, check over your bike, wash clothes, walk around, and talk to other campers. Bike touring alone or with one other person lets you have complete flexibility.

On the negative side, biking alone can be lonely. If you travel with one friend, compatibility is essential. For instance, you should both be content with the speed you are making, the distance you cover, even the food you eat.

You have to carry everything if you're on your own. There's no sag wagon to carry tent, sleeping bags, cooking gear, and spare parts. You'll have to use

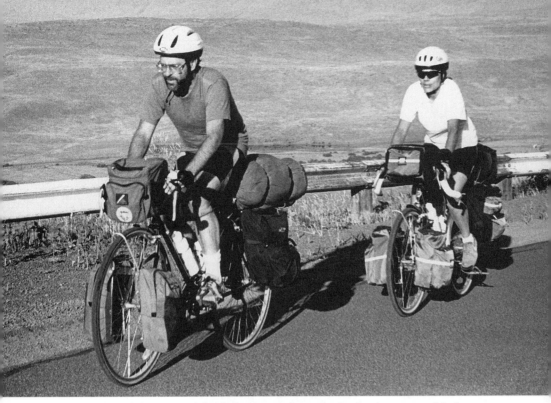

FIG. 10-3: On a bike tour with loaded panniers, keep the load as low as possible for stability and steering accuracy, as shown here. *Photo by Vera Jagendorf.*

carriers and panniers to carry everything on your bike (Fig. 10-3), which is, to me, a great way to travel. I like the idea of total self-sufficiency.

Packaged Tours

On a packaged tour, many details and chores are taken care of. You don't have to plan a route or be concerned about where you're going to sleep, or whether the campground will be full. Meals are planned and often cooked for you. You can bike empty (Figs. 10-4, 10-5, and 10-6), because most planned tours provide a sag wagon (Fig. 10-7) to carry your stuff. There is usually a skilled mechanic along.

On a packaged tour you can relax, forget about logistics, and concentrate on the pleasures around you, not the least of which are your fellow cyclists. At night, after a long day's ride, you will be surrounded by lots of people with whom to share adventures, conversation, and companionship (Fig. 10-8).

Of course it's more expensive to take a packaged bike tour than it is to go it alone. You pay for all the advantages. But if you want a highly sociable, hassle-free trip, then a packaged tour is the way to go.

See the list of packaged tour providers later in this chapter. Actually, there are so many of these providers that space forbids mentioning all of them.

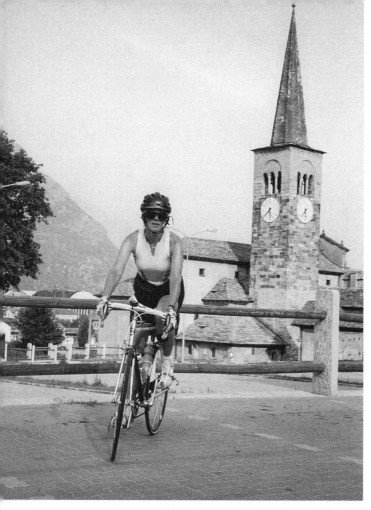

FIG. 10-4: One plus when on a guided, planned tour is the friendly people you share the ride with. *Courtesy Gerhard's Bicycle Odysseys.*

FIG. 10-5: A clearly enjoyable tour in France. *Courtesy Gerhard's Bicycle Odysseys.*

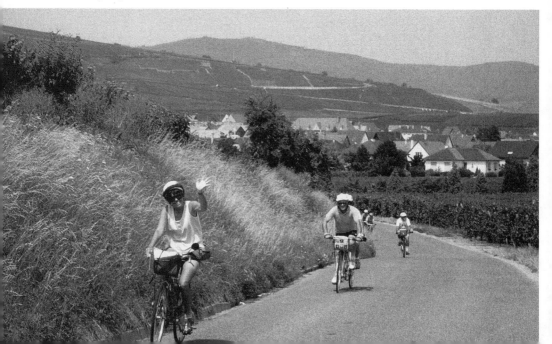

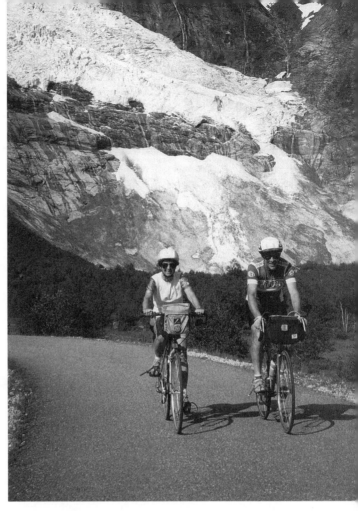

Fig. 10-6: On a tour in Austria, this couple can climb steep grades while their gear follows in a sag wagon. *Courtesy Gerhard's Bicycle Odysseys.*

Fig. 10-7: A sag wagon can carry an entire group's personal belongings, and the rider if he or she sags (hence the name "sag"). *Courtesy Paradise Pedalers.*

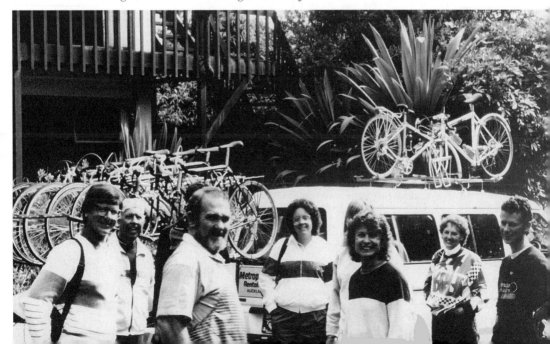

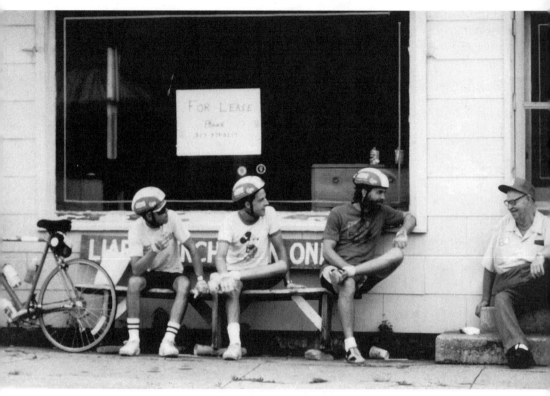

FIG. 10-8: Just sitting and chatting with a local on a ride break can be fun on a guided bike tour. *Courtesy Bob Firth and Tim Kneeland & Associates.*

Tours for specific regions, such as Vermont, California, and Oregon, for example, are run by local groups in these areas. Leaf through the advertising pages of bicycle magazines to find their names and those of providers of tour packages in these and other areas. New tour groups pop up almost daily, it seems, so any list I could provide would not be complete.

Campgrounds

Here are a few words of advice, hard-won by this writer, about campgrounds. First, try to get to one by 5:00 P.M. That gives you enough daylight hours to set up the tent, cook dinner, and relax over the campfire. Once we arrived at the campground well after dark, when the sky was moonless black. We set up the tent in the assigned site, we thought, but wondered why horses were whinnying outside the tent fly all night. Come dawn, we discovered our tent was pitched just outside the campground proper, in a private pasture devoted to horses, redolent with droppings.

Second, never take a "Sorry, all full" sign as applying to you. Many rangers, at least in state and county camps, are cyclists themselves, and they can always squeeze you in somewhere. Some campgrounds have "remote sites" you can bike right up to, far from car campers. County campgrounds quite often even have better facilities and are less crowded than state or national park campgrounds. Avoid private campgrounds like the plague. They are almost always overcrowded, jammed full of cars, trucks, campers, and six-wheeled Yuckabago monsters with all the comforts of "civilization" including bath, TV, furnace, and microwave. Select a campsite that's as far away from toilet and shower facilities as possible. The loudest, most obnoxious campers tend to cluster around the toilet shacks, as though deriving some comfort from the proximity of this most basic need. Besides, if you camp near these facilities, you'll hear running water, screen doors banging, and other noises all night long.

Food

You can of course buy a lot of excellent dried meals in camping goods stores. However, unless you're going off into wilderness where you can't shop for food, you won't need dried stuff on the road.

My advice is to check out the last town you come to before the camp of your choice, and shop there for dinner and breakfast foods. In some states, notably on both coasts, you can buy delicious fresh seafood: clams, crabs, oysters, bluefish, and lobsters in the East; salmon, shark steak, albacore, squid, and crabs in the West.

Bicycling Overseas

If you want to see the Orient, Tasmania, Tibet, Australia, or New Zealand, I recommend a package tour (see the list of tour providers later in this chapter). If you want to cycle in Europe, you have your choice of a package tour or planning one on your own. As I noted above, each approach has its advantages. Here are a few tips that can make your European trip more fun, if you are making your own arrangements.

Buy your bike in the United States. If you wait till you get to Europe to buy a bike, you're never going to have the time to debug it. Most new bikes need minor fine-tuning—such things as cable stretch and resultant brake and derailleur adjustment, for example. Minor, yes, but a major pain if neglected. If you buy your bike in this country (regardless of where it's made) from a good dealer, you can be assured the bike will have been thoroughly checked out. If you ride that bike for a few months, you will know it thoroughly and be aware of what it needs. Somewhere between Paris and Moscow is no place to discover that the bike is malfunctioning.

Predeclare anything and everything that's made outside the United States. If you don't, U.S. Customs may ask you to pay duty on these items, a cost that was included in your original purchase price. Then, on your return, just show that declaration to the customs agent and you're home free. To predeclare, take your foreign-made products, including serial numbers, to the U.S. Customs office at the airport, and with the customs agent, fill in the appropriate form. Make sure a Customs agent signs it. On the way back, flight attendants usually pass out Customs forms so you can list items you purchased abroad. List *everything* you bought and how much you paid for it. If you show this list to an agent, you'll get faster clearance through customs.

Check for any immunization shots you might need. See your travel agency, or a local branch of the U.S. Public Health Service. They're not necessary for most European countries, but if you're going to Africa, the Orient, or South America, you better check.

About your visa: If you're going to any of the Eastern bloc countries—or China—check your travel agent to make sure you have the proper visa, if one is needed.

About traveler's checks: For the best rate, compare traveler's-check cashing rates at your hotel with those at a local bank. Sometimes, hotels really charge a premium for such a service. Most U.S. international airports have a foreign currency exchange, where you should get at least $100 in the currency of the first country you're visiting. That way you can eat, drink, tip porters, and hire a cab, if necessary, as soon as you arrive.

About maps: Use Michelin maps if you're going to Europe. As you plan your route, you'll notice that the maps show roads labeled A, B, and C. The A roads are like our interstate highways, except that in Europe they may have no speed limit. It's not too healthy to bike on autobahns where the cars, trucks, and buses are whizzing along at 90 to 110 mph and up. B roads are the same as U.S. state highways, and these I would also avoid. If you want peace and quiet, use only the C roads, which are the equivalent of county roads in this country. European C roads are almost always paved and in good condition, with low traffic density. If you look closely at the map, you will also note that some roads, in some places, have chevrons or inverted V's on them. Each chevron denotes a 5 percent grade. Unless you want a back-busting climb, try to avoid three-chevron roads. Finer-scale Michelin maps show bike routes, many of which are far from highways. You'll share them with mopeds, but that's no problem. Europeans are used to bikes, and you'll be treated well.

For the United States, Rand McNally publishes a source book of maps and campsites that is a handy and compact guide to county, state, and national parks. It's available in bookstores. American Youth Hostels (AYH) publishes a compact list of hostels in this country and a list of affiliated hostel organizations in many foreign countries. The word "Youth" in AYH is a bit misleading. I've seen people of all ages staying at these hostels. Membership in the AYH is $20 for ages 18 to 59, under 18 it's $10, and for seniors (60 and over) it's $10.

County maps are absolutely invaluable. If you're going on a long trip, through several states, the county maps can fill up half of one of your panniers, and that is a problem. I buy the maps locally as I go and mail them home as I finish with them. That doesn't allow for much detailed trip planning, but I've never had problems figuring out a route, with the help of friendly natives. Maps are also available from Adventure Cycling (formerly Bikecentennial) to get you almost anyplace in the United States. What's so great about these maps is that they are designed for bicyclists and give you safe and convenient routes. For maps call Adventure Cycling at 1-800-933-1116, or write them at P.O. Box 8308, Missoula, MT 59807. Adventure Cycling also provides group tours.

Learn the language of the currency of the country or countries you'll be visiting, but don't ask how much something is if you can't understand the answer. Learn the basics of directions, how to order food, find a hotel, a campsite, a bed-and-breakfast place, or a youth hostel. Or you could use a hand-held electronic interpreter. They're available in many languages. Remember that campgrounds abound in Europe, and once you learn how to find them, you'll always have an inexpensive place to stay.

Airline bike fees: If you belong to the League of American Wheelmen and show your membership card, on at least four of the major airlines (as of this writing) you can bring your bike along at no charge. Call the L.A.W. at 1-800-288-BIKE for the cooperating airlines, or write the L.A.W at 190 West Ostend St., Suite 120, Baltimore, MD 21230-3755, for membership costs and privileges. If you are not an L.A.W. member, here is what it costs: A recent check with United Airlines (their prices are typical of at least domestic airlines) revealed that the flat-rate cost for carrying a bike on the plane is $50 for flights within the continental United States. For trips to Europe and Asia, there is no charge for carrying your bike.

The bike shipping box must be no larger than 69 inches long, 40 inches high, and 8.25 inches wide. Don't even think about trying to disguise your bike as something else to save money. The maximum size for any other package, according to United Airlines, is a total of 62 linear inches, which is the sum of length, height (doubled), and width (doubled). I don't think you can squeeze your bike into any combination of these dimensions. You could ship your bicycle via United Parcel Service if the total linear box measurement (height + width + width + length + length) equals no more than 130 inches. United Parcel Service is careful, but rough handling of baggage can occur with any carrier. If you have the time to ship via United Parcel Service, use the very sturdy and strong plastic bicycle box made by Pedal Pack. This box is 44 inches high, 11 inches wide, and 32 inches long, which adds up to 130 linear inches, the UPS maximum. The Pedal Pack container comes with foam lining, wheels, and sturdy case fasteners, one of which is lockable. The Pedal Pack costs $380, but is good insurance against damage to your costly bicycle. Reach Pedal Pack at 1-800-359-3096 or write them at P.O. Box 788, Porterville, CA 93258.

On overseas trips to Asia and Europe, I suggest you stow your laden panniers with the bike in the bike container. The only overseas restriction, other than the size limits noted above, is weight. The bike box with the bike, plus anything else you stuff inside it, can weigh no more than 70 pounds. You get to check one other bag onto the plane, but it must weigh no more than 50 pounds. On any flight, the airline will tag the bike container as fragile and include a disclaimer for damage. If you travel to South America, there may be additional costs or restrictions. Also check with the airline if you want to ship a tandem bike. You may not be able to if it does not meet dimensional restrictions.

Caution: I recommend you do not ride your bicycle from the airport to your hotel or campground if you have been flying longer than six hours. You will be tired and have jet lag, and also be stressed just looking for your first stopover in a strange place. In countries such as England where the cars travel on the "wrong" side of the road, you could, at first, find yourself riding into traffic, instead of with it, or automatically looking in the wrong direction for traffic clearance. So take a cab or bus to your first rest stop, sleep, rest up. You need to be alert and able to react quickly and accurately to road situations.

Pack your bike this way: Use a bike box you can get from a bike shop. Dealers throw them away, so you should have no problem. Or buy a container from the airline for $10, or invest in a Pedal Pack box (described above). Remove both wheels and place them next to the bike frame. If the container is long enough (and still meets airline dimension requirements), you could leave the rear wheel on the bike. Block the dropouts (where the wheel axle fits) with an old axle or a plastic dummy axle you can buy from a bike shop (save them for future trips) to keep the fork blades or rear stays from being bent in shipment. Remove the pedals and screw them in the cranks from the inside, or strap them to the frame. Remove the saddle with the seat post attached and lay it in the bike container. Remove the handlebars, drape them over the top tube, and tie them down parallel to the bike. Let some of the air out of the tires, because at flight altitudes a fully inflated tire could blow out in an unpressurized or lower-pressurized luggage compartment. There should be room in the bike box to stuff at least one set of loaded panniers, which may cut down on your carry-on bags. Put your tools and spare parts in the panniers you put in the bike box. I remember having a difficult time explaining to a security person at one airport that the long tube in my hand luggage was a bike pump. I had to disassemble the pump to prove it. If you have to explain your bike tools to a security guard, you could miss your flight if you're running late. That also goes for return trips from overseas, particularly from England, Sweden, France, Germany, and, above all, Switzerland.

Watch out for poison ivy in the eastern and midwestern United States, poison oak in the western United States, and poison sumac in the South. Look up these plants in botany books at your library, so you can recognize the leaves. Carry a tube of 0.5 percent hydrocortisone ointment in case you are infected. It's great for saddle sores, too, and does not require a prescription.

On train travel, remember, European trains usually have a baggage car in which you can put your bike, although there may be a small extra fare involved. You may have to put the bike aboard the baggage car yourself.

Do not carry Halt or Mace on your person or even in the bike box on an airplane!

Staying clean: There will come a day on a bike camping trip when your last six campsites were without showers and there were no lakes to bathe in. What I do is visit the first health club I come to in a larger city and give them a couple of bucks to use their shower. In fact, one such club was so bemused by our request they gave us free showers and even threw in the towels and soap.

Respect property: For example, if you're touring in the harvest season, in Europe especially, respect private property. This means not stopping to pick grapes from a vineyard or fruit from trees even though it's temptingly near. I have found that Europeans are pretty fussy about their property, but generous if you ask them. In Austria, for example, during the grape-harvesting season, I have waved from my bike to workers in the vineyards, who would wave back with a cluster of grapes in their hands, clearly offering me some. I didn't expect any grapes, but on a warm day, they were welcome.

Where to Ride and How to Get There

Here is a review of sources for bicycle touring and camping, state by state and for some foreign countries. First, for the United States, I wrote to the tourism departments of all 50 states for information on guides, maps, and suggestions on the best places to ride, as well as data on campgrounds and state parks. Most states were generous with data, maps, and other bicycle touring information. While I list state bicycle coordinators, remember that some states are yet to appoint one and those who are listed may no longer have that job. But a letter c/o the state bicycle coordinator should reach whoever fills that role. You will note that when I can, I give the bicycle coordinator's name, address, and phone first. Here's a summary of their replies.

ALABAMA: Bill Couch, Bicycle Coordinator, Urban Planning, 1409 Coliseum Blvd., Montgomery, AL 36130, phone 1-205-242-6089. For information on parks and camps, write the Bureau of Tourism and Travel, P.O. Box 4309, Dept. TIA, Montgomery, AL 36130-4309, phone 1-800-ALABAMA. State parks are located in nearly every part of the state.

ALASKA: Rich Poor, Bicycle Coordinator, 3132 Channel Dr., Juneau, AK 99801-7898. For maps contact DeLorme Mapping, Box 298, Freeport, ME 04032. Also write Alaska Division of Tourism, P.O. Box 110811, Juneau, AK 99811-0801, phone 1-907-465-2010. This state has an enormous area to explore. You might try the Kenai Peninsula, Kodiak Island (via ferry), Chugach State Park, Power Line Pass Trail, or the Bird Creek logging roads. Send for the booklet entitled "Alaska State Parks," which lists over 100 of them and tells where to write for more specific data, including maps. Bill Garry, Sup't., Chugach State Park, 2601 Commercial Drive, Anchorage, AK 99501.

ARIZONA: Steve Hancock, Arizona Bicycle Coordinator, Arizona Department of Transportation, 206 S. 17th Ave, Room 340B, Phoenix, AZ 85007, 602-255-7431. Maps, Arizona Department of Transportation, 1655 W. Jackson, Phoenix, AZ 85007. Phone 1-602-255-7498 for state and county maps. Also Arizona Office of Tourism, 1100 W. Washington St., Phoenix, AZ 85007, phone 1-602-542-8637.

ARKANSAS: Steve Weston, Bicycle Coordinator, Arkansas Department of Parks and Tourism, One Capitol Mall, Little Rock, AR 72201, phone 1-800-828-8974. For maps, Arkansas Transportation Department., P.O. Box 2261, Little Rock, AR 72203. Campgrounds include Devil's Den State Park in northwest Arkansas, Pea Ridge, Lost Valley, Buffalo River, and Bear Creek Mountain or Mt. Nebo State Park.

CALIFORNIA: Richard L. Blunden, Chief, Office of Bicycle Facilities, California Department of Transportation, 1120 N. Street, Room 4500, Sacramento, CA 95814. For maps and campground locations and reservations, write Department of Parks and Recreation California, P.O. Box 942896, Sacramento CA 94296-0001, and the California Office of Tourism, 1030 13th St., Suite 200, Sacramento, CA 95841, phone 1-800-TO-CALIF. In northern California good riding is available in these state parks: the Forest of Nisene Marks, Henry Cowell and Fall Creek Redwoods, Big Basin Redwoods, Butano, Annadel, Sugarloaf Ridge, Austin Creek, Armstrong Redwoods, Cow Mountain, Mt. Shasta, and Mt. Lassen. There are many more mountains, seashore areas, and scenic wilderness trails in that state that would fill up the rest of this book just to mention. Check with each park management for permission and maps. There are literally millions of acres of remote, beautiful, scenic wilderness available to you. Check the tour providers, professionally led tours, at the end this chapter. There are many such off-road tours offered by these organizations in California.

COLORADO: Nancy Cifelli, Bicycle Coordinator, Colorado Department of Highways, 4201 East Arkansas Avenue, Denver, CO 80222. Maps, Colorado Division of Parks and Outdoor Recreation, Room 618, 1313 Sherman St., Denver, CO 80203. Also Colorado Tourism Board, P.O. Box 38700, Denver, CO 80238, phone 1-800-COLORADO. Like California, Colorado is a bicycle tourist's and mountain biker's paradise. Lots and lots of trails and quiet mountain dirt roads are available in the Rockies in the high country of Colorado. The rangers are well-disposed toward bicyclists. With this in mind, pick a mountain that's within a state park or wildlife area and you should have no trouble. The famous Pearl Pass tour is a 17-mile jaunt, with a 3,835-foot vertical climb to the summit and an 18-mile, 4,915-foot drop to Aspen, and is well worth doing. Also the mountains around Crested Butte are famous for scenic trails.

CONNECTICUT: The state bicycle coordinator is Wayne DeCarli, Connecticut Department of Transportation, 24 Wolcott Hill Rd., Wethersfield CT 06109, phone 1-203-566-6450. Maps, Connecticut Department of Economic Development, 865 Brook St., Rocky Hill, CT 06067, phone 1-800-282-6863. My home state, and a great place to bicycle. Stop and visit the beautiful homes built by pioneer settlers in the early 1650s that could pass for mansions today.

DELAWARE: Elizabeth Holloway, Bicycle Coordinator, Delaware Department of Transportation, P.O. Box 778, Dover, DE 19903, phone 1-302-739-4318. Maps, same address, ask for free map index. Delaware Tourism Office, 99 Kings Highway, P.O. Box 1401, Dept. TIA, Dover, DE 19903, phone 1-800-441-8846.

DISTRICT OF COLUMBIA: Gene Abbott, Bicycle Coordinator, Department of Public Works, 2000 14th St., NW, 6th floor, Washington, DC 20010. Maps: Committee to Promote Washington, 1212 New York Ave., NW, #200, Washington, DC 20005, phone 1-202-724-4091; Office of Documents, Room 19, District Bldg., 14th St. and Pennsylvania Ave., NW, Washington, DC 20004.

FLORIDA: Dan Burden, State Bicycle Coordinator, Florida Department of Transportation, 605 Suwannee St., Mail Station 82, Tallahassee, FL 32399-0450. Maps: same address except Mail Station 12, phone 1-904-488-9220. Florida Division of Tourism, 126 W. Van Buren St., Tallahassee, FL 32301. For off-road bicycling, try the St. Marks National Wildlife Refuge, and trails paralleling rivers such as the Suwannee. There's not much in the way of mountains (the state is mostly flat) but there are hundreds of miles of great roads and sandy beaches to ride on. Try the island of Santa Rosa. For that area and other scenic bike routes, contact Gulf Islands National Seashore, 1801 Gulf Breeze Parkway, Gulf Breeze, FL 32561.

GEORGIA: Steve Yost, Bicycle Coordinator, Georgia Department of Transportation, #2 Capitol Square, Room 343, Atlanta, GA 30334, phone 1-404-656-5386. Maps, same address except Room 10, phone 1-404-656-5336. Also Georgia Department of Industry, Trade & Tourism, P.O. Box 1776, Dept. TIA, Atlanta, GA 30301, phone 1-800-VISIT-GA.

HAWAII: Ron Tsuzuki, State Bicycle Coordinator, Hawaii Department of Transportation, 7869 Punchbowl St., Honolulu, HI 96813, phone 1-808-548-3258. Maps, Hawaii Visitor's Bureau, 2270 Kalakaua Ave., Suite 801, Honolulu, HI 96815, phone 1-808-923-1811. State of Hawaii Department of Business, Economic Development & Tourism, P.O. Box 2359, Honolulu, HI 96804, phone 1-808-586-2423.

IDAHO: Charles Roundtree, Bicycle Coordinator, Idaho Department of Transportation, Box 7129, Boise, ID 83707, phone 1-208-334-8488. For maps and camping information, the Idaho Travel Council, 700 W. State St., Boise, ID 83720, phone 1-800-635-7820. For off-road riding there are many great trails in the Idaho back country. Sun Valley is a bicycling paradise, as is Clearwater National Forest. For more information on cycling in the hills or on the flats in Idaho write State Trails Coordinator, Idaho Department of Parks and Recreation, P.O. Box 83720, Boise, ID 83270-0065.

ILLINOIS: Craig Williams, State Bicycle Coordinator, Illinois Department. of Transportation, 2300 S. Dirksen Parkway, Room 110, Springfield, IL 62764, phone 1-217-782-3194. Maps, same address, phone 1-217-782-0834, for road and trail maps, including some 150 trails. Some of these trails are paved, most are dirt or rough stone. For camps and trail information, write to Dan M. Troemper, Public Information Officer, Lands and Historic Sites, Illinois Department of Conservation, Lincoln Tower Plaza, 524 S. Second St., Springfield, IL 62701-1787, or the Illinois Bureau of Tourism, 100 W. Randolph, Suite 3-400, Chicago, IL 60601, phone 1-800-223-0121.

INDIANA: Jim Stickler, Bike Coordinator, Indiana Department of Transportation, 100 N. Senate Ave., Indianapolis, IN 46204, phone 1-317-232-5526. Maps, same address, but phone 1-317-232-5115. Bikeway guidebooks: Hoosier Bikeway System Guidebooks, Indiana Division of Outdoor Recreation, 402 W. Washington, Room 271, Indianapolis, IN 46204, or Indiana Department of Tourism, One North Capitol, Suite 700, Indianapolis, IN 46204-2288, phone 1-800-289-6646.

IOWA: Nancy Burns, State Bicycle Coordinator, Iowa Department of Transportation, 800 Lincoln Way, Ames, IA 50010, phone 1-319-239-1621. Maps, Iowa Department of Transportation, same address. There are many miles of excellent, low-traffic country roads that offer scenic riding opportunities. Iowa Division of Tourism, 200 E. Grand Ave., Des Moines, IA 50309, phone 1-800-345-IOWA. Consider a very popular and major cycling event in that state called RAGBRAI. For information write Lois Peterson, RAGBRAI, P.O. Box 622, Des Moines, IA 50303-0622, phone 1-515-284-8282.

KANSAS: Mark Bechtel, State Bicycle Coordinator, Kansas Department of Transportation, 2nd floor, Thacher Bldg., 217 S.E. 4th, Topeka, KS 66063, phone 1-913-296-7448. Maps, Kansas Department of Transportation, Docking State Office Building, 8th floor, Topeka, KS 66612, phone 1-913-296-3841, or Kansas Tourism Division, 400 W. 8th St., 5th floor, Dept. DIS, Topeka, KS 66203-3009, phone 1-800-252-6727.

KENTUCKY: Dave Smith, Bicycle Coordinator, Transportation Department, Cabinet, State Office Building, 11th floor, Frankfort, KY 40622, phone 1-502-564-3730. Maps, Transportation Cabinet Department of Highways, 419 Ann St., Frankfort, KY 40622. Also Kentucky Department of Travel Development, 2200 Capitol Plaza Tower, Department DA, Frankfort, KY 40601, phone 1-800-225-TRIP.

LOUISIANA: Coan Bouch, Bicycle Coordinator, Louisiana Department of Transportation, P.O. Box 94245, Baton Rouge, LA 70804-9245, phone 1-504-356-1841. Maps, LA DOT, General Files Unit, P.O. Box 94245, Baton Rouge, LA 70804-9245. Louisiana Office of Tourism, Inquiry Department, P.O. Box 94291, LOT, Baton Rouge, LA 70804-9291, phone 1-800-33-GUMBO.

MAINE: Margaret Vandebroek, Bicycle Coordinator, DOT, State Office Building, Station 16, Augusta, ME 04333, for maps and biking info. This state has many scenic parks, and Acadia National Park, located on the state's coastline, has 16 miles of unpaved trails. Here you can enjoy the mountains and the coast simultaneously. For directions to parks and forest areas write Maine Publicity Bureau, 97 Winthrop St., Hallowell, ME 04347, or Maine Office of Tourism, 189 State St., Augusta, ME 04333, phone 1-800-533-9595.

MARYLAND: Jerry Stadd, Bicycle Coordinator, Maryland State Highway Administration, Room 218, 707 N. Calvert St., Baltimore, MD 21203-0717. Maps, State Highway Administration, Map Distribution Section, 2323 W. Joppa Rd., Brooklandville, MD 21022, phone 1-301-321-3518, or Maryland Tourism, 217 E. Redwood St., 9th floor, Baltimore, MD 21202, phone 1-800-543-1036. For parks and trail maps and information, also write Maryland National Park and Planning Commission, 8787 Georgia Ave., Silver Spring, MD 20907.

MASSACHUSETTS: Bicycle Coordinator (no name, position probably vacant at this writing), 10 Park Plaza, Room 4150, Boston, MA 02116, phone 1-617-973-8003. For information on biking contact Daniel O'Brien, Environmental Management, Department of Resource Conservation, 100 Cambridge St., Room 1401, Boston, MA 02202, phone 1-617-727-3160. At the same address, but ensconced on the 13th floor, Massachusetts Office of Travel and Tourism, phone 1-800-447-MASS. Lots of great rides in Massachusetts. I enjoyed the trip out to Cape Cod and rides around Provincetown, Cape Cod National Park, Nantucket, and Martha's Vineyard. Bicycles are allowed on hiking trails and fire roads within the Massachusetts forests and parks. The state has many scenic parks, some mountainous, others along the seashore. For information, write Gilbert A. Bliss, Director of Forests and Parks, 100 Cambridge St., Boston, MA 02202.

MICHIGAN: Terry Eldred, Nonmotorized Coordinator, Michigan Department of Transportation, P.O. Box 30050, Lansing, MI 48909, phone 1-517-373-9192. Maps and travel information, Michigan DOT, same address, or P.O. Box 30226, Lansing, MI 48909, phone 1-800-543-YES. This state has many miles of scenic dunes along Lake Michigan, and many state parks that have miles of trails that, if not challenging in terms of hills, do offer opportunities to pedal into the quiet rural countryside. For specifics, write also to Bill Tansil, Supervisor, Highways and Nonmotorized Planning, Michigan Department of Transportation, P.O. Box 30050, Lansing, MI 48909.

MINNESOTA: Cynthia McArthur, State Bicycle Safety Coordinator, 340 Coffey Hall, University of Minnesota, St. Paul, MN 55108. Maps, Minnesota Department of Transportation, Room B-20, St. Paul, MN 55155, phone 1-612-296-2216, or Minnesota Office of Tourism, 375 Jackson St., 250 Skyway Level, St. Paul, MN 55101, phone 1-800-657-3700.

MISSISSIPPI: J. E. Moak, Bicycle Coordinator, Mississippi Department of Transportation, 85-01, P.O. Box 1850, Jackson, MS 39215-1850, phone 1-601-944-9142. Maps, Mississippi Department of Transportation, P.O. Box 1850, Jackson, MS 39205. There are long-forgotten trails great for bicycle touring that run alongside the Mississippi River that Mark Twain must have seen at one time or another. Or you might try Natchez Trace, a path followed for generations by Natchez Indians and, later, British, Spanish, and French traders, but check with the Natchez Convention and Visitor's Bureau, P.O. Box 1485, Natchez, MS 39121-1485, phone 1-800-647-6724.

MISSOURI: Deborah Schnack, Trails Coordinator, Division of Parks, Recreation and Historic Preservation, P.O. Box 176, Jefferson City, MO 65102, phone 1-314-751-2479. Maps, Missouri Department of Natural Resources, same address, ask for highway, county, and state park maps. The Missouri Department of Natural Resources has approved bike trails in seven state parks, and more are being planned. The state parks that have approved trails are Castlewood, Graham Cave, Knob Noster, Lake of the Ozarks, Lake Wappapello, St. Joe, and Finger Lake State Park, which sounds to be the most promising, with over 70 miles of trails.

MONTANA: Dick Howell, Bicycle Coordinator, Montana Department of Highways, 2701 Prospect Ave., Helena, MT 59620, phone 1-406-444-6118. Maps and campground info, Travel Montana, 1424 9th Ave., Helena, MT 59620, phone 1-406-44-2654, and Montana Department of Transportation, same address as for Dick Howell, above. The state abounds with scenic areas that are state-managed and should be open to you. Montana is one of our largest states in geographical area, yet it is sparsely settled. Check also with the Montana Travel Promotion Bureau, Department of Commerce, 1424 9th Ave., Helena, MT 59620, and with Travel Montana, Room 259, Deer Lodge, MT 59722.

NEBRASKA: Derald Kohles, Bicycle Coordinator, Nebraska Department of Transportation, P.O. Box 94759, Lincoln, NE 68509, phone 1-402-471-4567. Maps, Nebraska Department of Roads, same address, and for maps and park and campground info, try Outdoor Education Division, Nebraska Game and Parks Commission, 2200 N. 33rd St., Lincoln, NE 68503, phone 1-402-471-5581. You can ride on hiking trails in their park system.

NEVADA: Kent Cooper, Bicycle Coordinator, Nevada Department of Transportation, 1263 S. Stewart St., Carson City, NV 89710. Maps, Nevada Department of Transportation, same address. Lots of on- and off-road trails in state and national parks. Much of the land in this state is publicly owned and well-suited for on- and off-road riding. For state park info write Nevada State Parks, 201 S. Fall Street, Room 119, Carson City, NV 89710.

NEW HAMPSHIRE: State Bicycle Coordinator, Department of Public Works, Hazen Drive, Concord, NH 03301, phone 1-603-271-3734. Maps, New Hampshire Office of Travel and Tourism, P.O. Box 856, Concord, NH 03302, phone 1-603-271-2666.

NEW JERSEY: William Feldman, Bicycle Coordinator, New Jersey Department of Transportation, 1035 Parkway Ave., CN600, Trenton, NJ 08625, phone 1-609-530-8062, for maps, info on parks, tour guides.

NEW MEXICO: James Kozak, Bicycle Coordinator, New Mexico State Highway Department, Planning Bureau, Advanced Planning Section, P.O. Box 1149, Santa Fe, NM 87504-1149, phone 1-505-827-5547. Maps, New Mexico Department of Travel and Tourism, 491 Old Santa Fe Trail, Santa Fe, NM 87503, phone 1-505-827-0291.

NEW YORK: For info on parks, write New York State Parks, Biking Information, Albany, NY 12238, phone 1-518-474-0456. Maps, New York Department of Transportation, Bldg. 4, Room 105, State Campus, Albany, NY 12232, phone 1-518-457-3555. The parks and trails around Lake George, the Catskills (shades of Rip van Winkle), the Finger Lake district, and the Adirondacks offer superb bicycling and scenery. For information on Finger Lake area riding, write Finger Lake State Park & Recreation Commission, Rte. 3, Trumansburg, NY 14886, and the New York State

Department of Commerce, Tourism Division, 99 Washington Ave., Albany, NY 12245.

NORTH CAROLINA: For maps and bicycle touring and campground information, contact Curtis Yates or Mary Meletiou, Bicycle Coordinators, North Carolina Department of Transportation, P.O. Box 25201, Raleigh, NC 27611, phone 1-919-733-2804. Great riding opportunities abound in this state, notably in the Blue Ridge Mountains in the western section, the Outer Banks area in the east, and the Pisgah National Forest.

NORTH DAKOTA: Norlyn Schmidt, Transportation Planner, North Dakota State Highway Department., 600 E. Boulevard Ave., Bismarck, ND 58501. Maps, North Dakota Tourism Promotion, Liberty Mutual Bldg., 604 E. Boulevard, Bismarck, ND 58505, and Bob Shannon, Transportation Planner, North Dakota State Highway Department, same address, as for Norlyn Schmidt, phone 1-701-224-2588.

OHIO: Sharon Todd, Bicycle Coordinator, Ohio Department of Transportation, 25 S. Front St., Room 418, Columbus, OH 43215, phone 1-644-8660. For maps and campground information write Ohio Department of Natural Resources, Division of Forestry, Fountain Square, Columbus, OH 43224. For road maps also contact the Ohio Department of Transportation, Map Sales, Room B-100, P.O. Box 899, Columbus, OH 43216, phone 1-614-466-4430, and the Ohio Division of Travel and Tourism, P.O. Box 1001, Columbus, OH 43266-0110, phone 1-800-BUCKEYE. There are good off-road trails in Pike, Richland Furnace, Perry, and Maumee state forests, and many miles of gravel back-country roads in the state forests. I recommend Shawnee, Tar Hollow, Zaleski, and Scioto Trail state forests for this type of riding.

OKLAHOMA: For maps and campground information, write Programs Coordinator, Planning and Development Division, State of Oklahoma, Tourism and Recreation Department, 50 Will Rogers Building, Oklahoma City, OK 73105. Road maps are available from the Oklahoma Department of Transportation, Reproduction Branch, Room 1N, 200 NE 21st St., Oklahoma City, OK 73112, phone 1-405-521-2588. For maps and campground information, also write Programs Coordinator, Planning and Development Division, State of Oklahoma, Tourism and Recreation Department, 50 Will Rogers Building, Oklahoma City, OK 73105. There's a title, but no name, of State Bicycle Coordinator, Oklahoma Department of Transportation, 200 NE 21st St., Oklahoma City, OK 73196, phone 1-405-521-2631. For camping and trail rides, look for parks and forests in the eastern and southeastern sections.

OREGON: Dick Unrein, Bikeway Program Manager, Room 200, Transportation Building, Salem OR 97310, phone 1-503-378-3432, or Bicycle Program Supervisor, 301 N. Adams, Eugene, OR 97402, phone 1-503-687-

5329. For maps, write Economic Development, Tourism, 775 Summer St., NE, Salem OR 97310, phone 1-800-547-7842, or Oregon Bicycling Guide, Oregon Department of Transportation, Highway Division, Salem, OR 97310, phone 1-503-378-3432. The state has so many state and national parks that I can only urge you to pick a park and take off. I prefer the western section of the state; the eastern section is flatter except for such outstanding mountain areas as the Sisters near Bend. The Umpquah National Forest in the west is an excellent example of a location for off-road riding. Get a fishing license, bring your trout rod (fishing regulations permit flies only, no live bait), and catch your dinner in the Umpquah River. Or try the Siskiyous, near Ashland, and in the summer you can bike down the mountain and attend the famous Shakespeare Festival in that city. There's an excellent campground about ten miles north of Ashland.

PENNSYLVANIA: Dave Bachman, Bicycle Coordinator, Pennsylvania Department of Transportation, Bureau for Highway Safety and Traffic Engineering, Room 203, P.O. Box 20478, Harrisburg, PA 17105-2047, phone 1-717-787-7350. For maps, off-road trails, and campground locations, write Pennsylvania Trails Coordinator, Pennsylvania Bureau of State Parks, P.O. Box 1467, Harrisburg, PA 17120. Ask also for lists of sources for National Parks and Trails information and the Pennsylvania Recreational Guide, which contains a map and list of state parks. The map also shows location of bicycle trails. For road maps, write Pennsylvania Department of Transportation, P.O. Box 2028, Harrisburg, PA 17105-2028, phone 1-717-787-6746. Bicycles are permitted on fire roads in state parks and forest lands. Lancaster County is the Pennsylvania Dutch country and offers very scenic routes for the bicycle tourist. Also write the Lancaster County Bicycle Club, Box 535, Lancaster, PA 17604, for their book of maps, at $7. Guided tours in the state are conducted by Four Seasons Cycling Tours, Box 203, Williamsburg, VA 23187, and Bucks County Bicycle Tours, 211 W. Callowhill Rd., Perkasie, PA 18944.

RHODE ISLAND: Constance V. Daniels, Bicycle Coordinator, Planning Division, Rhode Island Department of Transportation, Two Capitol Hill, State Office Building, Providence, RI 02903, phone 1-401-277-2694. Maps, Planning Division, Rhode Island Department of Transportation, same address. This little state has some excellent riding possibilities along the coast and in the forest and marshes of the southeastern section. For a good state map showing rural and back roads, write Rhode Island Department of Economic Development, Tourist Promotion Division, 7 Jackson Walkway, Providence, RI 02903. Also ask for the current visitor's guide to Rhode Island, and for info on these bike trails: Goddard State Park; Conanicut; Greenville area of Smithfield; Tiverton, Sakonnet, and Little Compton; Bellevue Avenue and Ocean Drive in Newport; and all of Block Island. The Rhode Island Bicycle Coalition has a "Metropolitan Providence Bicycle Map." Write the Coalition at P.O. Box 4781, Rumford, RI 02916.

SOUTH CAROLINA: Ron Carter, State Bicycle Coordinator, South Carolina Department of Parks, 1205 Pendleton St., E. A. Brown Building, Columbia, SC 29201, phone 1-803-734-0141. Ask for the Bicycle Guide to South Carolina. The guide is for the road biker, but it shows state parks and recreation areas. There are rugged mountains in the northwest, notably the Piedmont section, which offer great off-road riding in areas of scenic beauty. The coastal and central areas are mostly flat.

SOUTH DAKOTA: Craig McIntyre, Bicycle Coordinator, South Dakota Department of Transportation, 700 Broadway Ave. East, Pierre, SD 57501-2586, phone 1-605-773-3155. Maps and camping information, South Dakota Department of Tourism, 711 E. Wells Ave, Pierre, SD 57501, phone 1-800-843-1930. For road bikers, you will most likely find not much to look at.

TENNESSEE: William E. Jacobs, Bicycle Coordinator, Tennessee Department of Transportation, James K. Polk Building, Suite 700, 505 Deaderick St., Nashville, TN 37243-0349, phone 1-615-741-5310. For maps and information on state parks, write Tennessee State Parks, 7th floor, L&C Tower, 401 Church St., Nashville, TN 37243, phone 1-800-421-6683. Don Wick, Director of Information, Department of Tourist Development, sent five terrific maps of choice biking roads in the state. You might ask him for a set. He also noted that bears are common in the huge wilderness areas of eastern Tennessee in the Great Smoky Mountains National Park and in the 625,000 acres of the Cherokee National Forest. He feels it might be a good idea to avoid a bear-bike encounter in those areas. East of Chattanooga are lots of state parks with trails and fire roads. In the central area you can cruise along the Tennessee River. For a road trip, try the scenic Natchez Trace Parkway. Info on the parkway is available from Natchez Trace Parkway, RR1, NT-143, Tupelo, MS 38801. The western section is fairly flat. Also write Tennessee Department of Tourist Development, P.O. Box 23170, Nashville, TN 37202.

TEXAS: Paul Douglas, Bicycle Coordinator, State Department of Highways and Transportation, DeWitt C. Greer State Highway Building, 11th & Brazos, Austin, TX 78701-2483, phone 1-512-416-3125, or R. C. Hauser, Chief, Park Operations, Texas Parks and Wildlife Department, 4200 Smith School Rd., Austin, TX 78701. Mr. Hauser says, "The use of bicycles on trails and fire roads in Texas State Parks is prohibited with the exception of trails and fire roads that are specifically designated as hike and bike trails." Texas is so big it has just about every kind of bike riding there is. I like the Padre Islands (be sure to oil the chain every day when you ride in sand or through salt water), the forest region in the east, the hill country in the central region, and the back roads everywhere, once you are away from metro areas. I'd avoid the Panhandle, though, unless you like to eat wind-blown dust. For data on the hill country, write Kathryn Nichols at the same address as for Mr. Hauser, above. The Big Bend National Park is terrific for trail riding and camping. Write Big Bend National Park, TX 79834, for maps and info. Better have at least two water bottles on your frame in this desert country.

UTAH: For maps and campgrounds, write Kim Morris, Bicycle Coordinator, Utah Department of Transportation, 4501 S. 2700 West, Salt Lake City, UT 84119, phone 1-801-965-4390. This state is loaded with bicycle touring roads and trail rides. As with any hilly state, it is always advisable to check the contour lines of mountain area maps to be sure you can handle the grade. A few of the many areas to check are Bryce and Zion national parks, the Grand Canyon area, Yellowstone National Park (limited to paved trails), and the Great Salt Lake area. For a map of the Moab area Mountain Bike Trails, write Moab Visitor Center, 805 N. Main St., Highway 191, Moab, UT 84532. The Bureau of Land Management, Grand Resource Area, P.O. Box M, Moab, UT 84532, also has more data on this area. Deloy K. Peterson, of the Utah Transportation Planning Division, notes, "We do not have a state bicycle route system as none of our highways have any special provisions for bicyclists. You may ride at your own risk as part of the general traffic on any of our highways, except on portions of the Interstate system where paved frontage roads or nearby alternate routes are available. Areas where you may not ride on the Interstate are indicated in red on the enclosed highway map (I-84 from Tremoaton to Ogden and I-15 from Ogden to Nephi and in the Fillmore and Beaver areas). If you intend to ride at night you must have a white light in front, a red reflector in back, and reflectors or lights visible from each side for at least 500 feet. You must not have any siren or whistle mounted on your bike for a warning device. In planning your trip through Utah there are several things you need to consider. Outside of our urbanized area between Ogden and Provo, Utah is sparsely populated. It's a long way between towns and available services and you'll need to carry everything you will want between stops. Don't forget that much of Utah is desert, with summer daytime temperatures often above 100 degrees. Along many of our routes there not only are no services, there is no shelter and no drinking water either. In these areas be sure you carry plenty of water for the long distances involved.

"Utah is also crossed from north to south with mountain ranges, and some of our highways have long, steep grades. Be prepared for long climbs—and be sure your brakes are in good shape for the downhill runs on the other side. Most of Utah is at or above 5,000 feet above sea level.

Our air is 'thinner' than at lower altitudes and bikers from other areas generally find that they tire much more easily than they think they should because of the lower oxygen content. When (not 'if') this happens to you, don't try and fight it by keeping up your normal pace. It won't help. Stop and rest, then pace yourself at a slower rate until you get used to the altitude. You'll feel better and besides, Utah is too nice to rush through, anyway. Don't let all these grim-sounding things discourage you. Lots of bikers enjoy seeing Utah each year. Do remember them as you plan your trip. We want you to enjoy your visit with us, not just survive.

"Traffic on our highways shouldn't pose problems to experienced touring riders. However, if you are going to be in the urbanized area between Ogden and Provo, the peak traffic periods are between about 7:00 and 8:30 A.M., and 4:30 to 6:00 P.M. You'll probably want to avoid these times to miss having to try and find your way in a strange area and compete with the traffic.

"Our state highway map should provide basic route information to all the major points you might wish to visit. For greater detail, and more information about trails, scenic areas, elevations, etc., you might want to get the eight-map multipurpose map set published by the Utah Travel Council. These maps show more detail and are easy to use, with each of the maps being about the size of the highway map. The set costs $8.00, and is available from the Utah Travel Council, Council Hall, Salt Lake City, UT 84114. Our county maps are not helpful for bike trip planning, so don't bother to order them."

VERMONT: Joe Landry, Bicycle Coordinator, Agency of Transportation, 133 State St., Montpelier, VT 05602, phone 1-802-828-2657. For state and county maps, write Vermont Department of Tourism, same address. I've done a lot of biking in Vermont and I can tell you that roads in forest areas can be scenic and demanding. For information on off-road and trail riding, contact the Vermont Agency of Environmental Conservation, Department of Forests, Parks and Recreation, Montpelier, VT 05602. Ask for "Bicycling in Vermont" from the Recreation Division, Vermont Department of Forests, Parks and Recreation Agency of Environmental Conservation, Montpelier, VT 05602. For savoring the scenery and for camping out in state parks. I can heartily recommend Route 100, up the middle of the state. One campground in particular stands out vividly. It's on the road from Route 100 to Calvin Coolidge State Park. If you want to experience a 15 percent grade, that's it. If you have a low gear, you should be able to make it, but it will be slow. At least your rear wheel won't skid out from under you on the pavement. The back roads from Hanover down the Connecticut River and across to Vermont and down to Brattleboro are well worth taking. Despite state-imposed restrictions on trail riding, there are many challenging and rewarding trails to ride in this beautiful state. Mountain bikes are permitted on forest highways and other roads where motorized vehicles are permitted. There are thousands of miles of lightly traveled, unpaved back roads in Vermont that are quite suitable for bicycling. There are also two designated trails for off-road riding. These are the D&H Railroad ROW and the old Montpelier to Wells River Railroad ROW through Groton State Forest. Most Vermont state parks are very small units and for the most part are fragile environments, so stay on the trail.

VIRGINIA: Richard C. Lockwood and Phil Hopkins, Bicycle Coordinators, Virginia Department of Transportation, 1401 E. Broad St., Richmond, VA 23219, phone 1-804-786-2964 or 2985. For maps, write Virginia Department of Transportation, same address. For information on historic sites and places to visit, write Virginia Tourism, 901 Byrd Street, 19th Floor, Richmond, VA 23219, phone 1-800-VISIT-VA. Bicycles are permitted on all regular park roads and on all designated bicycle trails. There are lots of good back roads in scenic mountain areas, but hiking trails per se are off-limits to bicycles. The Blue Ridge section of the Appalachian chain, the Piedmont plains area, and the Shenandoah Valley are areas of interest. For more information, write Ronald D. Sutton, Commissioner, Department of Conservation and Economic Development, Division of Parks and Recreation, 1201 Washington Building, Capitol Square, Richmond, VA 23219.

WASHINGTON: Mike Dorkfeld, Bicycle Coordinator, Washington Department of Transportation, P.O. Box 47329, Olympia, WA 98504-7329, phone 1-206-753-6095. For maps write to Design Office, 2C11, Washington Department of Transportation, P.O. Box 47329, Olympia, WA 98504-7329, phone 1-206-753-6095. In late spring, summer, and autumn, when it finally stops raining, this state has just about everything an off-road cyclist could want. You like the mountains? Washington gives you Mount Rainier, Mount Baker, Mount Adam, the Cascades, the Olympics, and more. Do you like the seashore? She gives you Puget Sound plus hundreds of miles of ocean-hugging roads. For one great trip take the ferry from Seattle to an island, ride across, then take another ferry up to Vancouver, British Columbia. Do you like rivers? Try cycling along the Columbia River from Vancouver to the great Bonneville Dam. En route, cross the river into Oregon to view famous Multnomah Falls, a breathtaking view if ever there was one. Do you like the narrow, twisting trails of a rain forest? Within 20 miles of Seattle there's one you could get lost in if not careful. In some forests where biking is taboo there are former railroad paths, wagon trails, and other primitive roads that are like a trip back to the eighteenth century. Do you like volcanoes? Bike around Mount St. Helens. What is the state's attitude toward bikes on trails in state parks and forests? In answer to this query, William A. Bush, Chief, Research and Long-Range Planning, Parks and Recreation Commission, 7150 Clearwater Lane, MS KY-11, Olympia, WA 98504, sent me a copy of Chapter 352-20-WAC, regarding use of motor vehicles in state parks. Nowhere in this chapter is a bicycle of any kind mentioned. I can only conclude that there is no restriction on the use of mountain bikes.

Wheeled, operator-propelled equipment such as bicycles, tricycles, scooters, and skateboards are a traditional part of the visitors' recreational use of state parks. Families cycling along park roads and children riding tricycles and "big wheels" are common sights. Some state parks, such as Moran, are popular destinations for bicyclists. Bicycles are even frequently seen on pleasure boats for use as land transportation.

WEST VIRGINIA: Barry Warhoftig, Bicycle Coordinator, West Virginia Department of Transportation, 1900 Washington St. E., Charleston, WV 25305, phone 1-304-0444. For maps, write West Virginia Department of Highways, Planning Division, Map Section, Room 848, 1900 Washington St. E., Charleston, WV 25305. For information on parks and other recreational areas, write West Virginia Division of Tourism and Parks, 2101 Washington St. E., Charleston, WV 25305, phone 1-800-225-5982. West Virginia is a hilly state with lots of mountains. The state is teeming with road and off-road trails and ATB's are welcome, according to Nancy S. Buckingham, Information Representative, West Virginia Department of Commerce. For information on the Greenbrier River Trail and other West Virginia trails, write Nancy at the West Virginia Department of Commerce, 2101 Washington St. E., Charleston, WV 25305. She can also provide a map and listing of all the West Virginia state parks and campgrounds. For info and maps of national parks, write Chief, Eastern Mapping Center, U.S. Geological Survey, 12201 Sunrise Valley Drive, Reston, VA 22042. Or try the commercial tour group, the Elk River Touring Center, Slatyfork, WV 26291, and Blackwater Bikes, The Mountainside Outpost, P.O. Box 190, Davis, WV 26260. Or visit the Snowshoe Mountain Biking Center at the Snowshoe Mountain Resort, P.O. Box 10, Showshoe, WV 26209, phone 1-800-336-7009.

WISCONSIN: Catherine Ratte, Bicycle Coordinator, Wisconsin DOT, Box 7910, Madison, WI 53707, phone 1-608-267-3155. You might also send for the booklet that lists every state park, forest, trail, and recreation area, entitled "Wisconsin State Parks, Forests, Trails and Recreation Areas, Visitors Guide," from the Wisconsin Department of Natural Resources, Box 7921, Madison, WI 53707-7921. Bonnie Gruber, Bureau of Parks and Recreation, Box 7921, Madison, WI 53707, writes: "Enclosed is a review copy of Biking Wisconsin's State Park Trails. This is sold for $3.00 a copy at state parks and other Department of Natural Resources Offices, or for

$3.00 a copy plus $1.00 per order for postage and handling by mail or telephone (MasterCard or Visa) from the Bureau of Parks and Recreation, P.O. Box 7921, Madison, WI 53707, phone 1-608-266-2181. Also included is a list of our trails on former railroad grades. The trails listed as not for bicycling may be used by all-terrain bicycles, but are not surfaced for touring bikes. We also have detailed history/guide books about three trails—Military Ridge, Sugar River, and Bearskin. These are sold for $1.00 each, plus postage and handling, at those trails or the Bureau of Parks and Recreation. Off-road and wilderness trail bike riding is allowed in state parks except where posted. We do not keep a central list of what areas and trails are posted as not allowing bicycles. People interested in bicycling on other than designated bicycle trails should ask at the individual park before starting out. We are considering changing the rule so that bicycling would be prohibited except where posted. Such a change would not be effective until at least 1990. The primary reason for posting trails off-limits to bicycles is conflict with hikers. Silent bicycles coming from behind often startle hikers. The posted trails tend to be ones heavily used by hikers. On the bicycling trails on former railroad grades, bicyclists age 18 or older must have a daily or annual trail pass. These may be purchased at trail headquarters and other DNR offices, at some private businesses near the trails, or from trail rangers. Cyclists camping in the parks must pay campsite fees. Regular campsites are limited to a family with no more than two guests, or no more than five individuals age 7 or older. Many parks have group camp areas for larger groups; see the Visitors Guide. A Special Events Recreational Use License is required for events such as races and bike-a-thons. Forms are available from park superintendents. Sponsors of such an event must be a nonprofit organization and have liability insurance, and the event must be open to the public. An application must be reviewed by the DNR's Bureau of Legal Services before being approved or denied by the park superintendent. For more info write or call me at 1-608-267-7490."

This is one midwestern state that's far from flat, even though it has few mountains worthy of the name, aside from Rib Mountain up north. There's lots of scenic trail riding along the Mississippi River for hundreds of miles; miles of trails in picturesque Door County in the northeast, on Lake Michigan; and the cross-state trail following, in one section, an abandoned railway right-of-way from Kenosha in the east, near Lake Michigan, ending some 350 miles to the west, at La Crosse on the Mississippi.

Wyoming: Kelly Rounds, Bicycle Coordinator, Wyoming Department of Transportation, 5300 Bishop Blvd., P.O. Box 1708, Cheyenne, WY 82002-9019, phone 1-307-777-4180. For information on bike routes, maps and campgrounds, write to the Wyoming Travel Commission, Frank Norris Jr.

Travel Center, Cheyenne, WY 82002. For state maps contact the Public Affairs Office, Wyoming DOT, P.O. Box 1708, Cheyenne, WY 82002-9019, phone 1-307-777-4180. Yellowstone is in Wyoming and bicycles are OK there, but only on roads open to cars as well. This is also true in the Grand Tetons, judged by some to be the most beautiful of all mountain areas in the United States.

Books on National, Regional, and State Bike Trails

Here are just a few of the dozens and dozens of books that plan the route for you, point out areas of interest both scenic and historic, guide you to the best campsites, and more. Books like these roll so frequently off the press that I suggest if you can't find one here that covers the area of your interest check with your library, bookstore, or bike shop.

NICHOLAS CRANE. *Cycling in Europe.* Sparkford, Nr. Yeovil, Somerset, England: The Oxford Illustrated Press.

DON AND LOLLY SKILLMAN. *Pedalling Across America,* 150 pages. A diary of the joys, trials, tribulations, and rewards of their journey from Ashland, Oregon, to Virginia Beach, Virginia. Rewarding reading, with lots of sage advice, for anyone contemplating a bike trip across the United States. Brattleboro, VT: Vitesse Press.

ERIN AND BILL WOODS. *Bicycling the Backroads Around Puget Sound,* 206 pages. A guide to 54 recreational bicycling routes in the Puget Sound basins, from Olympia to the San Juans, from Port Orchard to the Cascades. Has maps and elevation profiles. Seattle, WA: The Mountaineers.

ERIN AND BILL WOODS. *Bicycling the Backroads of Northwest Washington,* 206 pages. Covers routes from Seattle north to lower British Columbia, the Hood Canal side of the Olympic Peninsula, Kitsap Peninsula, and Whidbey Island. Seattle, WA: The Mountaineers.

ERIN AND BILL WOODS. *Bicycling the Backroads Around Southwest Washington.* Gig Harbor to the Columbia River. Seattle, WA: The Mountaineers.

JOHN S. FREIDIN. *25 Bicycle Tours in Vermont,* 174 pages. Mapped and planned tours you can take in this beautiful state. Woodstock, VT: Backcountry Publications.

ERIC TOBEY AND RICHARD WOKLENBURG. *Northeast Bicycle Tours,* 282 pages. Covers 130 planned tours in New York and New England. Maps, location of bike shops, fun places to see and visit, mileage charts, campgrounds. New Canaan, CT: Tobey Publishing Company.

MICHAEL MCCOY. *Mountain Bike Adventures in the Northern Rockies.* ATB trips in Yellowstone, the Sawtooths, Jackson Hole, Sun Valley, Flathead River, the Black Hills, Idaho Panhandle, and the Bighorn Mountains. Covers 40 trips in the exhilaratingly beautiful and wild mountains of the West. Seattle, WA: The Mountaineers.

TOM KIRKENDALL. *Mountain Bike Adventures in Washington's Cascades and Olympics,* 222 pages. Covers over 1,000 miles of legal ATB trail and rural road rides in scenic mountain areas. Seattle, WA: The Mountaineers.

PAUL M. VAN AKEN, JR. *The California Bicycle Tour Atlas and Service.* Bike tours with maps, elevations, campgrounds—the works—the length and breadth of California. Berkeley, CA: Pacific Sports Actualities.

California Coastal Access Guide, 238 pages. If you like bicycling close to the water and camping next to the ocean, and you want to see the whales and other aquatic wildlife, this book is an excellent guide. Published by the University of California Press, for the California Coastal Commission.

MICHAEL H. FARNY. *New England Over the Handlebars,* 174 pages. From Maine to Connecticut, a thorough look at the best *road* bike tours in this historic, scenic part of the eastern states. Boston: Little, Brown.

DAVE GILBERT. *The American Bicycle Atlas,* 268 pages. Over 100 tours covered in detail. This book offers information on where to bike in the United States. New York: American Youth Hostels, Inc., E. P. Dutton.

PHILLIP N. JONES. *Bicycling the Backroads of Northwest Oregon.* Seattle, WA: The Mountaineers.

ERIC NEWBY. *Round Ireland in Low Gear,* 308 pages. Eric Newby and his wife, Wanda, rode their ATBs around Ireland, on the flats and up and down the mountains (hence the title). If you plan a bike trip to Ireland, read this book first. London: William Collins Sons.

RICHARD CRANE AND NICHOLAS CRANE. *Bicycles Up Kilimanjaro,* 156 pages. An ATB saga of a challenge with man and machine on Africa's highest mountain. Riding through snow and over ice can be fun. This book proves it. Sparkford, Nr. Yeovil, Somerset, England: The Oxford Illustrated Press.

THE NATIONAL PARK FOUNDATION. *The Complete Guide to America's National Parks.* Comprehensive data on all 360 U.S. national parks, including maps, mailing addresses, phone numbers, directions, permits, fees, facilities, regulations, weather, points of interest, and more. At $10 a copy, a real bargain. Cost is tax deductible as a contribution to the nonprofit chartered National Park Foundation, P.O. Box 57473, Washington, DC 20037, phone 1-202-785-4500.

HASSE BRUNELLE AND SHIRLEY SARVIS. *Cooking for Camp and Trail.* Camp fare is more than dehydrated foods, as this book will prove. San Francisco: The Sierra Club.

HASSE BRUNELLE AND WINNIE THOMAS. *Food for Knapsackers (and Other Trail Travelers)*. Take this book with you. Lots of excellent data on food, menus, preparation, nutrition, equipment, and recipes. San Francisco: The Sierra Club.

This is but a sampling of the dozens of such books covering almost every country on the globe. For bike touring guides to specific countries, again, see your library, bike store, or camping supply store.

Commercial Bicycle Tour Organizations

There are hundreds of commercial tour providers scattered throughout the United States. Many are small, local outfits, tucked away in a small town or rural location. Which is not to imply that these organizations do not provide a worthwhile service. They do, so far as I can determine. In fact, I believe local tour providers who offer regional tours are to be preferred over some big outfit located in a major city. The local providers know the area, the terrain, the best campsites, restaurants, and other facilities on a first-name basis.

On the other hand, if you want tours in foreign countries, the major tour groups offer the best value, in my opinion. They are usually well-capitalized, have clout with carriers, know the language and, customs problems, can provide visas and whatever else is needed to make your tour a happy, hassle-free vacation on two wheels. A stranded traveler you don't want to be.

Select a tour provider with at least three years' experience in the areas you want to go to, advertises in bicycle and travel publications, and can offer names of clients you can check with.

Here are a few of the professional tour organizers and providers that have been in business for at least three years, most for a lot longer, that appear to be well-financed and adequately staffed. For additional listings, see your travel agency or the classified ads in bicycle magazines, or ask your local bicycle shop for their own experience and referrals.

Tour Providers

These tour providers are but a small sampling of the dozens more such organizations that exist. For additional providers, please see the classified ads in the bicycle publications listed in the Bibliography. You can also subscribe to *Bicycle USA*, a monthly magazine devoted to bicycle touring, which lists many more providers. This is a publication of the League of American Wheelmen, the oldest bicycle club in the United States. Cost is $18 for an individual subscription. Send your subscription to *Bicycle USA*, 6707 Whitestone Rd., Suite 209, Baltimore, MD 21207, phone 1-301-944-3399.

If you would like a singles-only tour group, check with the provider of your choice listed below, because many such groups are available.

Adventure Center: 1311 63rd St., No. 200, Emeryville, CA 94608, phone 1-800-227-8747. Tasmania, Australia, Africa, South America, Thailand, Himalayas.

Adventure Cycling Association: 150 E. Pine St., P.O. Box 8308, Missoula, MT 59807-8308, phone 406-721-1776, FAX 406-721-8754. Criss-cross tours in the United States.

Alaska Bicycle Adventures: 2734 Iliamna Ave., Anchorage, AK 99517, 1-800-770-SAGA. Alaska railroad and glacier cruise.

American Youth Hostels, Inc.: P.O. Box 37613, Washington, DC 20013-7613, phone 1-202-783-6161. Send for their world tour catalog, which lists both U.S. and international tours.

Asian Pacific Adventures: Phone 1-213-935-3156, 1-800-825-1680. China, Nepal, Thailand, India, Malaysia, Indonesia, Pakistan, Vietnam, Cambodia, Laos.

Australian Outbike Tours: 1972 Lascanoas, Santa Barbara, CA 93105, phone 1-805-682-8458.

Back Country Excursions: R.F.D. 365, Limerick, ME 04048, phone 1-207-8189.

Backroads: 1516 5th St., Suite B, Berkeley, CA 94710-1740, phone 1-800-462-2848, FAX 1-510-527-1444. Europe, Asia, North America, the Pacific.

Bicycle Adventures: P.O. Box 7875, Olympia, WA 98507, phone 1-206-786-0989, 1-800-443-6060, FAX 1-206-786-9661. The premium tour group specializing in the Pacific Northwest. Very well-equipped on every front. Experienced group leaders. I suggest you start with their tour of Puget Sound's San Juan Islands. Offers bike tours for singles, which I think are a great idea! Has tours in Hawaii and in California's wine and redwood country.

Bike America: P.O. Box 29, Northfield, MN 55057, phone 1-507-663-1268. Major tour outfit, specializes in tours coast-to-coast in the United States, tours in various states.

Bike & Cruise: P.O. Box 69252, Portland, OR 97201, phone 1-503-226-1250. Puget Sound, Barbados, Martinique, Antigua, St. Thomas, Aruba, Curacao, Virgin Islands,

Bike Riders, Inc.: P.O. Box 254, Boston, MA 02113, phone 1-800-473-7040, FAX 1-617-723-2355. Italy, Prince Edward Island, Rhode Island, Massachusetts, Canada, Asia, Australia, New Zealand, Bali, Ireland, you name it and they go there, most likely. This is a major tour provider. Extremely well-organized and -equipped. Singles tours also; 106-page color catalog.

Brooks Country Cycling: 140 West 83rd St., New York, NY 10024, phone 1-212-8744-5151, FAX 1-212-874-5286. New England, France, Holland, Louisiana, North Carolina, Florida, Canada.

Canusa Cycling Tours: P.O. Box 45, Okotoks, Alberta, Canada T0L-1T0, phone 1-403-560-5859.

Ciclismo Classico: 65 Cady Lane, Woodstock, CT 06281, phone 1-800-866-7314, FAX 1-617-628-2041. Italy, Sardinia, Spain, Elba, Corsica.

Classic Adventures: P.O. Box 153, Hamlin, NY 14464-0153, phone 1-800-777-8090, 716-964-8488. Greece, Holland, France, Ireland, Scotland, Germany, Quebec, Nova Scotia, Prince Edward Island, Erie Canal, Virginia, Natchez Trace, Missouri.

Covered Bridges Bicycle Tours: P.O. Box 693, Saint John, New Brunswick, Canada E2L 4B3, phone 1-506-849-9028. New Brunswick, Nova Scotia, Prince Edward Island.

Cycle America: P.O. Box 485, Cannon Falls, MN 55009, phone 1-800-245-3263. United States coast-to-coast, Rockies, Texas, Bahamas, California, Grand Canyon, Minnesota, Wisconsin, Michigan, Ohio.

Cycling Through the Centuries: P.O. Box 877, San Antonio, FL 33576, 1-800-245-4226. Tours in Portugal, Spain, Denmark, England, and France.

EB Tours, West Virginia: Phone 1-800-231-9113.

Encompass Cycling Vacations: P.O. Box 3461, Madison, WI 53704, phone 1-608-249-4490. Also tours in southern states and the Midwest.

EuroBike Tours: P.O. Box 990, DeKalb, IL 60115, phone 1-800-321-6060, FAX 1-815-758-8851. Austria, Belgium, Denmark, England, France, Germany, Holland, Hungary, Ireland, Italy, Luxembourg, Portugal, Spain, Sweden, and Switzerland.

Europeds: 761 Lighthouse Ave., Monterey, CA 93940, phone 1-800-321-9552, FAX 1-408-655-4501. France, Spain, Costa Rica.

Excursions Extraordinaires: P.O. Box 3493, Eugene OR 97403, phone 1-800-678-2252, 1-503-484-0493. Oregon.

Gerhard's Bicycle Odysseys: P.O. Box 757, Portland, OR 97207, phone 1-503-223-2402. Switzerland, Ireland, Norway, Luxembourg, Germany, France, Austria, Czech Republic.

Goulash Tours: Box 2972, Kalamazoo, MI 49003, phone 1-616-349-8817. Moscow to St. Petersburg, other trips through Russia.

Green Mountain Two-Wheel: RR 2, Box 858, Woodstock, VT 05091, phone 1-802-457-3602.

Italian Cycling Center: 2117 Green St., Philadelphia, PA 19130-3110, phone 1-215-232-6772.

KoloTour: P.O. Box 1493, Dept. BG, Boulder Creek, CA 95006-1493, phone 1-800-524-7099. Czech Republic tours.

Lincoln Guide Service: 152 Lincoln Rd., Lincoln, MA 01773-0100, phone 1-617-259-1111.

NZ Pedal Tours: 522 29th Ave. S., Seattle, WA 98144, phone 1-206-323-2080, FAX 1-206-727-6597. New Zealand.

Paradise Bike Tours: P.O. Box 1726, Evergreen, CO 80439, phone 1-800-626-8271. Africa, Belize.

Rocky Mountain Cycle Tours: Box 1978-B3, Canmore, Alberta, Canada, T0L 0M0, phone 1-800-661-2453. Europe, Canadian Rockies, Hawaii.

Sobek Expeditions: Angels Camp, CA 95222. America's premier tour provider. Tours in the United States and abroad to just about any country you can name.

Steve Wineke: Halfway, OR 97834, phone 1-503-742-5722. A small but experienced local tour provider located in the scenic Hells Canyon district of eastern Oregon.

Student Hostelling Program: Ashfield Rd., Conway, MA 01341, phone 1-800-343-6132.

Timberline Bicycle Tours: 7975 E. Harvard, No. J, Denver, CO 80231, phone 1-303-759-3804. Glacier, Yellowstone, Colorado, Canadian Rockies, Oregon coast, Cascades, Puget Sound, California wine country, Sierras, Nova Scotia, Prince Edward Island.

Tim Kneeland & Associates: 200 Lake Washington Blvd., Suite 101, Seattle, WA 98122-6540, phone 1-206-322-4102, 1-800-433-0528, FAX 1-206-322-4509. Transcontinental rides, coast to coast, western United States, across Canada, England, Australia.

Ultimate Bicycle Tours: 1123 No. 1, Los Palos Dr., Salinas, CA 93901, phone 1-800-347-6136.

Van Gogh Bicycle Tours: P.O. Box 57, Winchester, MA 01890, phone 1-800-435-6192, FAX 1-617-721-0850. Holland.

Vermont Bicycle Touring: Box 711-JG, Bristol, VT 05443, phone 1-802-453-4811. *The* premium tour provider in New England, also conducts tours overseas. A very professional outfit, in business 17 years.

Vermont Country Cyclers: P.O. Box 145, Waterbury Center, VT 05677, phone 1-802-453-4811. United States, Canada, Europe, South Pacific.

Worldwide/Rocky Mountain Cycle Tours: P.O. Box 1978, Canmore, Alberta, Canada, T0L 0M0, phone 1-800-661-2453, FAX 1-403-678-4451. Hawaii, France, Italy, Germany, Austria, Switzerland, Norway, Canadian Rockies.

How to Carry a Load Safely on Your Bike

I am indebted to Jim Blackburn of Bell Sports for providing the material below, entitled "The Weight Factor," which he and Jim Gentes wrote, on weight distribution on a bicycle and how it affects bicycle handling and stability. As you read this material please refer to Fig. 10-10, which shows weight distribution, with low-rise carriers and panniers in front that keep load weights in the rear as low as possible.

The Weight Factor

If you must put weight on a bicycle, where is the best and safest place? We could not find comprehensive data on this important subject, so we decided to find out for ourselves. We approached our project in three basic, consecutive steps:

1. Research existing relevant data.
2. Test a bicycle loaded in various ways.
3. Construct the optimum system for carrying weight on a bicycle.

Most available material on how bicycles handle is concerned with their basic dynamics. Of particular interest is the acute relationship between rider and bicycle. The bicycle is stable only because of the rider's ability to constantly correct his line of direction. This led us to the realization that any weight should be carried in a position that will cause the least interference with the cyclist's ability to correct and balance the bicycle.

Test Procedures

Four panniers and a handlebar bag loaded with a total of 80 pounds of sand were used, and 17 different load combinations were tried. We do not recommend carrying this much weight. We went to what we considered the maximum for test purposes only. Each combination was run through a slalom course. If deemed stable enough, the loaded bike was ridden down a high-speed downhill course.

Characteristics considered were high-speed stability, standing and hill-climbing stability, cornering ability, and how well the bicycle tracked. Proper heel-to-bag clearance was always a consideration.

Our overall goal was to find the optimum weight position for maximum touring performance and safety. The testing was of a general nature. Different bicycles may show some variance from our test results. The following four tests proved to be the most interesting.

Test 1: *Large rear panniers with a large handlebar bag. No front carrier.*

This is the most commonly seen combination. With this setup most of the weight is behind the rear-wheel center axis. This in combination with a large, heavy handlebar bag tends to create a shimmy effect on the front wheel. The only way we could control this load was to keep the bike at a slow speed. We were unable to conduct the downhill portion of this test.

TEST 2: *Equal weight in front and rear panniers. Small handlebar bag.*

This system has become more popular recently. The bicycle weight proportion is kept constant, and severe changes in handling characteristics were not observed. There is a tendency to oversteer with 40 pounds of weight up front, but the feeling remains very solid. The results of this test were much better than those of Test 1.

Test 3: *Weight carried low on both front and rear panniers. Small handlebar bag.*

The basic assumption made here is that the lower the weight, the lower the center of gravity, and thus better handling. Not true! To gain necessary rotating heel clearance the rear bags must be placed behind the rear-wheel center axis. A whipping action occurs from the leverage effect of weight carried too far to the rear. The carrier must be heavier, being structurally larger, yet it cannot be as rigid. Each rotation of the crank arms creates an oscillation that is difficult for the rider to compensate for.

Placing weight low in front is much easier to accomplish. After trying several positions, we found that low and centered in the wheel works best for front weight. Overall, the low front/low rear combination does not handle well, and we do not recommend it.

Test 4: *Standard position for rear weight with low front weight. Small handlebar bag.*

Medium-size panniers mounted as far forward as possible on the rear carrier and medium-size bags mounted low on the front forks in the center of the wheel was by far the best system. This combination gave the best handling with heavy weight. The bicycle responds more slowly this way than it does with no weight at all, but in most cases is actually more stable. The result is similar to increasing the fork rake or head angle. Rotating heel clearance is maintained, and no frame whip was noted. Downhill runs were safe and steering felt secure.

Conclusions

Though our study emphasized performance and safety, some other factors must be taken into account. Most items will readily fit into pannier bags. Sleeping rolls and pads are usually attached to the top of the rack. A small, light handlebar bag is handy for personal items such as maps, cameras, snacks, or wallets. The bicycle's main triangle is an excellent place for weight, but is too limited a space. It is usual practice to carry water bottles and a frame pump here.

When weight is carried where the bicycle handles it best, your ride or tour is much more enjoyable and a great deal safer. Balanced weight distribution results in fewer mechanical failures, less tire wear, and fewer bothersome flat tires or broken spokes.

Recommendations

Of the 17 combinations tested, only two met our standards. Number 2, with medium-size panniers in front and rear, works well (Fig. 10-9). Number 4, with medium-size rear bags held at regular height and as far forward as possible combined with medium-size bags held securely in the low middle of the front wheel, was easily the best system of all (Fig. 10-10).

Now let's go to the health and happiness aspects of bicycling, including what it does for your sex life and for the prevention of aches and pains that come with an active life and the aging process.

References for the Weight Factor Section

People
Brown, Glenn, Designer/Engineer.
Gentes, Al, Mechanical Engineer, Lockheed Missile and Space Co.
Klein, Gary, Bicycle Frame Manufacturer/Engineer.

FIG. 10-9: A good way to balance the load on a bike trip is to keep carriers and panniers as low as possible. *Courtesy Bell Sports, Inc.*

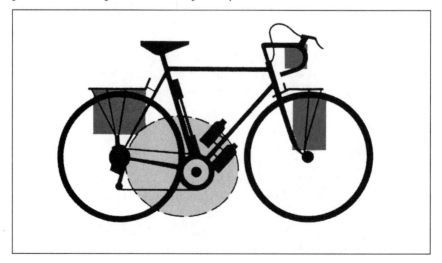

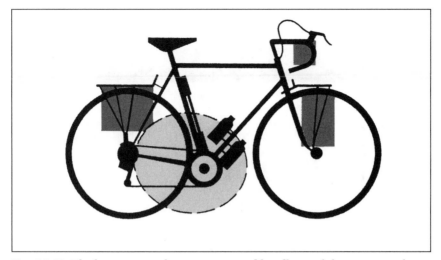

FIG. 10-10: The best way to achieve steering and handling stability is to use a low-rider front carrier as shown here. *Courtesy Bell Sports, Inc.*

Wilson, David Gordon, Professor, Mechanical Engineering, M.I.T., coauthor of *Bicycling Science.*
Wood, Phil, Mechanical Engineer, President, Phil Wood and Co.

Articles
"Dynamics of a Bicycle Non-gyroscopic Aspects." J. Liesang and A. R. Lee, *American Physics* 46: 130–32 F 78.
"Stability and Control of Motorcycles," R.E.S. Sharp, *Journal of Mechanical Engineering Science*, Vol. 13, No. 5, 1971.
"Steady State Cornering of Two-Wheeled Vehicles," A. L. Krauter, *Journal of Applied Mechanics* 40: 819–21 S 73.
"The Stability of the Bicycle," David E. H. Jones, *Physics Today* 23: 34–40 AP 70.

Book
Bicycling Science, Frank Rowland Witt with David Gordon Wilson, Cambridge, MA: M.I.T. Press.

CHAPTER ELEVEN

BICYCLING FOR A HAPPY, HEALTHY BODY

Bicycling is great exercise! It keeps your body flexible, your muscles firm, and your tummy taut. Best of all, cycling is a stress-free way to lifelong health. You can tailor a workout to fit your physical condition and age, without risk of overdoing it or of damage to joints or muscles. You can pedal slowly if you're just beginning a physical fitness program, or faster if you're already in good shape and want to stay that way. Bicycling strengthens your heart, helps reduce blood pressure if it's too high, improves the ability of your lungs to deliver oxygen to your muscles, and keeps your energy level up all day. Combined with a sensible diet, bicycling is a terrific way to lose weight and stay slender. Here's why bicycling is good for your heart, muscles, and lungs.

First, bicycling is second only to swimming as a calorie expender (see Table 11-1). But what kind of scenery do you see whizzing up and down a swimming pool? Biking is a lot more fun and more enjoyable than swimming, at least for me.

Weight Control

You can lose weight by combining a sensible low-calorie diet with cycling exercise. For example, let's say you weigh 180 pounds and you'd like to lose 30 pounds. If you have a sedentary job, you need about 15 calories per pound of body weight, or 2,700 calories a day ($15 \times 180 = 2,700$), just to keep your 180 pounds. If you ride a bike 10 miles per hour for one hour, you'll consume 360 to 420 of your unwanted calories (see Table 11-2). Of course, how many calories you burn depends on the energy you expend. For example, Table 11-2 shows that the faster you bicycle the more calories you use up. The table does not relate energy to hill climbing, but I am sure that if you go over the

TABLE 11-1: CALORIES USED BY TYPE OF EXERCISE

(Calories Expended per 20 Minutes)

TYPE OF EXERCISE	CALORIES USED
Swimming	240
Bicycling	220
Fast jogging	210
Handball	200
Rowing, kayaking, canoeing	180
Cross-country skiing	180
Downhill skiing	160
Tennis	160
Dancing	160
Vigorous gardening	140
Gym workouts, gymnastics	140
Walking briskly	100
Golfing (walking between holes)	90
Slow walking, sauntering, window shopping	60

TABLE 11-2: BICYCLE SPEED AND CALORIC USE

CALORIES PER HOUR	MILES PER HOUR
240–300	6
300–360	8
360–420	10
420–480	11
480–600	12
600–660	13

Rockies, for example, even at six miles per hour, you will burn energy at least at the 11-mph rate. If you keep the same pace into a stiff headwind you use more calories, and of course fewer calories if there's a breeze at your back. Drop your daily caloric intake to 2,500 and you'll save another 250 calories— that's a daily total reduction of 610 to 670 calories. Since each pound of body fat is equivalent to 3,500 calories, you need to lose over time 105,000 calories (30 × 3,500) to reach your target 150 pounds.

Diet plus biking can do it in about six months ([105,000 ÷ 600] ÷ 30 = 5.8). By then your heart will be stronger, your blood pressure down, energy level up, and you'll be able to ride your bike farther and faster than you ever thought possible. Compare your weight today with the ideal weight for your age and sex, shown in Table 11-3.

Pedal Exercise and Your Heart

Cycling helps make your heart stronger so it can pump more blood at a slower rate and so work less stressfully even when you're exercising hard.

TABLE 11-3: AVERAGE WEIGHT BY HEIGHT AND SEX

Height	Weight: Men	Weight: Women
4'10"		98–119
4'11"		101–122
5'0"		104–125
5'1"		107–128
5'2"	120–141	110–131
5'3"	123–144	113–134
5'4"	126–148	116–138
5'5"	129–152	119–142
5'6"	133–156	123–146
5'7"	137–161	127–150
5'8"	141–166	131–154
5'9"	145–166	131–154
5'10"	150–174	140–163
5'11"	154–179	144–168
6'0"	158–184	148–173
6'1"	162–189	
6'2"	167–194	
6'3"	171–199	

Many racing cyclists, for example, have a resting pulse rate as low as 45 beats per minute. If you have been sitting still while reading this book, stop now and measure your pulse rate. If it's much over 75 beats a minute it's working too hard for this sedentary activity. The higher the pulse rate the higher your blood pressure (not, of course, the only reason for high blood pressure). *Bicycling helps keep your blood pressure at a healthy low level.* It takes muscles to sustain the workout that drives your heartbeat up to your threshold aerobic rate for at least 30 minutes. Your heart should pump blood efficiently and at a high enough rate to reduce the buildup of fatty substances on artery walls (atherosclerosis) that contributes to high blood pressure. It's a good idea to have your blood pressure checked once in a while. As a ballpark figure, a blood pressure of 120/60 is great if you're under 30. If it's much over 160/95, ask your physician to set up an exercise regimen, using your bike, to bring it down. Blood pressure varies with age, so a pressure that's a health hazard at, say, 30 may be perfectly normal at age 50 or above.

A stress test at your local hospital is an excellent way to assure yourself that you can safely exercise for hours at your threshold aerobic level. In a stress test you're hooked up to an electrocardiogram (EKG) monitor. Then you start walking on a treadmill (Fig. 11-1). A physician or trained medtech watches the EKG readout. The treadmill is gradually sped up until your pace brings your heart rate to your maximum aerobic capacity. The EKG chart will spot any abnormalities in your heart as it pumps away at full blast.

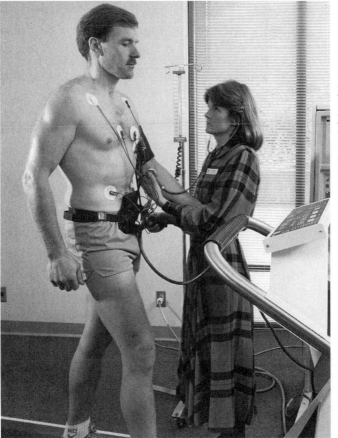

FIG. 11-1: Take a stress test at your local hospital to check your cardiovascular conditioning before you embark on vigorous bicycling. Here a medical technician is monitoring the subject's heart rate and blood pressure during the test.

Once you get a clean bill of health from such a stress test you can pedal away as hard as you wish *provided* you have built up the muscles needed to do it. See Table 11-4 for maximum/minimum aerobic heartbeat rates by age when exercising. You can keep tabs on your heart rate with a monitor you wear on your wrist (Fig. 11-2). This monitor is made by Polar CIC, Inc., 99 Seaview Blvd., Port Washington, NY 11050, phone 1-800-227-1314 (ask for

FIG. 11-2: On a bike or on an exerciser, use a heart monitor such as the Polar model shown here, so you know when you have reached your aerobic maximum.

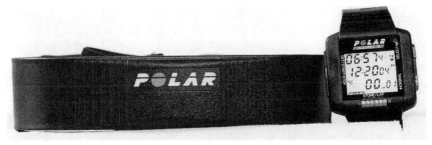

TABLE 11-4: MAXIMUM/MINIMUM SAFE AEROBIC HEARTBEAT RATE BY AGE

AGE	HEARTBEATS PER MINUTE (85%)	HEARTBEATS PER MINUTE (65%)
15	174	133
20	170	130
25	166	127
30	162	124
35	157	120
40	153	117
45	149	114
50	145	111
55	140	107
60	136	104
65	132	101
70	128	98
75	123	94
80	119	91
85	115	88

their article comparing palpated heart rates and heart rates using their monitor). You will be cheered to know that a study of college men showed that heart attack rates were 50 percent lower in men expending more than 2,000 calories a week in exercise than for men expending less than 500 calories a week.

Cycling Makes You Healthier (Maybe Even Wealthier and Wiser)

You can tailor exercise on your bike to match your level of physical fitness. First, find your level of fitness by consulting your doctor. Work your way up from a soft body to one with muscle and energy to spare. If you've just bought a bike but haven't engaged in regular physical exercise, start out by cycling slowly, say at a pedal cadence of 60 rpm (spinning a pedal 60 times per minute) on the flats. Stay off steep hills. Pedal for 20 or 30 minutes. Don't push it, or you could tear a muscle, which can be painful and keep you off the bike for a couple of weeks. In a half hour you should ride about three to four miles (pretty slow, but you'll be able to sustain more speed as you shape up).

If you've been ill with, say, the flu and have been bedridden or housebound, be aware that even if you *were* in good shape it takes twice as long to get back in shape as it did for you to lose your conditioning. For example, if you were laid up for two weeks it's going to take a month of steadily increasing workout to get back to your pre-illness physical condition. Please note, too, that you should *never* stop exercising, no matter what your age.

If you stop, you lose body strength fast. That's why there seems so little connection between athletic prowess as a youth and health and a long life when you get older.

Beginning a Bicycle Fitness Program

After a few weeks of daily slow and easy pedaling, gradually increase your pedal cadence to 70 rpm and try a few easy hills, say of no more than 5 percent grade (check your local highway or road department for the grade, if you wish). Now you're ready for an aerobically significant workout. There are two levels of aerobic activity, the maximum level and the threshold level. The maximum level is based on your age (assuming a reasonable level of physical fitness) and is a heartbeat rate that you should not exceed, certainly not without your doctor's approval. Calculate your maximum heart count by subtracting your age from 220. For example, if you're 30 years old, your maximum pulse rate will be 220 minus 30, or 190. Check this with your doctor. The threshold level is a heart rate you can safely maintain in exercise, and is generally taken to be 75 percent of your maximum rate, although some athletes prefer 85 percent. I'd stick to the lower, 75 percent rate. If your maximum heart rate for your age is 190 beats per minute, your threshold level would be 190 times 0.75, which is 142 beats per minute. If your pulse rate does not reach 142 beats per minute, you are not working hard enough to get the full health benefits from the time you spend exercising. If you're riding a stationary exerciser and reach your aerobic threshold, you should be bathed in sweat and feeling great after a 30-minute workout. I should point out that cycling is a *lot* easier on leg joints, particularly knees, than jogging. A less stressful exercise is swimming, but I can't say that does much for your leg muscles. At least it never has for mine. But if you grip the handlebars, bear down and pull up (slightly) as you ride, you'll strengthen and tone upper-body muscles as well as those of legs and thighs. You can buy a bike computer in most bike stores that will give you a readout of pedal cadence, mph, elapsed time, and trip and accumulated mileage.

Warmups and Stretches Before You Ride (Preventive Exercises)

Watch a cat when it wakes from a nap. Notice how it stretches one leg after the other. That's what you should do before you take off on a bike ride. Your muscles are made of intercrossed fibers. When you have been idle, these fibers tend to stick together. Unstick them before a ride, so muscle fibers don't "tear" and cause painful injuries. Warmups and stretches also increase blood supply to the muscles, along with the oxygen and nutrients your muscles need. Ease into warmups and stretches. Stretch slowly but firmly. If you feel pain as you stretch, slow down. If pain persists and increases, something is wrong. See your doctor to make sure nothing has been damaged. When you begin cycling take it easy for the first 5 to 10 minutes to give your heart time to pump blood and oxygen to your muscles.

Neck and shoulders: Road bikers are prone to neck pain because they ride hunched over the handlebars. Before riding, loosen neck muscles by rolling your head first one way, then the other way (Fig. 11-3).

Quadriceps and lower back: If you have ever experienced the painful cramps known as a charley horse you know what this pain can feel like when it comes from the quads. Avoid such pain by preride stretching (Fig. 11-4) to keep them supple. Assume the position in Fig. 11-4, lift your buttocks off the floor and twist your lower back. Hold for 10 seconds and repeat for the other side. You should feel the muscle in the top of your thigh and in the muscles of your lower back s-t-r-e-t-c-h as you make these moves.

Hamstrings: Lower-back pain often comes from a tight, tensed hamstring. Help prevent this pain by sitting on the floor, then drawing one leg up close to your body, with the foot placed against the opposite leg (Fig. 11-5). Stretch your arms forward to the foot of the outstretched leg as far as you can without a lot of pain. Hold for 10 seconds. Repeat with the other leg.

An excellent back support is made by WRS See Fig. 9-25 for more information.

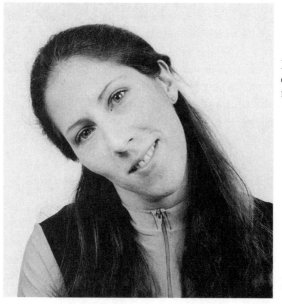

FIG. 11-3: Use this stretch exercise to loosen neck muscles.

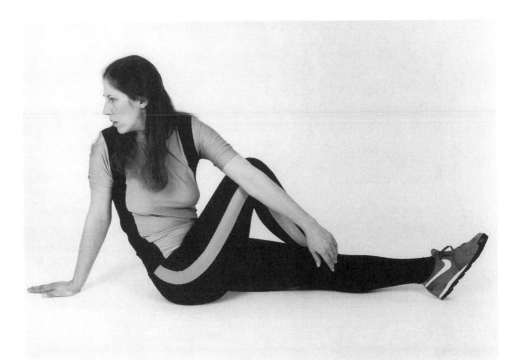

FIG. 11-4: Stretch your quads to prevent later strain and muscle pain.

FIG. 11-5: This hamstring stretch helps prevent lower-back pain.

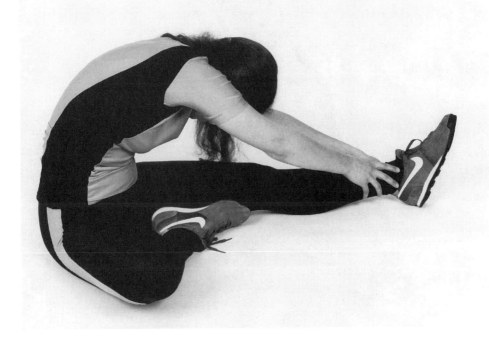

Calf and Achilles tendon: The Achilles tendon should be well stretched before any ride. Just grab the back of a chair (Fig. 11-6), place your feet as shown in Fig. 11-6, bend forward at the knee, hold for 15 seconds. Repeat with the other leg. You should feel definite stretching in the long muscle in the back of each leg as you perform this exercise.

Knee Problems

I am just going to cover the basics here, but if you have knee problems your best bet is to see a good orthopedic sports medicine physician as soon as possible. What you don't need is bone-to-bone contact from torn or worn cartilage, for example. Here are the four most common knee problems faced by bicyclists. As Fig. 11-7 shows, the knee joint is a sort of hinge between the two major bones of the leg, the femur, or thigh bone, and the tibia. The knee

FIG. 11-6: Stretch your Achilles tendon and calf for supple pedaling.

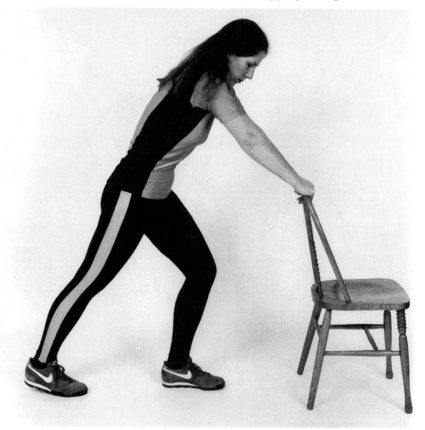

gives you a range of motion between squatting (flexion) and standing tall (extension). Your leg bones also articulate to permit rotational movement. Ligaments tie the upper and lower leg together and thus provide stability to the joint in all directions. The patella, a small oval disk of bone at the front of the knee, prevents the knee from overextending. Bone-to-bone contact of the femur and tibia (see Fig. 11-7) is prevented by a layer of cartilage between the bones. Frictionless movement of the knee joint is provided by bursae (fluid-filled sacs), which line the knee itself.

Patellar tendinitis relates to much pain felt just *below* the kneecap (the patellar). The pain is due to overstrain, as from pedaling in too high gear, particularly uphill. Tendons and ligaments become inflamed. In my case the pain occurs after I have been riding for a couple of hours. A solution that works for me is to ease the pressure on the affected leg, apply cold when I get home, and if necessary not ride for a couple of weeks.

FIG. 11-7: Cross-section of a knee shows some of the places where pain can occur.

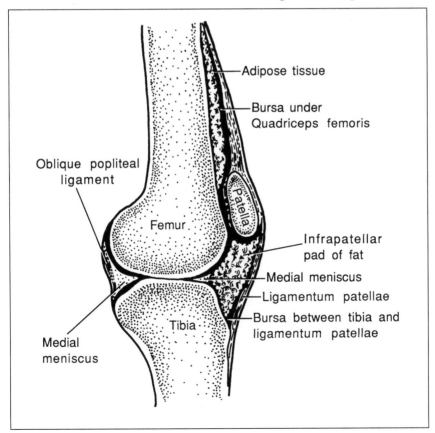

Chondromalacia brings pain to the *front* of the knee. It comes, like patellar tendinitis, from overuse. Sometimes you can feel pain when hiking, walking uphill, or just sitting still. Pain can also come from the side of the knee, usually the left side, or you could feel a grinding sensation in the joint. Eventually the cartilage can break down. Chondromalacia is a degenerative ailment that usually affects the cartilage behind the kneecap. This painful affliction can be caused by overstress, such as the use of too high a gear on a hill climb, or by too high a saddle, which can overextend the knee, which drives the patella against the femur. One solution is to see your sports medicine doctor for exercises that will strengthen thigh muscles, so the knee will have better support when stressed.

Iliotibial band injury can bring intense and continuous pain. The injury is usually due to inflammation of the tendon, caused again by overuse or by a genetic mechanical defect. If ice and anti-inflammatory drugs don't help, you may need surgery.

The hamstring is the tendon on the back side of your knee. Hamstring pain is reminiscent of muscle cramps. You may have your saddle up too high. Again, try ice therapy. And check the warmup stretch given earlier in this chapter.

For any of these knee problems, you might try an Ultra-Active Patellar knee support (Fig. 9-26). The support comes in four sizes from small to extra-large. Available from your bike shop or call WRS SportsMed at 1-800-299-3366 for a local outlet.

Other Physical Problems

Now that you have read and passed the course on Knees 101, let's look at other sources of pain that can afflict bicyclists.

Numb hands are a common complaint of bicyclists. The numb feeling is caused by compression of the hands and of the nerves in the hands. Try changing hand position on dropped handlebars, or shift your weight off your hands or from the palm of your hands up near the base of your fingers. Steer with one hand while you shake the wrist of your other hand, and repeat with the opposite hand, to get blood flowing in your palms.

Carpal tunnel syndrome is an injury to the median nerve that traverses the palm of your hand. If you have persistent swelling and pain in the palm you could have this problem. Carpal tunnel syndrome is most likely in people between 30 and 60 and is five times more common among women than among men. If you are wakened at night by pain, tingling, and numbness in the palm of your hand, carpal tunnel syndrome may be the culprit. As you may guess, carpal tunnel syndrome can afflict dedicated bicyclists who put in long hours gripping the handlebars. If you suspect carpal tunnel syndrome you should see a physician who can do an electromyogram (EMG), in which electrical impulses are sent down the median nerve. You can get some relief from this type of pressure-generated pain with a pair of bike riding gloves designed for carpal tunnel syndrome patients (Fig. 9-29). For more information on these gloves and where they can be purchased write A. Robert Spitzer, M.D., at 3535 W. Thirteen Mile Road, Suite 305, Royal Oak, MI 48073, phone 1-313-551-0615. Dr. Spitzer is a specialist in neurological disorders who designed these gloves. His gloves are padded, except where the median nerve runs through the palm of your hand. The idea is to relieve pressure on this sensitive area. (The white dots in Fig. 9-29 are my own doing just to show the area of pressure relief.)

Neck and shoulder pain can be crippling on a long bike ride. The pain is more common on road bike dropped handlebars than on mountain bike flat handlebars, because on downturned handlebars you have to tilt your head back while your torso leans forward, so you can see the road ahead. Neck and shoulder pain and tension can be a real bother from this tilt position. Relieve this pressure on neck and shoulder muscles by moving the stem up until it is about an inch below the saddle, thereby reducing the bend in your neck. You might also try a shorter stem, which will let you assume a more upright riding position, which won't be as aerodynamic as your old crouch lean, but hey, you want to keep riding without pain. Also use stretch exercises before and after riding, as described earlier in this chapter. Another good way to relieve the type of neck pain associated with the head tilt position is to install a new product, a forward viewing mirror called a Windcheeta (Figs. 8-14 and 8-15). This unit uses two mirrors, one to show a view of the road ahead, the other to reflect that view up to you.

Saddle sores (aka hurting bums) are quite common among bicyclists. New cyclists on a long trip seem particularly prone to this affliction. What happens is that your "sit bones" (aka ischial tuberosities) and your thighs are moving vigorously and even rubbing on the saddle. Shorts lined in the crotch area with a protective layer of soft leather such as chamois can be a big help in preventing skin chafing. Don't wear underwear under cycling shorts, because it can bunch up and cause more chafing. Talcum power can help when applied to your crotch area. If you develop sores and boils be sure to wash the area frequently with warm water and soap to kill skin bacteria. I also recommend you use one of the chafe-resistant saddle covers made by WRS

SportsMed, or switch to a leather saddle that will eventually conform to your body dimensions.

Male bottom problems include, besides those I just mentioned, blood in the semen after a long hard ride. While you should see your doctor about this, don't be too alarmed. Blood in the semen is rare but does occur after a long hard ride. But it can also indicate a prostate problem, so see your urologist about it.

If you have prostatitis, characterized by a swollen prostate and difficulty in urinating, long bike rides can worsen the condition and bring on additional symptoms. If you have had prostate surgery, such as a transurethral resection (TURP), a sort of roto-rooting of the urethra so urine can flow more readily and without urine retention, you should not ride your bicycle for a couple of weeks. There is, however, no medical evidence that bicycling *causes* prostate problems, though it can worsen an existing problem. Warm baths, padded cycling shorts, and a saddle that takes pressure away from the crotch can be helpful. Don't let prostate problems keep you from bicycling! However, if you are 50 or over you should have an annual check for prostate cancer by a urologist, which should include a PSA (prostate-specific antigen) blood test that can reveal the presence of cancer cells. If further tests reveal such cancer, and you have your prostate removed (and have the nerve-sparing procedure that keeps your sex life alive), there is no reason not to start bicycling again a few months after the surgery. Your author can testify both to the efficacy of the nerve-sparing procedure and, once healing is complete, to the ability to keep right on pedaling!

Women and Bicycling

Women need a different shape and size of saddle than men need. Many women, for example, experience pubic-area pain on a saddle that is really designed for men, which comes on most bicycles. Women have sit bones about a half-inch farther apart than men's sit bones, so women need a saddle that's wider in the rear. Women also need a saddle with a shorter nose that reduces pressure on the pubic bone, particularly when riding with road bike dropped handlebars. You might also move the saddle so it is flat, parallel to the ground, and not tilting upward. Switch to a saddle with a gel area that absorbs road shock and that is about seven inches across the rear.

Pregnant women can ride, even strenuously, during the first two trimesters of pregnancy after checking with the doctor. Ride on a mountain bike so you ride in a more upright position than on your road bike. If morning sickness during early pregnancy is a problem, eat more calories before you ride and drink water copiously as you ride. Active women who are in good shape also seem to have easier deliveries than less active women. However, if pregnancy interferes with reaching the handlebars I suggest it's time to stop until the baby is born. You could also use a baby jogger (Fig. 11-8) as you get back in shape after childbirth.

Bicycling and Cancer

Now there's a really nasty word. The question is, can bicycling reduce the likelihood of cancer? Bicycling can indeed reduce stress. But you need to know when you are stressed, or what life situations can raise your stress to cancer-causing levels and then take steps to change your life.

FIG. 11-8: Run with your child with a racing buggy.

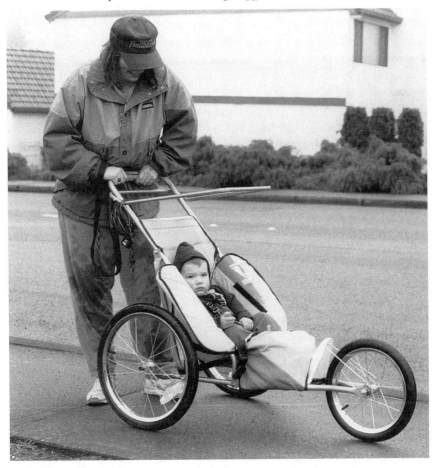

Muscles Protect Your Joints

When I started biking regularly, way back in the olden days, the mid-1960s, my right knee hurt a lot. This knee had been injured in a football accident in high school many years before. The pain became so intense I consulted an orthopedic surgeon, who determined, after X-ray and arthroscopic examination, that I had torn a major knee cartilage. My doctor said that if I wanted to avoid becoming a cripple in my old age I should give up cycling. So I did, with great reluctance. I went out and bought a good pair of shoe roller skates, the kind with plastic wheels, and began roller skating to work. He hadn't said anything about not skating.

Each day I skated past the *Chicago Tribune* office. Finally one of my reporter friends spotted this stock exchange executive in a business suit on his skates and ran a short story with a photo about this phenomenon. My orthopedist phoned that day and advised that, all things considered, I was, after all, better off on the bike. Those were the days before sports medicine had become a medical specialty and before doctors realized that strong muscle tissue around bad knees can compensate for such knee damage as mine. So I hung up the skates, got back on the bike, and eventually found that by cycling gently, and with more pressure from my good left leg, I built up supportive muscles around the right knee and the pain disappeared.

I should add that cycling leads to balanced muscles, so that use, or lack of use, of one set of muscles won't lead to painful tears in another set. For example, I was back on the bike after nearly a month off from a bad case of flu. It was springtime, and I tucked in behind a lovely young woman dressed in cycling togs. She must have seen me, because she began to speed up a bit. No woman was going to leave *me* behind, no sirree. So I stayed with her. The next day was filled with pain, which lasted two weeks and kept me off the bike during that period. What happened was that the adductor muscles, which control the twist or turning of the leg, were torn by the undue stress of my admittedly chauvinistic behavior. They were not strong enough to compensate for the stronger muscles that pushed my leg up and down. It took over two months to build up all my leg muscles so they were equally strong.

Bicycling and Your Sex Life

When I first began long-distance touring about 20 years ago I thought that by the end of an 80-mile day I would be too worn out to even think about, much yet actually have, a sex life. Well, folks, I can only say that once one is in good physical shape, both parts of that last sentence are untrue. The feeling of well-being after a day on the saddle extended well into the evening. Medical research indicates that men in good physical condition show a greater rise in testosterone levels after vigorous exercise than do nonathletic males. Keith Kingbay, one of the most knowledgeable bicycle experts I have ever met, reported in an issue of the *League of American Wheelmen Journal* about a 117-year-old man in Kuala Lumpur, Malaysia, who cycled 27 miles to "pay the fine of a 40-year-old woman who was imprisoned for living with him out of wedlock." They were both Moslems. He had been married 17 times, she was married and so could not marry him, but later did so after a divorce. There's a moral here, somewhere.

Cycling Slows Age-Related Osteoporosis

As you age, calcium tends to leave your bones, so they become more brittle and break easily. I had X-rays taken a few years ago and my doctor remarked that I had the hip bone density of a twenty-five-year-old, though I was well over 50 at the time. He felt that my cycling had slowed or even prevented undue calcium loss that would have made these bones less dense, more brittle.

The Wind and You

On a bike the wind speed is the speed you're traveling less the speed of the wind from your back. Thus, if the wind is from the west at 20 mph and you're traveling west at 20 mph, the windchill index (see Table 11-5) is canceled and the air temperature is the same as that read by the thermometer. If you're traveling east at 20 mph into a 20-mph wind (unlikely as this may be) the effective wind speed is 40 mph. The shaded area in Table 11-5 is the temperatures that are definitely unsafe. Add more clothing, watch for skin freezing, stop and take shelter if necessary.

Remember that as you bicycle your body generates about eight times as much heat as it does when standing still. Which is why you can be shivery cold waiting on the corner for a bus, but comfortably warm on a bike at the same outdoor temperature, even though you are creating a windchill factor as you speed through the air. And when you stop at a red light, for example, the heat you have generated on the bike ride keeps you warm until you get moving again. Remember, too, that black absorbs more solar energy than lighter colors. A black sweater, for example, will feel warm to the touch on the side facing the sun but feel cold on the other side. In the summer heat, though, wear light-colored clothing. Sometimes, on a very hot summer day, noncyclist friends ask how I can bike in such humid heat. I simply tell them that the wind I create cools my body. I also point out that I drink a lot of water on hot days, which translates into perspiration, which cools by what

TABLE 11-5: WIND AND TEMPERATURE COMBINATIONS

WIND SPEED (MPH)	¢ THERMOMETER READING (DEGREES FAHRENHEIT)						
	50	40	30	20	10	0	−10
	WINDCHILL TEMPERATURE (DEGREES FAHRENHEIT)						
0	50	40	30	20	10	0	−10
5	48	37	27	16	6	−5	−15
10	40	28	16	4	−9	−24	−33
15	36	22	9	−5	−18	−32	−45
20	32	18	4	−10	−25	−39	−53
25	30	16	0	−15	−29	−44	−59
30	28	13	−2	−18	−33	−48	−63
35	27	11	−4	−20	−35	−51	−67
40	26	10	−6	−21	−37	−53	−69

physicists call the "latent heat of evaporation." Check this for yourself. Put a few drops of isopropyl alcohol on the back of your hand, wave your hand around, and feel the cooling effect as the alcohol evaporates. This is not to suggest, though, that you should drink alcoholic beverages as you cycle along. Water is just fine, and a lot better for you.

Cold Damage Symptoms

As you bike in cold weather be aware that your nose and ears have less blood supply than other parts of your body. These and other exposed areas, such as cheeks, are susceptible to frostbite. Watch for numbness that persists in these areas. Sudden tingling following such numbness signals the onset of frostbite. Stop, remove a glove, and place your warm hand over the frostbite area until tingling stops. Use Helmuffs (Fig. 11-9) from Mountain Safety Research, which Velcro-fasten to your helmet.

Feet can get cold, too. In cold weather wear the heaviest socks you can find and add bike booties over your shoes. In extreme cold weather try electrically heated inserts, using a rechargeable battery (see Fig. 9-35), which works for me (available from sporting goods outlets). Protect your hands with long-fingered cycling gloves, or in very cold weather, down-filled gloves used by cross-country skiers.

I won't take bad weather for an excuse not to ride your bike. Even if you live in the so-called Temperate Zone, where the winter temperature can drop well below zero degrees Fahrenheit, you can still get a good workout on a bike exerciser. Excellent machines are on the market on which you can mount your bike and pedal away while watching TV. There's even a model with rollers that

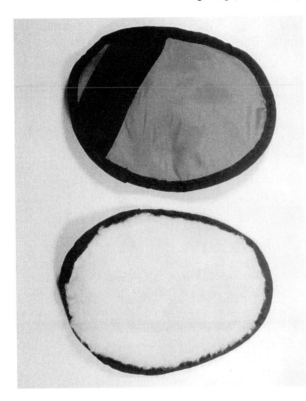

FIG. 11-9: Keep your ears warm in cold weather with Hell-muffs, which can be Velcro-fastened to your bike helmet.

grip the rim flats of wheels with knobby fat tires so you don't have to change to a smooth tread fat tire when you mount the bike on this trainer.

The Air You Breathe

There are many substances in the air that can harm your lungs. I won't give you a lecture on smoking except for one little incident that occurred to me way back in the dark ages, even before health warnings appeared on cigarette packages. As the editor of *Air Engineering,* a professional journal in air pollution, I met with the then U.S. surgeon general just before I testified before a Senate subcommittee considering air pollution control regulations. As we talked he kept glancing nervously over at a desk clock, which seemed to me to say he wanted to be elsewhere. At 11 o'clock he leaped up, walked rapidly to a desk across the room, reached in, extracted a cigarette, lit it, and began to puff away. He said he was trying to quit and allowed himself only one fag per hour. He talked to me about the relationship between smoking and lung cancer, bronchitis, high blood pressure, and heart diseases and showed me some slides of emphysematic lung tissue. When he finished I threw my own pack of cigarettes in his waste basket and never smoked again.

Do not ride during a thermal inversion, where cold air blankets warm air and natural wind ventilation is low. In an inversion, industrial, automotive, and other pollutants are trapped and concentrated and can cause lung problems. Such inversions are more frequent in basin cities surrounded by mountains, such as Denver, Los Angeles, and Mexico City. But inversions can occur in Chicago, New York, and any city where natural ventilation from wind movement drops in idle air. If you have to ride where the air is polluted, a mask, such as the one by W.R.S. SportsMed shown in Fig. 11-10, can filter out airborne dust particles. But no mask, short of a military-type gas mask, can filter harmful gases such as the carbon monoxide from auto exhaust. But this mask is a healthy filter if you have to cycle through dust kicked up by cyclists in front of you, or by cars on a dry, dusty dirt road or trail.

Altitude

As you pedal up a mountain pass, you will lose some of your ability to transfer muscle power to "go power" up to about 5,000 feet, after which you acclimate to reduced oxygen power. If you have a heart problem, use the same commonsense precautions you would take when riding at sea level. In fact, the reduced air pressure at higher altitudes lets arteries open wider, result-

FIG. 11-10: Protect your lungs against airborne dust particles with a cyclist's mask that filters them out of the air you breathe.

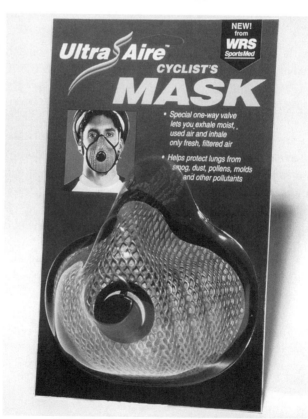

ing in less blood flow resistance, so the heart can pump more blood with less effort. If the high altitude gives you mountain sickness (something like seasickness) take it easy, rest a lot, and drink lots of fluid. At higher altitudes the air is also drier, so fluid intake is important. Also, as elevation increases so does solar intensity, so use sunblock, and cover exposed skin. If you ride in New Zealand and in the south of Chile and Argentina please remember that ozone depletion in these southern climes increases ultraviolet radiation, which can cause skin cancer.

Asthma

Asthma need not keep you from enjoying the healthy outdoor exercise of bicycling, unless your symptoms are severe. I suggest you carry whatever medication your physician has described for your asthma and use it if symptoms develop as you ride. Just remember that with bicycling, as with any strenuous sport, your muscles will call for more oxygen, and as they do you will have to breathe deeper and faster, which may aggravate your asthma. Cold, altitude, and auto fumes can also trigger reactions.

Physical Difficulties

Physical difficulties need not keep you from enjoying life on a bicycle. I will never forget the time I bicycled with a group 400 miles across Wisconsin, from Racine on Lake Michigan to LaCrosse on the Mississippi River. One of the riders was a middle-aged man who had only one leg. He rode a heavy three-speed bike and carried some clothes in a metal wire basket fastened to a carrier over his rear wheel. That man stayed right with us. He was an inspiration to the people who thought they were weak.

You can modify a road or mountain bike for a one-legged cyclist by adding a toe clip and strap to the one pedal he or she can use. Just be sure the strap is loose enough to permit the foot to be removed in an emergency. But the toe clip and strap will let the rider pull up and then push down on the pedal.

Back Pain

Back pain is rare among avid bicyclists. If you bike a lot you build up muscles that support the back and the rest of your body. But if you do have a lower-back problem you should see your doctor, who can, if necessary, prescribe drugs, along with a regimen of physical therapy. But beware of doctors who tell you not to ride your bike again, and who do not probe and poke your body or make an anatomical diagnosis.

Sometimes, though, something may click in your back as you bend or stoop to pick something up off the floor, or rise energetically and bounce out of bed first thing in the morning. Most of us have experienced the resulting lower-back pain, which can be excruciating for a short time. Just take it easy, roll rather than bounce off the bed, stoop slowly, and bend at the knees to lift a heavy object.

For persistent back pain you might try a WRS SportsMed back support (see Fig. 9-25), designed to be used with active sports such as bicycling. Reach WRS at 1-800-299-3366. If sitting upright on a bicycle saddle hurts your back, try riding a recumbent, such as the Linear (Fig. 11-11), which offers excellent back support along with a more upright position. See your bike shop for more information about this and other recumbents.

If you need motivation to get up, get going, and keep moving, read a new book by Kara Leverte Farley and Sheila M. Curry entitled *Get Motivated!* Here's a motivational guide that will spur you onward to exercise. The authors know what motivation is. Sheila M. Curry is a former collegiate field hockey and lacrosse player, an experienced sailor, and an avid sports fan. Kara

FIG. 11-11: You can pedal even with a back problem when you ride on a recumbent such as this Linear model, which offers excellent seating posture and support for your back.

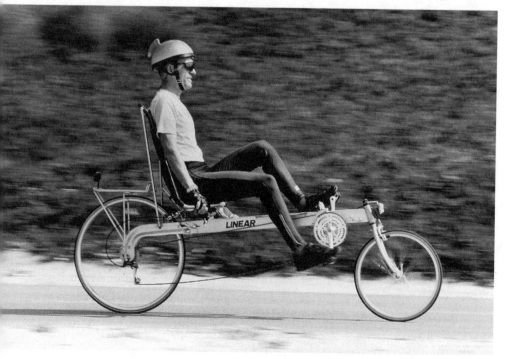

Leverte Farley is a former tennis instructor and a regular runner who has competed in two New York City marathons. Both Curry and Farley live in New York City. Their book is published by Fireside Books, a division of Simon & Schuster, Inc.

Diet for Endurance and Health

Since I am not a dietitian, I asked Lonnie Isaacson of Camas, Washington, to write the following section on the relationship between diet and sport. Her qualifications are listed at the end of this section. Isaacson begins with this quotation by Cathy Ellis, former winner of the women's division of the 2,930-mile Race Across America: *"Nutrition is the single most important factor in being able to finish the race."*

Here is what Isaacson has to say about food and health.

The Importance of What You Eat

Whether you are a recreational or a competitive cyclist, you can perform better and be more healthy with good nutrition. Food has much more than energy to stop your hunger. Within food are six nutrients: carbohydrates, protein, fats, vitamins, minerals, and water. All are necessary in certain amounts for your body to run well.

A good starting point to meet your nutrient needs is to choose a variety of foods based on the U.S.D.A. food pyramid guide (Fig. 11-12). It is no coincidence that the largest portion of the pyramid contains foods rich in complex carbohydrates such as grains (breads, cereals, rice, pasta), legumes (dried beans, split peas, lentils), vegetables, and fruits. I recommend that 65 percent of your food calories be in the carbohydrate family. As Fig. 11-12 shows, much smaller portions of the food pyramid are protein-rich foods such as milk, meats, fish, poultry, and eggs. If you are a vegetarian, find your protein in nuts, seeds, legumes, and grains. Remember that just 15 percent of your total food calories should be from protein sources. The most concentrated source of calories is fats. As you can see in Fig. 11-12, fats are in the smallest portion of the pyramid. Be aware that fats are present in many protein sources and are also added to many foods. I recommend that no more than 20 percent of your total food intake be fats.

Carbohydrates

You will see references to carbohydrates in articles about sports training, usually called "carbo-loading." This is because carbohydrates are the best

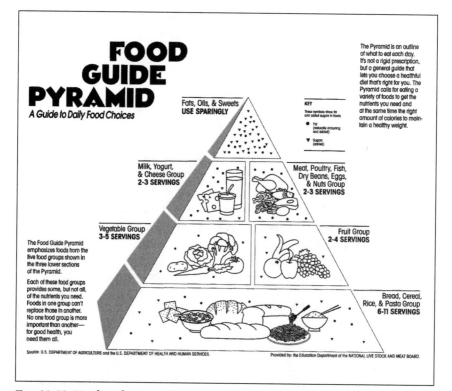

FIG. 11-12: Food guide pyramid suggests a daily diet that gives you all the nutrients you need to stay healthy.

source of energy for your body. You digest carbohydrates into glucose. This glucose is either burned for energy or stored for future use. Some glucose that is not needed immediately for energy is stored as glycogen in muscles and in the liver. Although your body burns mostly fat for fuel during light activities, intense exercise requires glycogen for energy. Your muscle glycogen is used as a readily available source of energy when you are cycling. However, the amount of time you can exercise is determined by the amount of glycogen you have stored. When you run out of muscle glycogen, you "hit the wall" and become too fatigued to continue. Cyclists call this energy drop the "bonks." Training exercise will increase your muscle's ability to store glycogen by 20 to 50 percent, but you must still eat foods with adequate carbohydrates to fill these muscle stores to capacity. Even with adequate muscle glycogen, cyclists can still bonk when their liver glycogen is depleted.

Liver glycogen is used by the brain for food. Failure to eat enough carbohydrates before an intense physical effort can result in depleted liver glycogen. The symptoms are weakness, lack of coordination, and inability to concentrate. So obviously your athletic prowess and success depends on how much and when you consume carbohydrates. To build muscle mass you must first meet your body's energy needs by eating enough carbohydrates to "spare" your proteins for tissue needs. A minimum of 500 to 800 grams (17.64 to 28.22 ounces) of carbohydrates per day for minimum muscle glycogen stores is ideal for cyclists who train exhaustively on successive days or who compete in prolonged endurance events. For example, one slice of bread or a half-cup of cooked grain contains about 15 grams (.529 ounces) of carbohydrates.

Protein

Unlike carbohydrates, proteins are not an ideal source of energy. Proteins cannot be converted into muscle glycogen. However, proteins are digested into amino acids, which are used as building blocks for muscles, red blood cells, other tissues, and hormones. Athletes require a small increase in protein, which can easily be provided by four to six ounces of protein-rich foods such as lean meats, chicken, fish, and dried beans. For vegetarians, it is essential that grains be combined with legumes or milk, or that legumes be combined with seeds or milk at each meal so that an adequate combination of amino acids be available for building and repairing body tissues. If you are a vegetarian, have your diet evaluated by a dietitian for sufficient protein, iron, zinc, calcium, vitamins B_{12}, and D, and riboflavin. Because the importance of proteins may have been overestimated by athletes, it is important not to minimize their significance. Besides amino acids, meats also contribute to sizeable amounts of iron, zinc, and B vitamins to your body. But remember, excessive protein intake, either with high-protein foods or with amino acid and protein supplements, is unnecessary, does not increase your muscle mass or your athletic performance, and may even be detrimental to health and athletic performance.

Fats

Fats supply more than twice as many calories by weight as protein or carbohydrate. In distance cycling, your body can burn fat for fuel, thus sparing your muscle glycogen. But your body has more fat stored than you will ever need in a race event, so hold the line on your fat intake, especially saturated fats. Saturated fats are in animal fats and hydrogenated vegetable oils (look at the ingredients label of packaged meals and on containers of margarine). For this reason, the use of lean meats (flank, loin, round), fish, and poultry with the skin removed is recommended if you eat meat. Fats can be used for up to 20 percent of total energy. Excess fats beyond what you need for energy will be stored as body fat. Also, excessive fat has been identified as a risk factor in several forms of cancer.

Eating less fat, saturated fat, and cholesterol has been shown to reduce the risk of heart attacks and strokes. Cyclists are not immune to heart attacks and strokes. Although regular exercise has been shown to increase the level of HDL or "good cholesterol," a family history of heart disease and an elevated cholesterol level may require evaluation by a physician and dietary counseling by a dietitian. Ideally, blood tests will show a cholesterol level below 200 mg and an HDL level greater than 40 mg for men and 50 mg for women.

Vitamins and Minerals

Vitamins and minerals play an important role in metabolizing carbohydrates, proteins, and fats, and in muscle functions. Get your vitamins and minerals from a wide variety of wholesome foods, rather than from supplements (pills) for several reasons:

1. You need to eat well regardless of whether you take supplements.
2. You won't have to worry about toxic excesses or imbalances of vitamins or minerals when you get them from food.
3. There is no evidence that taking vitamin or mineral supplements (or any ergogenic acids) improves athletic performance or builds muscles.

Most cyclists receive sufficient vitamins and minerals because of the large quantity of food they eat. But if you need the reassurance of dietary supplements, take a multivitamin mineral supplement containing the RDA (recommended daily allowance) of these supplements.

Water

The most important nutrient for an athlete is water. It is the nutrient needed in the largest quantity and it is the most essential for health. Think of water this way: When you exercise, heat is produced in the body. This heat is dissipated through sweat. To prevent dehydration you must match fluid intake with fluid loss. Dehydration can lead to less muscle strength, less endurance, poor coordination, and the risk of cramps, heat exhaustion, and life-threatening heat stroke. Some individuals can lose up to eight pounds of sweat per hour. Each pound lost must be replaced with two cups of fluid. Athletes also need to drink enough fluids during exercise to minimize weight loss from dehydration. Do not wait to drink water until you get thirsty, because thirst alone won't tell you when your body needs water. Develop the habit of fluid intake at regular intervals, whether you feel thirsty or not. One way to tell when you need more water is to check your urine. If urine is light-colored, you are drinking sufficient water, but if it's dark-colored and scant, you need more water.

Remember that if you exercise for one hour or less in moderate temperatures, cool water is your best fluid replacement. But when you exercise for more than an hour, or in high heat or humidity, you may benefit from a commercial sports drink containing electrolytes and carbohydrates to meet your needs. A 6 to 8 percent glucose, glucose polymer, or sucrose with a small amount of sodium are absorbed quickly and help maintain blood glucose levels during exercise. Note: beer is *not* a sports drink! Beer has a dehydrating effect.

Not All Foods Are Equal

For maximum nutrition power, here are food recommendations:

1. Eat 4 to 6 lean meats, fish, poultry, or legumes per day.
2. Select vegetables with nutrition power, such as spinach, kale, Swiss chard, broccoli, tomato, asparagus, cauliflower, cabbage, and green pepper.
3. Eat fruits such as oranges, grapefruit, kiwi, apricots, cantaloupe, and strawberries. Add other fruits for variety to a total of four servings per day. Bananas help you recover from exercise because they are high in fiber and have lots of potassium and carbohydrate.
4. Drink two cups of 1 percent or nonfat milk, or use yogurt or low or nonfat cheeses if you cannot tolerate milk products, or take a calcium supplement.
5. Be very sparing in your use of fats, oils, and salad dressings.
6. Eat whole-grain bread, rice, pasta, and cereal for your basic energy needs.

Body Composition

Most cyclists perform at their best when they achieve a high strength-to-weight ratio. However, you need to know how much of your weight is lean body mass, rather than fat tissue, because fats simply add pounds to your body without contributing to body strength. Male athletes should ideally have a body fat value of 5 to 12 percent, female athletes 10 to 20 percent. Body fat values greater than 26 percent for men and 29 percent for women put one at risk for certain chronic diseases. Body fat values below 4 percent for men and 10 percent for women indicate possible eating disorders. Tests to measure body fat vary from the expensive but accurate underwater weighing technique to the economical and less precise skinfold measurements and bioimpedance analysis. For the underwater method, try a research or university medical school hospital and be ready to pay $500 or so. The other, less pricey measurements can be done by a licensed clinical dietitian.

If these measurements show that you need to adjust your body fat, make this adjustment far, far in advance of intense training or competition. Combine a well-balanced low-fat intake with exercise for a slow adjustment to your desired results. Avoid rapid weight loss, which can deplete your glycogen stores and leave you feeling chronically tired and performing poorly.

Pre-Exercise or Competition Diet

A poor training diet cannot be compensated for by a good pre-event meal. Start with the recommendations above for good daily nutrition. But maximize glycogen storage to prepare for an event of more than 90 minutes of continuous activity by slowly increasing carbohydrates to 800 grams (29.22 ounces) each day for at least three days before the event. Workouts during the week before competition need to taper into a complete day of rest before the event. As noted earlier, this is called carbohydrate (carbo) loading and has been recommended by sports nutritionists for the past decade for healthy adult athletes in distance events.

Depending on your individual preference, two to six hours before the event eat a meal containing 85 to 200 grams (3 to 7 ounces) of carbohydrate. Doesn't seem like much, does it? Well, the fact is that carbohydrates are a relatively small part of most foods, and for 200 grams of carbohydrate you may need, for example, seven or eight slices of bread. For specifics on what is in foods, I recommend you read *Nancy Clark's Sports Nutrition Guidebook* (see references at the end of this chapter), which contains charts breaking down the components of most common foods. Common choices are bagels, fruit, cereal, pasta, rice, baked potatoes, and popcorn (not the movie theater variety). Choose familiar, comforting foods that you know do not cause an upset stomach. Some athletes with precompetition jitters choose a liquid meal supplement, such as fluids containing a small amount of carbohydrate, drunk 5 to 10 minutes before the event (but the drink should be comfortable to the stomach). Prepare for hot-weather cycling by drinking two to three cups of cool water before taking off.

During Competition

For events of less than one hour in a moderate temperature, drink 5 to 8 ounces of water every 15 minutes. For longer events use carbohydrate and fluid replacement drinks to maintain normal blood sugar. Without liquid replenishment you may become fuzzy and lose your competitive edge. So chow down 24 grams of carbohydrates (.85 ounces) every 30 minutes. Get used to these feedings during practice sessions. For events longer than six hours drink sports liquids or eat foods containing electrolytes, especially sodium. On extra-long trips, cross-country or off-road, try peanut butter sandwiches, cookies, and granola bars.

After Competition

If you drink adequate fluids during a cycling event, your weight after cycling will be the same as your weight when you began. Carbohydrate, fluid, and electrolyte replacement is essential and vital, so pay attention to your postevent meal. Ideally, begin to replace carbohydrates within 15 to 30 minutes after exercise. Juices, bananas, oranges, and grapefruit are good choices. Research shows that glycogen stores will build to a higher level if you eat up to 600 grams (21 ounces) of carbohydrate within the first several hours after a long, intensive workout. Never skip breakfast after a morning cycling workout. Eat the same high-quality foods that you ate during training to refuel your body during recovery.

ABOUT THE AUTHOR

Lonnie Isaacson, M.Ed., R.D., C.D., is a registered dietitian. She completed her master's in nutrition from Tufts University and her dietetic internship at the Frances Stern Nutrition Center in Boston. With 22 years of experience in universities, public health, and community programs, she specializes in helping individuals transform their eating habits for optimal health and fitness. She is currently in private practice at the McLoughlin Family Practice Clinic in Vancouver, Washington.

If you're healthy and have that old competitive spirit, check out the next chapter, which covers the racing scene from road to off-road to the oval- track events. You'll even find tips on how to watch the Tour de France or any other bike race.

References

Sports and Health

Bloomfield, John, Fricker, Peter A., and Fitch, Kenneth D., *Textbook of Science and Medicine in Sport.* Human Kinetics, P.O. Box 5076, Champaign, IL 61825-5076, 1992.

Bouchard, Claude, Shephard, Roy J., and Stephens, Thomas, *Physical Activity, Fitness, and Health.* Human Kinetics, P.O. Box 5076, Champaign, IL 61825-5076, 1994.

Costa, D. Margaret, and Guthrie, Sharon R. *Women and Sport.* Human Kinetics, P.O. Box 5076, Champaign, IL 61825-5076, 1994.

Journal of Aging and Physical Activity. A quarterly publication of Human Kinetics, P.O. Box 5076, Champaign, IL 61825-5076.

Journal of Sport Rehabilitation. A quarterly publication of Human Kinetics, P.O. Box 5076, Champaign, IL 61825-5076.

Sport Science Review. An annual publication of Human Kinetics, P.O. Box 5076, Champaign, IL 61825-5076.

Fuel for Your Body

Clark, Nancy. *Nancy Clark's Sports Nutrition Guidebook.* Champaign, IL: Leisure Press, 1990.

Clark, Nancy, et al. "Feeding the Ultra Endurance Athlete: Practical Tips and a Case Study," *J. Amer. Dietetic Assoc.* 92(10): 1258–62, October 1992.

"Position of The American Dietetic Association and The Canadian Dietetic Association; Nutrition for Physical Fitness and Athletic Performance for Adults." *J. Amer. Dietetic Assoc.* 93.6: 691–96, June 1993.

Tribole, Evelyn. *Eating on the Run.* Human Kinetics, P.O. Box 5076, Champaign, IL 61825-5076, 1992.

CHAPTER TWELVE

AN OVERVIEW OF BICYCLE RACING

In this chapter we will briefly explore the world of bicycle racing, on the road, on the track, and on the off-road trail. Let's start with road racing.

Bicycle racing is on the rise in North America. A growing league of U.S. pros are competing for prize money internationally. Some are ranked among the best racing cyclists in the world.

And they are winning big. As a case in point, consider the history of the Tour de France (Fig. 12-1). This isn't a race for just anybody. Only 150 of the

FIG. 12-1: The 1991 Tour de France race. Foreground, left to right: Ronan Persec and Greg LeMond. *Photo by John Kelly, Courtesy Giro Sports, Inc.*

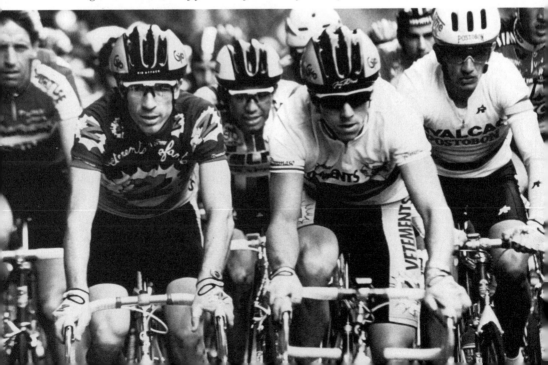

best cyclists in the world can participate, and only by invitation. Since the Tour was first held in 1903, no cyclist from the United States was invited to race until Jacques Boyer competed in 1981. Americans have been there ever since, and in 1986, Greg LeMond became the first American in history to win the Tour de France.

An Uncertain Future

But U.S. bicycle racing may still have a way to go before it can really compare to the quality and popularity of its European counterpart. Part of the problem is the lack of a large spectator following for the sport here in North America. The attention of fans draws media coverage, and with that comes the all-important financial contribution of corporate sponsors. It all comes down to money, because without sponsorship a young athlete may be unable to finance his training and buy the expensive equipment it takes to compete. Many promising careers have foundered when the demands of getting an education and making a living interfered with the necessity of pursuing a long training program.

Things are different in many European countries. In Italy, where cycling has long been a way of life and racing is something of a national obsession, bicycle racing is well-funded by proceeds from the national lottery. In Russia and other eastern European nations, racers were paid professionals, whose education, athletic training, and salary were provided by the state. Unfortunately, such support has been eroded due to the political and economic changes in these countries.

A Sport of Strategy and Wits

American audiences may be uninterested in bicycle racing for a good reason: Most of us simply don't understand racing's subtleties. To the uninitiated, the likely winner of a race should be the cyclist who can outrun all competitors in a mad dash from start to finish. That may be true for the final 200 meters before the finish line. But what happens over the tens or even hundreds of kilometers before the sprint can make the outcome impossible to predict. Sprinters break from the pack in bursts of speed, only to "blow up" from overexertion and get "reeled in" by the riders behind them. Alliances between rivals and petty rivalries between teammates disrupt carefully laid strategies, making for a constant flux in race leadership. Racing demands intensive effort, it's true, but success also depends upon reason, teamwork, and chance.

The enjoyment of racing events, like winning strategy, depends upon understanding of wind resistance. Wind resistance upon a cyclist's body increases as the square of his speed. So if a rider doubles his speed, he quadruples the wind resistance he has to fight against. Simply put, this means that the lead rider has to work harder to stay up front, while those behind him can use his slipstream to take shelter from the wind and conserve their strength. Good riders learn how to glue themselves to the rear wheels of those in the lead, coming as close as they can without touching. This is called "drafting," and it acts like a tow on the rider who follows behind.

A racer would quickly become exhausted by the effort it takes to "pull" if he tried to hold the lead for long periods of time. If you watch closely during a race you can see riders trading the lead back and forth. Together, two can maintain a higher speed than either could alone, a fact that makes for odd alliances at times.

Road races begin in a massed start, with all racers taking off from the line at once. The pack, or "peloton," as it is called, soon sets a fast pace, with the best riders and strongest teams bunched up in front. Somewhere along the course, one or more of the riders will attempt to "break" from the peloton. When this happens, those in a position to do so may draft off the rider who is making a break, taking a gamble that the lead rider has a good chance of creating and holding a commanding lead. The two, three, or more riders who form the breakaway could be bitter rivals, but cooperation may be their only key to success. They will have to take turns pulling each other in order to set a faster pace than the pack. In doing so, they create a gap that subsequent breaks or individuals will not be able to close.

What happens next depends largely on the support of their teams. It's common for teammates to agree before the race to split the prize if one of their members wins. They will let their rider with the best chance to win join in the attack while they attempt to keep others from catching up. The team takes up as much space as it can at the head of the pack and dawdles along, with elbows held out to stop the passage of riders around the side. Blocking is also used in a breakaway, when someone wants to slow progress and give a hand to a teammate who is trying to catch up. In this case, a rider in second position can let a gap form between himself and the leader, who will have to slow without someone to pull for him.

Two teammates can try to wear out a rival sprinter by repeatedly pulling away from the break. The sprinter can't afford to be left behind, especially if the end of the race is near. He'll have to jump the gap several times, thereby losing his "snap," the ability to accelerate quickly, as the end approaches. Good sprinters will have strategies of their own and will try to draft off somebody else until the moment when they can jump for the finish line. A teammate can help with a "leadout," pulling the sprinter along at his fastest pace, which sets up the sprinter for a jump at even greater speed.

With everything that's involved, it's obvious that much of a top rider's success depends upon the strength and cooperation of his teammates. Usually, only the most powerful teams can put a rider across the finish line in first place. At the same time, intrateam rivalries between some of the best racers in the world can crop up as they eye an individual chance to win.

This was made clear by the stormy relations between Bernard Hinault and Greg LeMond, members of La View Claire team during the 1986 Tour de France. Hinault, one of three cyclists who have won the Tour five times, was racing his last professional season. It was his final chance for an unprecedented sixth win. But for LeMond, 1986 was to be his year, his best hope to win the Tour himself. Little love was lost between the two. LeMond publicly leveled barbs at Hinault during the race, charging that the Frenchman had repeatedly joined breaks to win. In spite of the friction, La Vie Claire had a string of victories to its credit, a clear testament to the strength of this powerful racing team.

Watching Road Races

Following the action in a road race can present a bit of a challenge. Road races may cover hundreds of miles, and unless they are televised, it can be difficult to catch anything more than the finish. But don't be daunted. You can still see plenty of racing action if you do some careful planning. Find the best spots to watch the race and learn the itinerary so you can time your arrival and departures at a few locations along the route as the riders press on.

Criteriums

Luckily, watching some road races won't require any frenetic activity on your part. The criterium is the most common road race in North America. It's a massed-start event, in which riders have to complete several laps of a tortuous circuit through city streets. Frequent corners place a premium on a racer's bike-handling skills and make this a race for thrill-seekers, whether on the course or at the sidelines. Packs of riders funnel into the corners at breakneck speed and surge out together in a sprint for the next corner. It's not a spectator event for the faint of heart: Be prepared to see frequent pile-ups as riders jostle each other through the turns.

Good criterium riders can negotiate corners at full speed. In the early laps, riders of varying talents will mix up in the pack, slowing the pace in the turns. The better racers will begin to put some distance between themselves and the pack as the race warms up. Free of the peloton, they can lean harder and pedal farther into each turn without breaking. While other racers are just slowing to enter the turn, the breakaway group will already be sprinting up the course. They will also build speed and conserve energy by drafting off each other, a practice that's impossible in the chaos of the pack.

To watch a criterium to best advantage, try to find a place with close views of a spot promising fast action and stay there. The racers will pass by with some frequency, depending on the length of the circuit they have to complete. It will help to study the layout of the course ahead of time. Scout it out on foot or bike and look for overpasses or balconies where you can get an overview of the course below. Get there early, because you will want to be close to the street. Criteriums usually draw boisterous, cheering crowds, adding an element of excitement that is missing from many racing events.

Time Trials

Time trials are held in two broad categories, either for a set distance, such as 40 or 100 kilometers, or for a set time, commonly 1 or 24 hours. The objective in racing time trials is straightforward: to set the fastest time for the field. Riders start out from the line with a few minutes' break between themselves and the next racer. Depending on the size of the field, this process can take several hours and the race may take much of the day to complete.

Sometimes called the "race of truth," the individual time trial is a lonesome test of athletic prowess. There is no other competitor besides the clock. It's a long-distance endurance race, demonstrating little in the way of strategy. The time-trial racer can't use his head to better his position or play off the rivalries of others. He can't stick to somebody else's wheel to take a rest and protect his lead. It is supreme effort, and an ability to ignore the inevitable pain, that makes for success in the time trial.

Road Races

This is the classic form of the genre, covering a varied terrain over a course that is 100 miles or more in length. Road races can be laid out in one large loop, over several laps of a circuit, or one way from start to finish, in which case it's called a point-to-point race. Road racing combines the tactics, athletic ability, and skill needed to win all other racing events. A road racer must have the superior handling skills of a criterium rider, the endurance of a time trialist, the quick jump of a sprinter, and the power of a good hill climber, like Mark Engleman in Fig. 12-2, shown "climbing the wall" during the Mogul Bismark in 1992. The road racer has to combine all these talents and make up for any deficiencies by using his head. That's probably the main reason such a mystique surrounds the great road-racing champions of the world, while many other riders who excel in their own right go largely unnoticed. The champion road racer represents the athletic ideal.

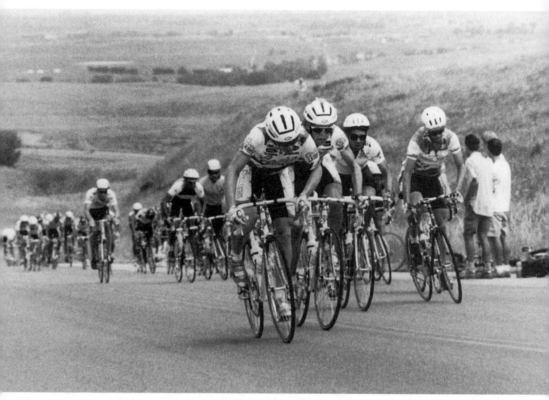

FIG. 12-2: Mark Engleman "climbs the wall" up a steep hill during the 1992 Mogul Bismark. *Photo © Beth Schneider.*

Following a Stage Race: The Tour de France

Often, point-to-point races, criteriums, and time trials are combined in a single event lasting several days, which is called a stage race. The Tour de France is unquestionably the world's most famous example, although none of its stages are criteriums, and most of the races are point-to-point. There are similar races in the United States.

The commotion and air of festivity that inevitably surrounds a stage race, such as the Tour de France, are good reasons to see this type of race. You will see some of the world's best racers compete. Let's take a look, for example, at how to follow a stage race as a spectator, with the Tour de France as an example.

A Gypsy-like caravan of support vehicles, dignitaries, journalists, and hordes of fans winds its way through the French countryside, descending upon each little town in the Tour's path. The natives, who have anxiously been awaiting this economic boon for some time, greet the entourage as if the circus has just come to town. The carnival atmosphere runs especially high in the stage towns, where the race finishes each day and the riders try to catch some sleep. These will be some of the best spots to soak up the ambience. After watching the winning sprint into town, you may find a chance to mingle with the racers in the cafés later that night. In the morning, you can catch the excitement of the massed start that begins another day of racing.

The Tour is unbelievably long. It circles the perimeter of the country, from the Atlantic lowlands and the Normandy coast to the high passes of the Alps and Pyrenees. It won't be possible to see the whole race, but even if you only see part of it you will still be visiting some of the world's most beautiful countryside.

Because of the distances you will have to cover, you should give a lot of thought to how you will travel. Traveling by bike is an obvious choice, because it will get you closest to the action. The race's route tends to be closed to automobile traffic for several hours before the peloton even makes its appearance. During this time, automobile traffic jams up on either side of the route, while the numerous fans riding bikes are given free access.

The big problem with traveling by bike is the great distance involved. Unless you are a marathon rider yourself, you probably won't have the stamina to finish the average 125 miles that the race covers each day. However, the French train system provides extensive service, is inexpensive by U.S. standards, and is accommodating to passengers with bikes. The drawback is that the train will not provide access to many areas that the Tour visits, and some of these may be the least-visited and most charming regions of the French countryside. One solution is to rent a car when necessary, and to ride your bike and the train when feasible. Study the route thoroughly so you can select good locations to watch the race. Several of the French cycling magazines, and the national sports paper, *L'Equipe*, publish route maps giving detailed information on the race's schedule. From these you can learn what times the peloton is expected to pass certain locations along the way. To know where the hot spots are, it helps to know how a stage race is scored. The winner is determined by comparing every rider's cumulative time for the whole series of stages. A race leader is recognized daily as the rider holding the lowest overall time at the end of each stage. In the Tour de France, this rider is awarded a yellow jersey, which he wears until his position is overtaken by another racer. Another element of competition is introduced by awarding bonuses, called *primes* (pronounced "preems"), to riders who win sprints at designated locations along the route. A rider may try for the green points jersey, which is awarded to the one who collects the most primes at these locations. Or, if he is a strong climber, a rider may attempt to capture the red-spotted mountain jersey by accumulating points at designated areas on the mountain passes.

By studying the route guide carefully, you can find the spots where primes will be awarded. Capturing primes is a focus of fierce competition between the front-runners, so you can expect some exciting sprints at these locations. Mountain passes in general are some of the best spots for viewing the race, because the peloton spreads out as the climb gets tougher, and you can see more than just a flash of the riders as they go by. The long hills give a commanding view of the race, and there is an air of intense excitement as the fans urge the tiring racers on. The sight of unparalleled mountain scenery may alone be worth the trip. For these, as for all other good viewing locations, you must find your spot and stake your claim to it very early. The French take their cycling very seriously; the crush will be tremendous, but well worth it.

There are dozens of road, track, time trial, and other races in the United States and in France, Italy, Japan, Australia, Germany, South Africa, Austria, and Ireland. For specific race titles, locations, and dates, ask for the media guide from the United States Cycling Federation, One Olympic Plaza, Colorado Springs, CO 80809, phone 1-719-578-4581, FAX 1-719-578-4596.

How to Watch Track Events

Track racing generally doesn't bring into play the same range of tactics that can make road racing so unpredictable. But the track still holds mass appeal, since spectators can watch the whole event in one place. Enjoying the track events will take a sharper eye, but once you catch on to the intricacies, you will find the action just as intense as anything the road race can offer.

If you are lucky enough to live near a velodrome, you can catch a number of track races every spring and summer. Local tracks will boost a variety of events and classes of riders. Races during international events, such as the World Cycling Championships or the Olympic Games, usually get fair to good television coverage. Here's a sample of the track races you can see at these events.

The Sprint

This is something of the aristocrat of cycle racing, requiring tactics more akin to those of chess than to those of a flat-out athletic performance. In the sprint, two riders (sometimes three at local events) try to beat each other to the end of 1,000 meters, or three laps of a 333-meter track. What makes this race interesting is that the riders' times are recorded only for the final 200 meters of the race.

"What's the sense in that?" you're asking. "Why not just give the riders a rolling start and time them in a 200-meter dash?" You hear the starting gun, and something even weirder happens. These people aren't racing, they are standing on their pedals, trying to hold their bikes still! And why are they staring at each other, as if waiting for something to happen?

The answer, once again, lies in the principle of wind resistance. Should either rider jump from the starting line at the sound of the gun, he immediately places himself at a disadvantage. The other racer can simply fall into the slipstream behind the leader and get a free ride for most of the race. In the last 200 meters he will jump into a sprint, easily defeating the exhausted front-runner.

A very explosive starter may have an advantage in the sprint if he can immediately establish a lead that can't be closed. Then the other rider can't draft his way around the course. But this requires great endurance on the part of the leader, and good sprinters aren't necessarily strong on endurance. He's also unlikely to get a good time this way, since he's bound to be tired once he reaches the final 200 meters. It's more likely that the two riders will be equally matched, and will try to trick each other into making a jump, whether by "trackstanding," as described above, or by "soft-pedaling" around the track for a while, until one rider makes his move and the real race begins. Current world record times for the 200-meter sprint are hovering near 45 mph.

The Pursuit

In this event, two riders or two four-person teams start on opposite sides of the track. For 4,000 meters they "pursue" each other around the track, but unless someone dumps his or her bike, it's not likely that anybody will ever be caught. The real object is to set the best time, and speeds are high from the very start. There's little in the way of tactics or finesse here: It's all-out effort and athletic ability that make the difference. World-record times for the individual pursuit top 30 mph, while the team event is a bit faster, since riders can take advantage of drafting to increase their speed.

Time Trials

Time trials (Fig. 12-3) are also a common sight at track events. A typical individual time trial is a 1,000-meter race known as the "Kilo." World-class times for the Kilo are around one minute, or a little better than 35 mph. A particularly grueling race is the one-hour time trial, where a cyclist races for one hour in an attempt to cover the most ground he can. In 1984, Francesco Moser of Italy set a world-record time of 51.151 kilometers in Mexico City, maintaining an incredible average speed of 32 mph for one hour.

Another brutal test of high-speed endurance is the team time trial. This

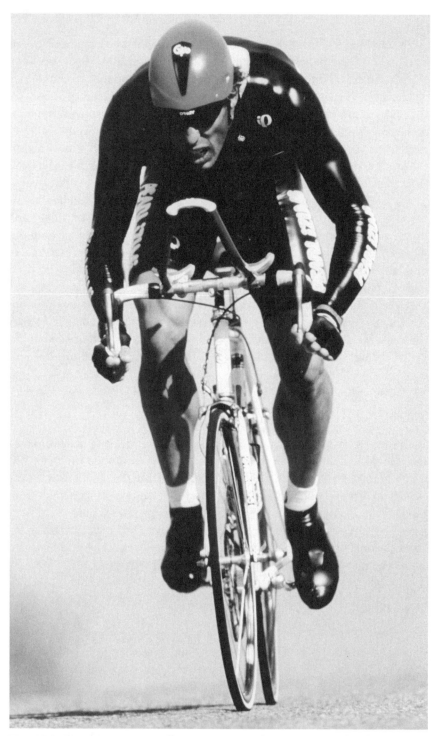

FIG. 12-3: Ray Browning goes all out in a time trial, a race against the clock. *Photo by John Kelly, Courtesy Giro Sports, Inc.*

race is 100 kilometers long, with world-class times approaching 120 minutes. That's an average speed of a little over 30 mph—for two full hours! Racers are able to keep this pace up for so long only through intense concentration and perfectly orchestrated movements. Each rider in a four-person team takes turns pulling for about 30 to at most 45 seconds. He barely assumes lead position before "pulling off" to the side, letting his teammates pass by only inches away. Then he falls back to the end of the line to take a rest. In another minute and a half he has to be ready to do it again. The movements must be performed flawlessly, since any disruption in the concentration of the group will mean a loss in efficiency and time.

Points Race

This is one of the few massed-start races held on a track. The constant action, the continuous buzz of 30 riders flying around the track in a group, and the potential for crashes make this a more exciting event than other track races. But it's a difficult race to follow because the winner isn't necessarily the first rider to cross the line. Instead, points are earned by placing in a few lead positions each time the pack completes a specified number of laps. The winner is the rider who chalks up the most points by the end. As a rider, keeping track of the tally is a difficult task. For a spectator it's impossible. But, the frequent sprints are sure to bring you to your feet, time after time. You'll just have to enjoy the action, and wait for the end to find out who wins.

Other Track Events

Another massed-start race is the scratch race. It follows the same procedure as the points race, without the award of primes. So the scratch is a simple race to the finish over a course from 3 to 10 miles in length. If the "chase rule" is applied, the competition will intensify. This rule requires all riders leading the pack to take up the chase on a break, or face being disqualified.

Yet another massed-start race is the miss-and-out, sometimes known as devil-take-the-hindmost. This is an elimination event, in which the last rider over the line at the end of each lap, or with the completion of several laps, is dropped from the race. The race continues either to the last rider or to a sprint between a designated number of survivors.

A remnant of the nineteenth-century six-day race survives in the Madison. "Six-day race" is still a common name for this event, but it has been scaled down considerably from the time when racers really did ride continuously for six days without relief, trying to cover the longest distance for the field. These days, the six-day involves teams of two to three riders who relieve each other after every few laps. The relief rider is pushed onto the track from a standing start, and is then shot into the thick of the race by a grasp of the hand and swing of his teammate's arm. Madisons are run for a set time, rarely longer than a few hours, or for a set distance, usually about 10 miles. The Madison is a popular race on the European continent, where, owing to its place of origin (in New York City's old Madison Square Garden) it's sometimes called *l'Américaine.*

Racing for the Adventurous

The races described above form the core of the classic European racing circuit. Purists would argue that membership in the club comes to an end right there. Nonetheless, some super-endurance races are finding favor with a new breed of racer, and aficionados swear that these races are the ultimate tests of physical and mental stamina. The purists countercharge that the speed, finesse, and intellectual challenge of road racing are absent in marathon events. They say that this is no sport at all, but rather a plodding, long-distance exercise in self-punishment. Let's take a look at two of these ultra-endurance races: the bicycle marathon, and an even more brutal spinoff, the triathlon.

The Marathon

This race might be thought of as a very long time trial. It's hard to say where road races end and marathons begin, but the 24-hour time trial, a race with record times over 500 miles, is probably as good a place as any to make the distinction. In races lasting more than a full day, the racer's individual talent and his exercise of tactics in the pack bear less and less relationship to the outcome. The longer it goes on, the more a marathon race become a measure of raw courage and pure endurance.

Marathon racing can ravage a racer's body and psyche. Perhaps no race illustrates this better than an ultramarathon event called the Race Across America, or RAAM. The RAAM covers over 3,000 miles from Pacific to Atlantic coasts. The average finisher makes the crossing with about two hours of sleep per night and consumes 8,000 or more calories every day. But many of the starters never even see the Atlantic shoreline. Lack of sleep and physical exhaustion result in a dropout rate of 40 percent.

For those who do complete it, the RAAM can be a harrowing, even dangerous experience. Many competitors report having vivid hallucinations and late-night conversations with imagined companions, common symptoms of long-term sleep deprivation. Inexplicable accidents have also occurred.

Shelby Hayden-Clifton was just 130 miles from the finish line in 1986 when she rode over an embankment and fractured two neck vertebrae. She had just slept two hours, and reportedly had no idea why she crashed. "It just happened," she said, indicating that she may have had a blackout. Luckily, she fully recovered and is riding again. A Canadian cyclist, Wayne Philips, was not so fortunate in the 1985 RAAM. He was paralyzed by a hit-and-run driver near Tucumcari, New Mexico, an accident made doubly tragic by his decision to race without a support vehicle. Philips wanted to show that a rider could finish the race unassisted.

It's not mandatory that all riders be accompanied by a support vehicle in the RAAM. Racers have also adopted high-tech solutions in the quest for faster times. One of the biggest problems with marathon riding is that it fully depletes the body's glycogen, a source of stored energy, forcing it to use fats for fuel (see Chapter 11 for excellent data on foods and cycling, written by a professional licensed dietitian). Burning fat is less efficient and eventually leads to fatigue and a crawling pace. Many RAAM contestants now use liquid food that is high in carbohydrates to replenish blood sugar and ensure continued muscle activity. They have also used the findings of sleep research to determine the most beneficial time to sleep each night. Judging by the shrinking record times, the effort is getting results. But the price of it all is getting a little high. It's estimated that the average contestant in the 1985 RAAM spent at least $15,000 in an attempt to split a $20,000 purse.

The Triathlon

This is surely one of the most intense athletic events of modern times, bordering on gladiatorial. Those who can summon the reserves to make it to the finish line are as likely to collapse from exhaustion as to raise their hands in the victory salute. Those who are champions definitely operate on a different level.

To be fair, you wouldn't have to kill yourself to finish a triathlon. Most triathlons feature swims of 0.5 to 1 mile, bike races that average 25 miles, and final foot runs of 5 to 15 miles. So most local triathlons are within the athletic ability of the average person of good to excellent physical fitness. But then there are the real gonzo events, such as the Ironman Triathlon, usually held in Hawaii every year. The Ironman includes a 2.4-mile ocean swim and a 112-mile bike race, capped off by a 26.2-mile run. All of this happens in 90-degree tropical heat, most of it on a highway that winds through blistering-hot fields of volcanic rock. The champs can do it in nine to ten hours. In case that's not enough for you, there's always the Ultraman. This is a two-day event that starts with a 6-mile swim and a 100-mile ride on the first day, and finishes with another 168-mile ride and a 52.4 mile run on the second, definitely not a race for the average fitness buff.

Bicycle racing is a fairly glamorous activity. Certainly it's a beautiful sport, but it's also one of the most physically demanding. If by chance my description of bicycle racing has stirred your interest to participate directly, I will be pleased.

Glossary of Racing Terms

Attack: An aggressive acceleration taken to open a lead on other riders.

Blocking: Attempting to slow the progress of the pack in order to assist a breakaway group to create and secure a lead.

Blow up: To be unable to maintain a fast pace due to overexertion.

Break, breakaway: A rider or group of riders who sprint away from the pack.

Bridge, bridge a gap: An attempt to catch up with a breakaway.

Chaser: A rider who tries to bridge a gap.

Drafting: Taking advantage of the slipstream created by another cyclist by riding close to his rear wheel. Also called wheelsucking, sitting-in, and riding in tow.

Field sprint: A mass sprint toward the finish line by the front of the pack.

Jam: A period of hard pedaling. Also called hammering.

Jump: To accelerate rapidly, as in a sprint.

Leadout: A tactic where one cyclist rides at his fastest pace to help a teammate in tow. The second rider then jumps around the first at an even faster pace to sprint toward the finish line.

Mass start: A race that begins with all riders leaving the starting line in a group.

Motorpace: A training method in which a rider follows a motorcycle or other vehicle that breaks the wind. Also a race in which riders are motorpaced.

Peloton: The main group of riders in a race. Also called bunch, group, and pack.

Prime: A bonus awarded to the first rider to reach a specified point on the course or to the leader at a specified lap during a race.

Pull: To ride at the front of the group.

Pull off: To leave the front of a group so the next rider in line can take the lead.

Reel in: Action in which the peloton overtakes a breakaway attempt.

Snap: The ability to accelerate quickly.

Soft-pedal: To pedal without applying power.

Trackstanding: A tactic used during sprint races to foil an opponent's attempt to sit-in. Cyclists try to hold their bikes in place until one or both riders break into a sprint. Sometimes called jockeying.

Velodrome: A banked track where bicycle races are held.

Velodromes in the United States

The list of U.S. velodromes is still relatively small, but if you live near one of the tracks listed below I encourage you to see what they have to offer. Some of these tracks may be inactive at times. For more information, and to find exact locations, ask local bike shops or local bike clubs.

7-Eleven Olympic Velodrome, California State University, Carson, California.

7-Eleven Olympic Training Center Velodrome, Colorado Springs, Colorado.

Alket Velodrome, Houston, Texas.

Alpenrose Velodrome, Alpenrose Dairy, Portland, Oregon.

Balboa Park Velodrome, Morely Field, San Diego, California.

Baton Rouge Velodrome, Baton Rouge, Louisiana.

Brian Piccolo Park Velodrome, Cooper City, Florida.

Brown Deer Velodrome, Milwaukee, Wisconsin.

Dick Lane Velodrome, East Point, Georgia.

Dorais Velodrome, Detroit, Michigan.

Edward Rudolph–Meadow Hill Park Velodrome, Northbrook, Illinois.

Encino Velodrome, Encino, California.

Hellyer Park Velodrome, San Jose, California.

Kissena Velodrome, Lynbrook, New York.

Lehigh County Velodrome, Emmaus, Pennsylvania.

Major Taylor Velodrome, Indianapolis, Indiana.

Marymoor County Park Velodrome, Redmond, Washington.

National Sports Velodrome, Blaine, Minnesota.

Olympic Velodrome, Carson, California.

St. Louis Velodrome, St. Louis, Missouri.

San Diego Velodrome, San Diego, California.

Shakopee Velodrome, Shakopee, Minnesota.

Washington Park Velodrome, Kenosha, Wisconsin.

The United States Cycling Federation is in charge of road, track, and mountain bicycle racing in the United States. It licenses amateur racing cyclists. For more information on racing in your state, contact the state USCF district representative (see Table 12-1).

TABLE 12-1: USCF District Representatives

District	Name	Phone
Alabama/Mississippi—01	Jeannette Marsh PO Box 2435, Mississippi State, MS 39762	(601) 325-8199
Alaska—02	Paul Roberts PO Box 111095, Anchorage, AK 99511	(907) 344-1436
Arizona—03	Albert Hopper PO Box ABC, Bisbee, AZ 85603	(602) 432-5795
Arkansas—04	Steve Shepard 2720 Charter Oak Rd., Little Rock, AR 72207	(501) 225-6077
California/Nevada North—05 (incl. zip code 893-898, 936-961)	Lee Maniscaico 1153 Delaware St., Berkeley, CA 94072	(510) 526-5983
California/Central—06 (incl. zip code 930-935, 900-919)	Jan Luke 438 Dolores St., Wilmington, CA 90744	(310) 835-8388
California/Nevada South—07 (incl. zip code 890-892, 919-929)	Jan Luke 438 Dolores St., Wilmington, CA 90744	(303) 835-8388
Colorado—08	Yvonne Van Gent 1135A South Oneida, Denver, CO 80224	(303) 757-1892
Connecticut—09	Tom Vinson 157 Everett St., Wollaston, MA 02170	(617) 328-8704
Florida—10	Joel Goldmacher 1134A E. Fletcher Ave., Tampa, FL 33612	(813) 632-9224
Georgia—11	Joel Goldmacher 1134A E. Fletcher Ave., Tampa, FL 33612	(813) 632-9224
Hawaii—12	Gib Richards 14-I Kaslala Pl., Wabiaw, HI 96786	(808) 621-2004
Idaho—13	Richard Nystrom 4480 Silver Lake Rd., Buhl, ID 83316	(208) 543-6332
Illinois—14 (incl. zip codes 419, 463-464, 600-629)	Nestor Evancevich 419 Linden Ave., Wilmette, IL 60091	(708) 251-6021

TABLE 12-1: USCF DISTRICT REPRESENTATIVES (CONT.)

DISTRICT	NAME	PHONE
Indiana/Kentucky—15 (incl. zip codes 400-429, 460-462, 465-479)	Nestor Evancevich 419 Linden Ave., Wilmette, IL 60091	(708) 251-6021
Iowa—16	Lucy J. Wall 2335 S. 22nd St., Marion, IA 52302	(319) 373-1112
Kansas—17	Mike Hudson 1361 Medford, Topeka, KS 66604	(913) 235-0428
Louisiana—18	Lorrie Hebert 605 Parkview Dr., New Iberia, LA 70360	(318) 367-6226
Maine/New Hampshire—19	Tom Vinson 157 Everett St., Wollaston, MA 02170	(617) 328-8704
Maryland/Delaware—20	Bing Topper 3082 Scottsborough Way, Riva, MD 21140	(410) 721-8593
Massachusetts/Rhode Island—21	Tom Vinson 157 Everett St., Wollaston, MA 02170	(617) 328-8704
Michigan—22	Reg Modlin 1770 Waverly, Trenton, MI 48183	(313) 675-3539
Minnesota/Dakota East—23	David Hogan 2216 E. 34th St., Minneapolis, MN 55407	(612) 729-0810
Minnesota /Dakota West—24	Lucy Williamson 225 Johnson, Laramie WY 82070	(307) 742-4763
Missouri—25	Michael Murray 4454 Lindell Blvd., #31, St. Louis, MO 63108	(314) 652-9939
Montana—26	Don Arthur 205 Sunny View Lane, Kalispell, MT 59901	(406) 752-4100
Nebraska—27	Richard Thompson 1825 Radial Hwy., N.W. #4, Omaha, NE 68104	(402) 551-7428
New Jersey—28	Cindy Donnelly 416 Catherine St., Somerville, NJ 08876	(908) 725-8245
New Mexico—29	Paula Higgins 2801 Florida, NE, Albuquerque, NM 87110	(505) 884-1880
New York North—30 (incl. zip codes 120-123, 128-149)	Holda Monaghan 42 Robins Rd., New Rochelle, NY 10801	(914) 632-3755
New York South—31 (incl. zip codes 100-119, 124-127)	Hilda Monaghan 42 Robins Rd., New Rochelle, NY 10801	(914) 632-3755

TABLE 12-1: USCF DISTRICT REPRESENTATIVES (CONT.)

DISTRICT	NAME	PHONE
North Carolina—32	David Poole	(704) 788-2972
	260 Brookwood Ave., #1D, Concord, NC 28025	
Ohio/West Virginia—33	Tym Tyler	(614) 890-4145
	6124 Freeman Rd., Westerville, OH 43081	
Oklahoma—34	Walt Hoppensteadt	(918) 588-7555
	967 E. 36th Place, Tulsa, OK 74105	
Oregon—35	Candi Murray	(503) 667-6220
	4318 S.E. 8th Ct., Gresham, OR 97080	
Pennsylvania—36	Judy Miller	(215) 866-4051
	1605 Cardinal Dr., Bethlehem, PA 18015	
South Carolina—37	Joe Sullivan	(803) 239-1404
	PO Box 2860, Greenville, SC 29602	
Tennessee—38	Harry Williamson	(615) 842-2554
	8340 Gann Rd., Hixon, TN 37343-1234	
Texas—39	Gary Stephenson	(915) 692-7566
	1809 S. Willis St., Abilene, TX 79605	
Utah—40	Del Brown	(801) 392-4019
	1375 E. 4225 S., Ogden, UT 84403-2550	
Vermont—41	Tom Vinson	(617) 328-8704
	157 Everett St., Wollaston, MA 02170	
Virginia/Washington, D.C.—42	Gerald Teeuwen	(804) 547-7905
	946 Shillelagh Rd., Chesapeake, VA 23323	
Washington—43	Gino Lisiecki	(509) 838-3707
	1012 W. 23rd Ave., Spokane, WA 99203	
Wisconsin—44	Nestor Evancevich	(708) 251-6021
	419 Linden Ave., Wilmette, IL 60091	
Wyoming/Dakota West—45	Lucy Williamson	(307) 742-4763
(incl. zip codes 575-577, 585-588)	225 Johnson, Laramie, WY 82070	

Professional Bicycle Racing

For information on professional bicycle racing in the United States, write the *National Cycling League (NCL)*, One Times Square, New York, NY 10036, phone 1-212-944-8170 or 1-917-871-7478. Professional NCL teams are: *Houston Outlaws*, 4400 Memorial Drive, Suite 3098, Houston, TX 77007; *New York Gotham Ghosts*, Suite 2R, 358 E. 19th St., New York, NY 10033; *Miami Wheelers*, 3850 Hollywood Blvd., #300, Hollywood, FL 33021; *Pittsburgh Power*, 800 Vinial St., Suite D, Pittsburgh, PA 12512; *Los Angeles Wings*, 11245 Vanower St., N. Hollywood, CA 91605; *San Diego Zoom*, 1035 Lake Ridge Rd., San Marcos, CA 92069; *Portland Thunder*, 600 Mayer Building, 1130 SW Morrison St., Portland, OR 97205-2217; *Seattle Cyclones*, 800 Fairview North, Seattle, WA 98103.

Racing Your Mountain Bicycle: Words of Wisdom from Sara

I asked Sara Ballantyne to write about the world of mountain bicycle racing. Sara is a multitalented athlete who enjoys mountain climbing, snow skiing, and mountain running during the off-season. Sara has been the NORBA (National Off-Road Bicycle Association) World Champion in 1987, 1988, and 1989, European World Champion in 1988 and 1989, number two in the World Championship NORBA Senior Cross-Country event in Durango, Colorado.

"Ten seconds riders! 5, 4, 3, 2, 1, GO!" Tensions and heart rates are high as the racer tries strenuously to be the first to lock into his pedals and maintain the lead. Sometimes I wish I had a normal "8-to-5" job when I wake up (for the umpteenth time in the morning), my stomach a ball of knots, nervous energy flowing through my body in preparation for another day of mountain bike racing. But all it takes is jumping onto my mountain bike and riding off into the cool breeze of the early morning, spinning effortlessly through the gorgeous surrounding mountains, to realize why I do what I do. I can't think of any other job I'd rather have. I love mountain bike racing and feel fortunate that I can make a living at it. It enables me to travel to many parts of the United States as well as Europe, New Zealand, Australia, Japan, and who knows where else. I find ever-increasing numbers of people are discovering how much fun mountain bicycle racing can be. I love the feeling I get from competing and pushing myself to new limits all the time. I'm continually meeting new and interesting people. It's also exciting to have an influence on other novice riders while at the same time helping the sport grow. I can't quite figure out exactly what it is about mountain biking that turns so many people on. Is it that primitive desire to be a

kid again and get all muddy out in the wilderness? Is it the continual obstacles we encounter out there while riding, and the creativity it takes to
get around or over them? Is it those "out-of-body" experiences we may get
on those all-day rides? I only know that the bug has hit me hard and is here
to stay awhile.

Today there are many choices of mountain bike races. The sport has
grown tremendously, both from a standpoint of participation and in its technology. In the early days, on single-speed bikes, the objective was to get
downhill the fastest. A heavy weight was no consideration. In fact, the heavier the bike, the better. Bikes today are much lighter and have steeper frame
angles, shorter chain stays, and shorter wheelbases. This new geometry lets
the mountain bicycles of today go faster and negotiate turns and obstacles
at speeds impossible with the single-speed clunker of yesteryear. Now you
can choose a combination of 21 gears, instead of no gear at all.

NORBA

Before I get into racing techniques, I would like to comment briefly on a
recent change in the governing body of off-road racing. Up to 1989,
NORBA was owned by the American Bicycle Association. Today the United
States Cycling Federation (USCF) owns NORBA. The USCF now over-
sees both road racing and off-road racing. I see no major change in off-road
racing from this switch in ownership. However, this change is a sign that
the growing sport of mountain bike racing will have the guidance and the
requirements for orderly conduct the USCF has long brought to bicycle
racing events.

NORBA rules and guidelines, however, remain virtually unchanged.
Self-sufficiency and individual ability are still stressed. In other words, the
rider must know how to change a flat tire, piece back a busted derailleur,
reconnect a broken chain, or handle whatever other problems arise while
racing. This translates into carrying a spare tube, pump, patch kit, chain
tool, Allen wrenches, and good karma. It is guaranteed that no one will come
along driving a support vehicle. In fact, if a racer does take outside assistance for any kind of mechanical problem, or changes bikes during the race,
he will be disqualified. A racer must know his bike intimately. He must be
prepared to deal with whatever mishap may occur. I know of stories where
sticks or rocks, caught up in the drive train, demolished a racer's rear derailleur, forcing the rider to create a single rear speed because he no longer
had shifting capability. This self-reliance rule is what separates mountain
bike racers from road racers. In fact, mountain bike racing is a much more
individual sport than road racing. There are few, if any, team tactics in
mountain biking. The terrain doesn't allow for this. Riding on a dirt two-

wheel-drive road, then through stream beds, then back to a narrow single track is not uncommon. Having to negotiate rocks and fallen trees in your path makes a pack situation (where riders in a team help each other beat other team riders) difficult if not impossible. The surrounding aspens and pine trees dictate where the rider's path will be, rather than the team tactics of road racing. So the rule for traveling through these areas may be single file. The racer must always be prepared for anything or anybody on the course. It makes life very exciting for both racer and spectator. Each rider seems to have his own style of riding. You may have a two-minute lead on the rest of the pack and seem to have the race in the bag when you hit a rock a little too hard and "uh-oh" . . . next thing you know the lead racers are passing you by! It's all part of mountain bike racing.

Race Categories

As of 1989, the categories of racing are:
1. Beginner (formerly known as Novice), a first-timer.
2. Intermediate (formerly Sport), experienced amateur rider.
3. Expert (remained the same), very advanced amateur rider.
4. Super (formerly Pro/Am), elite top level amateur.

1. The Hill Climb

These races are often mass-started with your category (as designated above). Men and women are in their own class. Every race promoter decides on the distance of the hill climb. I have seen them as long as 13 miles (for example, Whistler, British Columbia—elevation gain 5,280 feet!) and as short as a quarter mile. Racers tend to spread out quickly as each rider battles for more oxygen as the elevation increases. Promoters may decide to have a time-trial hill climb, in which each racer pushes himself to the limit against the clock. Some say, "If you can still stand at the finish line, you haven't pushed hard enough!"

Hill climb techniques: The rider's position on the bike varies with the grade of the climb. For instance, to prevent the rear wheel from slipping, it may be necessary to remain seated on the bike. Over loose, rough sections, the rider should keep momentum up while concentrating on a smooth, round pedal stroke to maintain forward power. Bikes with shorter wheelbases and steeper angles tend to climb better, but lose comfort downhill. Be prepared for a much friskier ride and quicker responses from your bike. It's like comparing a Jaguar cruising down a mountain road to a Lincoln Continental on the same road. The Jag will have a quicker response, the Lincoln will be comfortable, more laid-back, not as aggressive.

2. The Downhills

These races are done in time-trial fashion. Each racer has his own start. The quickest time to the bottom wins. Ride your bike as if you were riding a horse. Let what's underneath you absorb the shock. Think of skiing—same thing. You bend your knees to absorb the bumps and undulations on the slope. On a mountain bike you can stand up on your pedals, off the saddle (Fig. 12-4). Grasp the handlebars with your arms slightly bent (Fig. 12-5). Relax and focus on what's up ahead, pick your line, just as if you're picking the smoothest, most efficient line around the moguls on a ski slope. Angulate with your knees (Fig. 12-6), depending on which way the slope of the hill is leaning. This allows you to always be over the balance point of your bike. I can't help but feel that the winter skiers and former motorcycle racers in the mountain biking groups have a distinct advantage over other racers in the way they handle their bikes, the lines they choose, and the confidence they exhibit at high rates of speed down the hill.

I prefer my handlebars to be around 21 to 22 inches across. This for me

FIG. 12-4: For balance and control you can get up off the saddle and balance on the pedals.

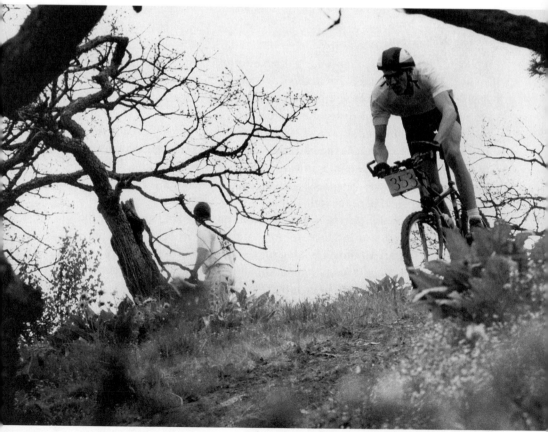

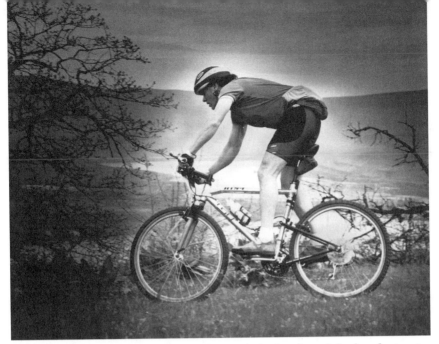

FIG. 12-5: Or balance with arms slightly bent to help absorb road shock and yet maintain steering control.

FIG. 12-6: Downhill, you can angulate with your knees, depending on which way the trail turns.

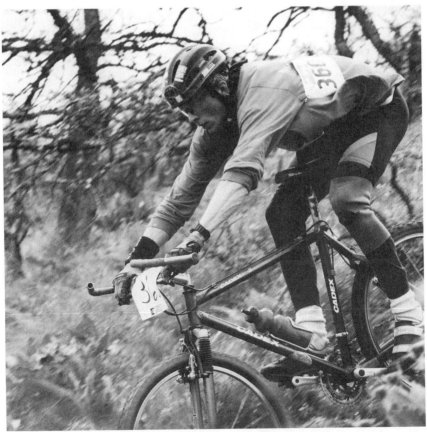

is shoulder width. Shorter handlebars inhibit my breathing. Wider handlebars feel awkward and unbalanced when descending,

I recommend toe clips. They give you more power per stroke and prevent your foot from slipping off the pedal. Some beginner riders may feel frightened of the "locked-in" feeling, especially while traveling over technical (spell that terribly difficult, treacherous terrain) rocky sections. However, the toe clips don't need to be clamped tightly across the foot. I usually ride with mine loose and only secure them when I know that I will not be dismounting during a course.

Warmups are important: Warming up properly before a hill climb (Fig. 12-7) is also very important to ensure optimum performance. Generally speaking, the shorter the race, the longer I warm up. For me, it takes a good hour before my body starts responding to fast speeds. I also recommend a good session of stretching or yoga in the morning. Whatever it takes for you to relax and allow only positive energy into your body can only translate into

FIG. 12-7: On uphill runs, get your weight back over the rear wheel for good traction.

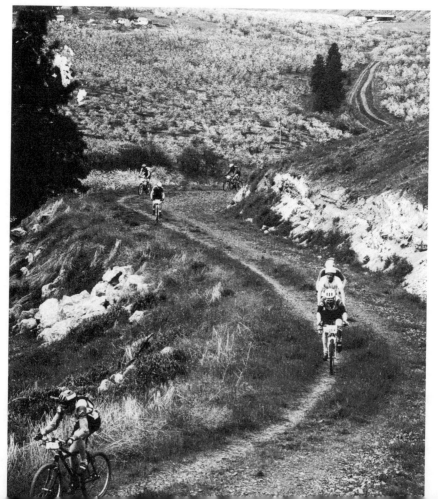

a good race for you. The body is very adaptable and once it gets into a certain routine I find mine actually craving it, or reminding me if I have neglected certain things, such as stretching.

I remember my first ride on the infamous Slickrock trail in Moab, Utah. I woke up the next morning with my body feeling as if I had just finished a game of football with the Refrigerator and someone had taken a sledgehammer to my forearms. After much more experience and time on my mountain bike, I found, using the above tips, that my body was a much happier unit!

3. The Cross-Country Race

This is my favorite race. This is the real test of mountain biking, because a racer must be a good overall bike handler and be in top aerobic shape to win. Usually the course is from one starting point to a different finishing area (point to point). Or the race may start and end at the same location— one big loop of any length. The rider never crosses the same part of the course twice, which requires top-notch concentration for the unknown. Always preride a race course if possible. Knowing what to expect and how to pace yourself can only help your performance. I also like to have short goals while racing in the back country for several hours. For instance, I play games—I tell myself that "I know at the top of this hill, it will be flat and I can recover," or, "If I make it around this corner and up that hill, it's home free." But not like the Little Engine That Could, "I think I can, I think I can." Once the mind starts defeating itself, the body soon follows and performance plummets. Instead of "I think I can" try "I know I can." It really works!

Gearing for the cross-country course depends on the individual rider's strength. Choose gears that allow you to spin efficiently with a relatively high cadence. Pushing hard gears will give you nothing but knee pain down the road. For my smallest gear in front (chainring) I use a 24-tooth. In the rear I use a 28-tooth cog. This can usually get me up anything in Colorado and if I need something easier than this, I'm better off dismounting and running my bike up the hill. Again, this is all personal preference.

4. The Circuit Race

A circuit race is one in which the racers ride around a closed course several times, usually more than 2 miles but less than 10 miles per lap. Since you will be doing a multitude of laps, perhaps it is a good time, early on in the race, to observe the faster riders ahead of you. What are their weak points? If I notice that someone ahead of me is slower on the flats than I am, I pick an opportune time to pass him there, try to catch him off guard so that when I go by him it is already too late for him to respond. This is a great trick to pull on someone right before the finish line. It usually demoralizes him so badly that he just gives up as I ride by him, trying not to smile too much! Or, if a competitor is floundering through a short technical section, try dismounting your bike and running by him. I remember one time trying to finesse my way through some shin-deep mudholes when the top male rider ran by me as if I were going backward. From then on, I did the same—even though it meant taking the chance of getting my shoes sucked off in the process!

5. Dual Slalom

In a dual slalom, just as in skiing, the rider must negotiate and go around "gates." The rider is usually matched up against another rider in a similar course, side by side. The winner is the first across an imaginary finish line with the least dirt on the body—that is, with no wipeouts. The adrenaline is high when you wait behind the gate, hearing the countdown, trying to get out of the start position just a bit faster than your opponent. I find it's the one who is the most levelheaded, who handles his or her bike most smoothly and with the most finesse, who takes the straightest line around the gates, and who makes it across the finish line with no falls will have the quickest time of the day.

The dual slalom is not only a real gas to do but it also improves your bike-handling skills tremendously. It teaches you how to take corners at high rates of speed, which translates to other areas of racing such as the downhill or cross-country course. I found that by applying a bit more pressure on your back brake and a little less in the front, you can pull off a move called the "brody," which will impress all former BMX racers. This move swings your rear tire around much quicker, rather than your having to steer the wheel around. Some riders like to compete in the dual slalom without toe clips. This enables you to drop your foot to the inside of your turn, providing almost a pivot point and something by which to turn around. Plus it's a good safety backup in case you feel yourself going down. You may be able to bounce back up and still maintain that clean image we all strive for when we cross that finish line.

6. Observed Trials

This competition is not considered racing—in the aerobic sense, that is. This involves a single rider going over obstacles such as stumps (Fig. 12-8), boulders, logs (Fig. 12-9), and holes in the ground. This all happens within

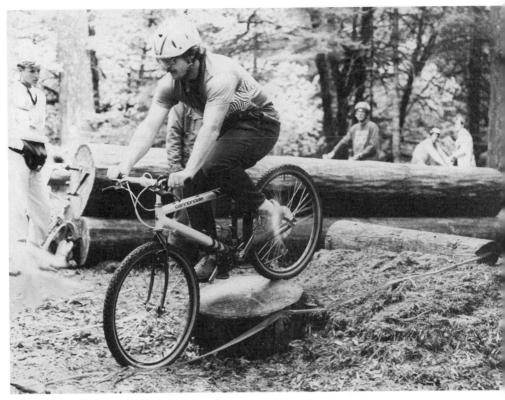

FIG. 12-8: Trials meets can take you over stumps.

FIG. 12-9: Another trials obstacle, a fairly major one, is a big log.

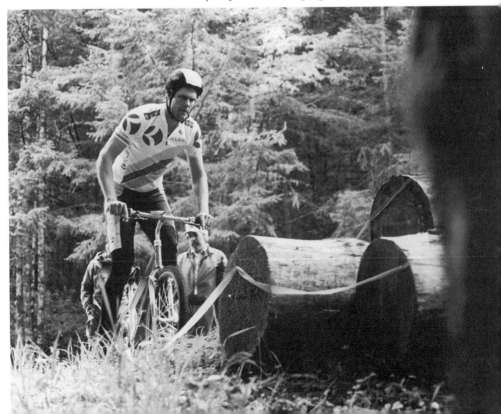

a 10- to 20-yard distance! There is no time involved. There is, rather, a scoring system in which the rider accumulates points by "dabbing" or touching his or her foot off the pedal onto the ground. There are usually 6 to 10 different sections that the rider must complete 2 to 3 times. The rider moves from one trials section to the other with a little scorecard (which always reminds me of playing putt-putt when I was a little kid). Each section has a judge who watches you carefully and lets you know how many points you have accumulated in one section—the maximum being 5 points per section. The rider with the fewest points is declared the winner. Today there are several different observed trials categories to enter:

1. Novice stock bike.
2. Intermediate stock bike.
3. Expert stock bike.

A stock bike has a few criteria to meet, such as a minimum of a 40-inch wheelbase, a rear derailleur with two or more gears, and no skid plate (a device that goes under the bottom bracket and allows the bike to roll smoothly over logs instead of the chainring hitting). Other categories are:

1. Novice modified bike.
2. Intermediate modified bike.
3. Expert modified bike.

These are the bikes that people call "trials bikes." They generally have a minimum of a 20-inch diameter wheel. Other than that guideline, each trials bike could be very different.

The trials rider is not allowed to practice the sections before competing but can walk through the sections to get an idea of what line to ride.

Equipment Used in Off-Road Racing

1. A helmet. Always wear one! To me not wearing a helmet is the same as not wearing your seatbelt while driving a car. They make such lightweight helmets now that you hardly even notice they are on your head. It only takes one rock against the head to prohibit you from ever riding again. Check to make sure they are A.N.S.I. approved (a standard all racing helmets must pass—see Fig.2-1). There should be a sticker inside every helmet stating this. I recommend the LT 700 helmet.
2. Gloves. These not only provide extra cushioning for those long, rocky descents but also add protection for the palms of your hands in case of a fall.

3. Glasses. You can choose now between different colored lenses—and it does make a difference! I like the orange or yellow lens when it is partly cloudy. Otherwise I find that shadows are a factor when riding through woods. Clear lenses are good for muddy courses or rainy days. Gray or darker lenses are better for bright days where the rider will be out in the open with direct sunlight.

4. Shoes. Most racers nowadays wear cleated shoes. These shoes, along with toe clips, provide a tight fit into the pedal, allowing the optimum power from each stroke. Also, a stiffer shoe will provide a better platform to push against, translating into a more efficient, powerful pedal stroke—as opposed to riding in your tennis shoes where more energy is lost due to the excess flexibility in the shoe.

Remember this, though. My theory has always been that 80 percent of your performance is yourself and 20 percent is the bike! I received my first mountain bike as a Christmas present about four years ago. It was a lower-end model priced around $450. The following spring, we went to Moab, Utah. This was where the bug bit me. I was amazed at what these two-wheeled vehicles could roll over and the constant abuse they took over the sandstone crags. It was incredible what those knobby tires could grip, as if we were actually climbing with sticky rubber shoes over and around these prehistoric land sculptures. These bikes were built for this treatment. They were still in one piece after every ride. When I returned to Colorado in May, I decided to enter a local race, feeling very primed from my ventures on Slickrock and other infamous trails in Utah. I was mentally ready and psyched (and a bit nervous) for my first race. It worked! I beat most of the top-level women, who were riding $1,500 bikes, when I was a rank beginner.

Training

Which brings me to another issue in racing, and that is the homework it requires—or rather training. I train with a heart monitor (see Fig. 11-2) and find it beneficial. What's even better is to include a VO2 Max Test. Usually at universities you can pay to have these done or be a guinea pig for an exercise physiology major. These tests tell you your maximum heart rate and many other interesting facts about your body that are useful for training correctly and efficiently. The combination of the heart monitor and VO2 test gives you guidelines on how hard you should be training day to day. The following is a general workout week for me during race season:

Sunday: Race.
Monday: Recovery day. Easy spin, one to one and a half hours. Low heart rate.

Tuesday: Intervals. Speed work. High heart rate.
Wednesday: Long distance, 3 to 5 hours. Medium heart rate.
Thursday: Sprints. Same as Tuesday.
Friday: Easy day. Get body ready, relaxed.
Saturday: Race.

It is important during the days before a race to make sure your body is well-hydrated and properly tanked up. A good indication of this is checking your urine. Yellow, dark urine is good indication of being dehydrated—unless you take a lot of vitamins, your urine should be clear when you are well-hydrated. On longer races, I take Power Bars or fig bars or dried fruit. I need to eat every couple of hours, or my performance goes downhill and I'm not enjoying life much either. I always race with two full water bottles—unless it's a very short race (less than one hour). The morning of a race what I eat depends on the length of the course. If it is a hill climb, I tend to eat lighter, like a bowl of cereal with fruit. For a longer cross-country event, I'll eat one to two hours beforehand and eat a bigger breakfast, such as pancakes. I begin eating about one hour into the race to keep my blood sugar level high and to avoid bonking. When your car runs out of gas, it doesn't run, and our bodies are certainly the same!

If you are still fascinated with all this preparation and work, I suggest you ride down to your local bike shop and find a race in your area to enter. Why not? There is nothing to lose and you may even have some fun at it. In fact, I haven't met a rider yet who hasn't enjoyed a first attempt at racing. I guarantee you'll be at the dinner table that same evening sharing tall tales with other fellow "mudheads" about the day's adventures. Watch out—it's contagious!

All racers must have a current NORBA license to enter. All shapes and sizes are encouraged to enter. You can obtain an application at the race or write to NORBA at One Olympic Plaza, Colorado Springs, CO 80909, phone 1-719-578-4717, FAX 1-719-578-4628.

Tandems

I had the opportunity to ride a 150-mile off-road race in southern California called the Dodge 150—Desert-to-Sea. This was a race open to both single mountain bikes and tandems. We (Gary Fisher and I) opted for the latter, and what a day was in store for us! We rode from Palm Springs to Dana Point, traversing the San Gabriel and Santa Ana mountains. Granted most of it was on fire roads—thank God!—but we did have a short 5-mile section of technical single track, with 90-degree switchback turns and rocky gullies. I must admit this took some creative thinking since our Fisher tandems did not have a bungy cord in the middle or any other device that would allow the bike to fold itself in half in order to master these abrupt turns! So we planned for me, "the stoker" (person behind the driver), to run ahead (I was wearing road cleats, not exactly the most comfortable things to run in!). I'm not quite sure how Gary maneuvered the tandem around the tight turns, but when I threw a quick glimpse over my shoulder, while running uncomfortably down the rocks, it was a funny sight to see! The rear wheels were bouncing off the ground and Gary was whooping and hollering. Or was that cussing and swearing I heard?

Anyway, tandems can move very fast on the road because of all the momentum you have. Only one person breaks the wind. We were averaging speeds of 45 mph at times on the pavement with slick tires pumped up to 100 psi. When we returned to the dirt roads, we pulled over at the designated aid station and changed back to our Fisher FatTracks (knobby off-road tires) at 40 to 50 psi.

It is a very different feeling to be the stoker and relinquish all control and vision to the person in front. It is just like sitting on the backseat of a motorcycle or a toboggan where you must lean with the driver for a smooth ride.

There aren't many tandems in mountain bike races. Technical terrain plus the long wheelbase of the tandem makes off-road mountain bicycle tandemming quite difficult. Tandems operate much better on wide-open roads where tight turns and large obstacles are not encountered. There are, however, specific mountain bicycle tandem races where the courses are outlined specifically for tandems.

NORBA

The National Off-Road Bicycle Association (*NORBA*) says that it is: "The national governing body for mountain bike racing in the United States with approximately 23,000 licensed members participating in over 500 sanctioned events nationwide. Each year, more than 33,000 new riders participate in this unique sport which originated in the United States." For more information about racing rules, classification program, trail riding, and special events, send for the 66-page *Competition Guide,* which costs five dollars. Ask NORBA for the name and address of the NORBA local official in your state. (NORBA'S address was given earlier in this chapter.)

NORBA offers the following tips for mountain bike racing, which I have excerpted from their *Competition Guide:*

- At the race your bike should be in top condition. Bring a variety of cog sets and chainrings, spare tubes and tires, and an extra wheel.

- Keep your chain clean and well-lubricated. Chain damage is a major problem with mountain bikes. Replace it whenever it shows signs of wear, stretch, and damage to avoid a long walk home (see Chapter 4 for chain maintenance).
- Bring six feet of rope along so you can hang your bike (not the judges) from a tree branch if it needs work. Bring your tool kit too.
- Bring heavy-duty plastic packing tape. Use it for rimstrips, boots for fractured tires, and repacking your bike for the trip home.
- Drink lots of water, starting 72 hours *before* a race. Carry a water bottle with or near you at all times.
- Avoid "snakebite" tube punctures. Sprinkle talcum powder around the tube and in the tire.
- Avoid chain slap on a downhill race by removing two links from your chain.
- Before a race, look at your tire seating. Check where the tire hooks into the rim for proper seating. Check the tire for embedded foreign objects and remove them.
- Check tire pressure before a race. Use the tire pressure noted on the tire sidewall.
- Avoid last-minute hassles by pre-entering a race. Make sure your entry is for the correct race and that the date, time, and location of the race have not been changed.

Human-Powered Vehicles and the Continuing Quest for Speed

Radical change hasn't exactly been a watchword in bicycle design. Few truly dramatic changes have been attempted since the safety bike with pneumatic tires first hit the racks nearly a century ago. Developments in technology and new, lightweight materials have certainly altered the way the traditional bicycle performs and handles. We can go farther, faster, in greater comfort than ever before. Modifications in design and componentry have also made off-road travel by bike possible. Yet, it looks as if the upright diamond-shaped frame with spoked wheels and a chain-driven gear system will be the design of choice for some time to come.

Such longevity and versatility certainly attest to what a simple and sensible machine this really is. Consider, for example, the following stories of human-powered speed.

On July 20, 1985, John Howard set a new motor-paced speed record of 152.284 mph. Howard is a well-known U.S. amateur cycling champion, as well as a Race Across America veteran and Ironman Triathlon winner. He set this pace riding in the slipstream of a race car on the table-smooth surface of the Bonneville Salt Flats. His bike was a $10,000 motorcyclelike machine with fat tires and a single 390-inch gear (see Chapter 5 for a discussion of gear ratios; the average touring bike has around a 100-inch high gear) driven by three sprockets and two chains. Traveling forward 111 feet with each turn of the crank, the bike had to be towed to 60 mph before Howard reached a pedal cadence fast enough to keep it moving. To most people, even 60 mph on a bike would seem a little suicidal. But Howard was eager for another try after his rear tire suddenly deflated and the bike began to fishtail at 150 mph!

So, you say, how practical is a bike that goes 150 mph, especially when it needs a race car to get it started? Not too practical, I'll admit. But some people are working on alternatives that are more down-to-earth. In May 1986, a specially designed bike called the Easy Racer reached an incredible speed of 65.484 mph. Its designers collected a $15,000 prize for being the first to surpass the 65-mph mark in a human-powered machine unassisted by a pace vehicle.

The Easy Racer could be the shape of things to come in human-powered transportation. It still rides on two wheels, but the configuration of the traditional bike has disappeared. The rider sits in a semiprone position, something like sitting in an easy chair. The semiprone position is more aerodynamically efficient because it reduces the frontal area of the bike. The Easy Racer is also encased with a complete fairing of Kevlar to reduce drag. Better aerodynamics and a more comfortable seating posture allow a rider to go farther with less energy expenditure and less physical discomfort.

The success of the Easy Racer team represents over a decade of work to set new land speed records for bicycles. The process was given a great boost when the International Human Powered Vehicle Association (IHPVA) was formed in 1974. The IHPVA was originally created to provide official recognition for speed records then being set on altered and redesigned bicycles. Many people felt at the time of the IHPVA's founding that the current governing bodies had stifled development through excessive restrictions on design. Currently, the IHPVA holds annual races to test and stimulate further developments in human-powered transport.

Early record-setters were usually standard racing bikes enclosed in lightweight fairings. This design took advantage of the more powerful pedal stroke that is possible in the upright posture. However, because of their height and large frontal area, these vehicles were disadvantaged aerodynamically. IHPVA rules stated only that vehicles entered in competition could have no energy source besides that provided by the riders. A very creative process of design and product refinement followed the association's ruling.

IHPVA meets tend to be colorful events. The race is unique because it's a design competition as much as an athletic competition. Vehicles of all descriptions, from bikes with fairings to three-person tricycles and quadricycles, compete together. Many vehicles use a prone or recumbent riding position. The Vector, a quadricycle entered in the 1979 competition, used three riders in prone positions who all pedaled with their feet. But, while the front rider steered with his hands, the others also turned handgrips attached to the pedals immediately in front of them. It's estimated that this produced 12.5 percent more power than cranks turned by foot pedals alone.

Will these innovators develop the human-powered commuter machine of the future? It's possible, but many problems still have to be worked out. Some form of recumbent bicycle is likely to emerge as the most viable option. A two-wheeled vehicle is more stable when cornering than either the tricycle or the quadricycle. The semiprone position is most comfortable, and makes the rider more visible in traffic than a prone-position vehicle. A lightweight fairing is likely too, since reduced drag can increase speed by several mile per hour. The fairing will also protect the rider from the weather and allow cargo to be carried inside, two matters of some importance to the average commuter.

However, use of fairing has several drawbacks. Sidewinds can knock the bike on its side. The cyclist also needs assistance to get seated inside. Both problems could be solved by using small outrigger wheels that are dropped or pulled in when necessary. A bigger problem is the vehicle's poor performance in climbing hills. The upright position is still the best for hill climbing because the rider can apply body weight to the pedals for added power. This and other problems are sure to consume a lot of time and human energy before they can be solved.

Flying into the Future

In the meantime, another competition is underway in the realm of human-powered aviation. Many will remember Bryan Allen's crossing of the English Channel in the human-powered plane called the *Gossamer Albatross.* That flight not only made aviation history, it also brought the $200,000 Kremer prize for human-powered flight to its designer, Paul MacCready. MacCready and Allen's feat was compared to that of other aviation pioneers, and the *Gossamer Albatross* appropriately took its place beside the *Kitty Hawk* in the Smithsonian Institute.

But MacCready didn't put his prodigious talent to rest with the *Gossamer Albatross.* He went on to develop several more planes, among them the *Bionic Bat,* which uses human power along with energy from pedaling that is stored in a battery. The *Bionic Bat* won another Kremer prize, and MacCready went on to become president of the IHPVA. Later, the *Gossamer Albatross's* distance record was beaten by a plane called the *Eagle.* The *Eagle's*

M.I.T. designers say it's a forerunner of another human-powered plane named *Daedalus*, after the father of Icarus, whose ill-fated flight is one of the most famous stories in Greek mythology. As you may have seen on the television coverage of this event, the *Daedalus* did make the 69 miles from the Greek mainland to the island of Crete, just.

Whether any of these developments will leave a mark on the future of transportation, or whether inventions like the *Bionic Bat* and the Easy Racer bike will become the curiosity pieces of some future age, may depend upon our determination to carry the process forward. Reserves of fossil fuels are limited, and as the growing problem of acid rain shows, we may be forced to reconsider our practice of burning oil and coal long before these fuels are depleted forever. At least for traveling short distances, we already have the means to create clean, efficient, and healthy forms of human-powered transportation. What's needed now is a vigorous application of human ingenuity.

Speaking of ingenuity, the next chapter takes up the birth of bicycling from the crotch-numbing Draisene to the high-wheeler and to the development of today's modern multi-speeed bicycles.

CHAPTER THIRTEEN

BICYCLING, THE FAD THAT GREW

I like to think that the sexual revolution began back in 1867 and that it was all due to the beginning of the large-scale production of bicycles. Two-wheelers certainly did get young folks away from the beady eyes of family supervision, let couples romance far from the madding crowd, and gave women as well as men a new form of low-cost transportation. Moralists forecast dire consequences for the newfound freedom that came with the bicycle. But millions found pleasure in this economical mode of transportation that ate no fodder, did not need the services of a veterinary surgeon, cost no more than a good horse, and did not require a costly saddle or a barn at night. Early bicycles were heavy, clumsy, cumbersome, and with the rider up high, somewhat hazardous (Fig. 13-1). Yet the bike boom continued.

By 1875 bicycling was virtually an infatuation with the American public. By 1885 factories were working around the clock to meet the demand for bicycles. By 1895 over two million Americans had bought a bicycle, one for every 27 people, man, woman, and child, even though a bike cost from $50 to $150, a hefty 12 to 33 percent of the then per capita $420 annual income.

But in 1902 Henry Ford struck what was almost a death blow to the bicycle industry in the United States. Americans simply forsook the two-wheeler for the four-wheeled Tin Lizzie, and the automotive industry was off and running. In the late 1960s, however, an emphasis on health, fostered by President John F. Kennedy, led Americans to take a long, hard look at the relationship between exercise, health, happiness, and longevity. Riding a bicycle became more than a nostalgic return to childhood, it became the "in" thing to do and boomers bought them and rode them by the millions. In 1974, in fact, bicycles outsold cars—11 million bikes versus 9 million new cars. By 1993 almost 100 million Americans owned bikes and were riding them to work, on cross-country trips in this country and abroad, and on

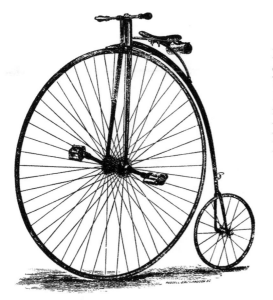

FIG. 13-1: An 1881 Standard Columbia high-wheel bicycle, made by Pope Manufacturing in Hartford, Connecticut. This type of bicycle was also known as a Penny Farthing and an Ordinary.

mountain trails. And by 1993 an entire new service industry was well out of swaddling clothes and into a healthy economic life, the packaged bike-touring business, which today is taking tourists on two wheels all over the world on planned tours.

Back in the 1890s, lifestyles, even clothing styles, changed dramatically to meet the special needs of this new mode of transportation. It became apparent to women, for example, that a dress down to the floor, restrictive body gadgets, and other clothing impedimenta were going to be unsafe for cycling. Riding sidesaddle might have been feasible, more or less, on a horse, but not on a bicycle. So women changed to clothing styles that gave freedom to legs, such as baggy clothing (Fig. 13-2), which became the fashion, along with social clubs that fostered an interest in bicycling (Fig. 13-3). Even the military adopted bicycles as a quick way to move troops (Fig. 13-4). Soon postmen (Fig. 13-5) were riding bicycles on their appointed rounds.

By 1890 men were racing high-wheelers at velodromes (Fig. 13-6), both sexes were riding them on trails, roads, and canal towpaths, to the terror of horses and the anger of barge towmen (Fig. 13-7), and occasionally doing an "endo" over the front of a high-wheeler (Fig. 13-8). Women were riding down country roads in odd-looking contraptions such as the tricycle in Fig. 13-9. In 1896, Margaret Valentine LeLong rode her bicycle from Chicago to San Francisco, no mean feat considering her primitive, heavy bicycle, the rough roads, the two major mountain ranges, and the desert between them that she had to cross. My hat is off to that lady, may she be remembered forever!

Bicycling reached such a height of popularity by 1890 that it took over 400

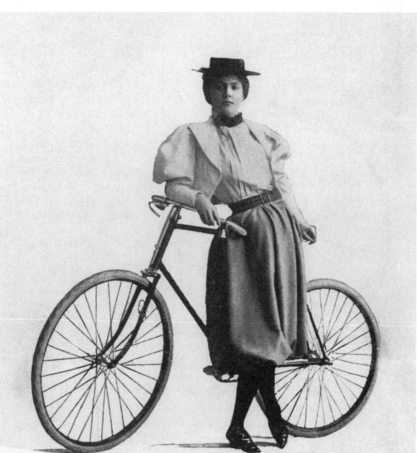

FIG. 13-2: When women began to ride "men's" bicycles with a top tube frame, back in the late 1890s, their clothing styles had to change to pantaloons or baggy knickers. *Bettmann Archive.*

FIG. 13-3: High society embraced bicycling with fervor, starting indoor riding rinks. Here members of New York's Michaux Cycle Club enjoy the pleasures of indoor cycling in a ballroom atmosphere. *Bettmann Archive.*

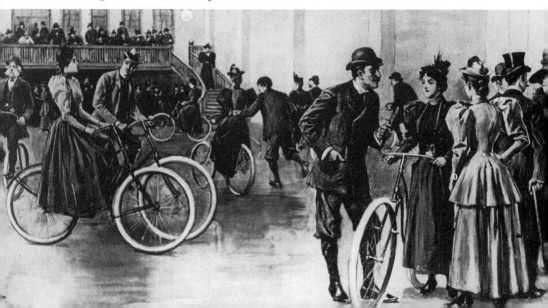

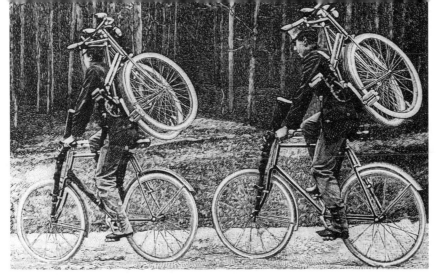

FIG. 13-4: French soldiers of the 1890s carried 23-pound folding bikes on maneuvers. Note the rifle strapped to the fork.

FIG. 13-5: This French postcard commemorates the days when postmen made their daily rounds on a bicycle. The locale is a country lane near Aix-en-Provence, in the south of France. In the background is what appears to be Montaigne San Victoire, near the atelier of the famous artist Paul Cézanne (1839–1906), in which your author found this card.

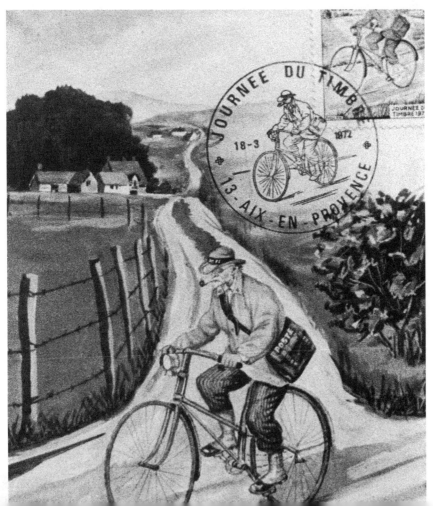

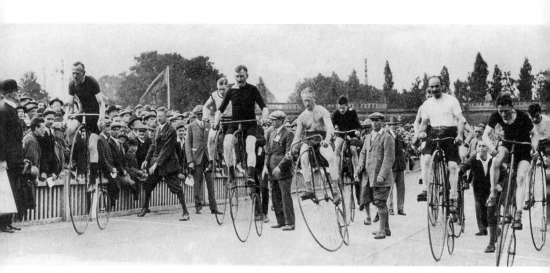

FIG. 13-6: The competitive instinct of every sport found its way to bicycles, as this high-wheeler race on a velodrome of the early 1890s shows. *Bettmann Archive.*

FIG. 13-7: Bicyclists of the 1890s spooked horses and mules much as they do now. Here mules pulling a barge on the Erie Canal bolt off the trail as the unusual sight of a high-wheeler scares them. The bargemen, as you can see, were rather upset by this event.

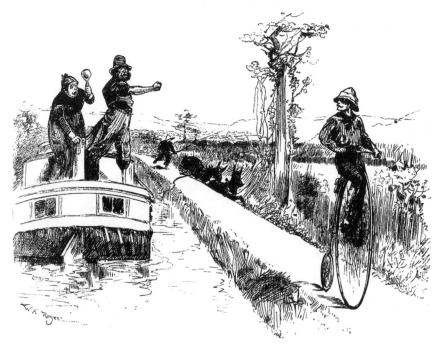

AN EPISODE OF TOW-PATH RIDING.

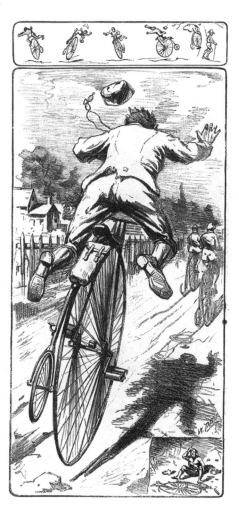

FIG. 13-8: High-wheelers were unstable machines that could propel the rider over the handlebars if they hit even a small obstruction in the road.

FIG. 13-9: Designers came up with many unusual designs for self-propelled vehicles, such as this Oldreive's tricycle or "iron horse" in which the rider sat in a chair next to the front wheel and pushed down on rod-mounted pedals. *Bettmann Archive.*

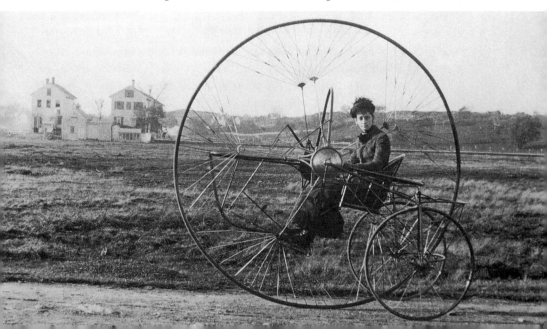

bicycle manufacturers in the United States alone to meet the demand. Enthusiasts of this new sport spent so much money on these metal steeds that they had little left to spend on other goods, to the consternation of businessmen. By 1896 the sale of watches and jewelry had dropped precipitously, for example, and as a status symbol were replaced by the more fashionable bicycle. Piano sales fell as people turned to their bicycles, although a hit tune of the era contained the words "Daisy, Daisy, give me your answer true . . . for you'd look sweet, upon the seat, of a bicycle built for two." Attendance at theatrical performances dropped, because, I like to think, people spent their money on bikes and their energy on riding them so that by curtain time they were too tired to go out.

In 1896 bicycles were truly big business, akin to the auto industry today. To quote from the February 1896 issue of *Outing*, a magazine devoted the leisure activities of the wealthy:

> The cycle trade is now one of the chief industries of the world. Its ramifications are beyond ordinary comprehension. Its prosperity contributes in no small degree to that of the steel, wire, rubber and leather markets. Time was when the spider web monsters, now nearly extinct, were built in one story annexes to English and American machine shops; now a single patented type of a jointless wood rim, one of the minor parts of a modern bicycle, is the sole product of an English factory covering over two acres of ground. A decade ago the American steel tube industry was unprofitable. The production of this essential part of cycle construction has, during the past two years, been unequal to the demand, and even now every high-grade tube mill in this country is working night and day on orders that will keep them busy throughout the year . . . prices will be very generally maintained, and the number of riders, of both sexes, will be at least doubled.

Bicycles of the 1890s were heavy and cumbersome compared to the lightweight bicycles of today. Metallurgy in those days did not produce bike tubing that combined lightness with the strength and durability of the tubing used in modern bikes. To reach racing speeds riders had to wind up to quite high crank revolutions per minute. A. A. Zimmerman, a famous racer of the 1890s, could sustain a cadence of 140 rpms, which on a modern bicycle would have him whizzing along at around 48 mph if he had a 116-inch gear.

Development of the Bicycle

The earliest known depiction of a two-wheeler is in a stained-glass window in a church built in 1637, in Stokes-on-Poges, England (Fig. 13-10). I find it hard to believe that this kick-along bike was just a creation of the fertile mind and talent of an artist. Surely someone, somewhere in that village, must have built one, but there is to date no trace of it. It took another 154 years for a

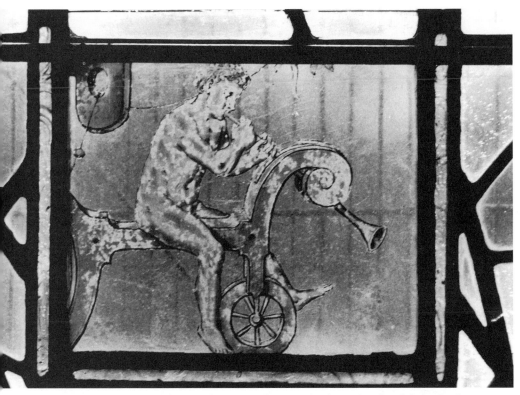

FIG. 13-10: The earliest known depiction of a two-wheeler is this detail from the famous stained-glass window in a 1637 church in Stokes-on-Poges, England. *Courtesy Pierre Maissaneuve.*

somewhat similar model to appear. In 1791 such a bike was built by a Frenchman. It was called a "celerifere," meaning fast feet. I found an actual sample of this machine on display in the Technical Museum on a visit to Milan, Italy (Fig. 13-11).

Only 26 years later, in 1817, a more comfortable-steering version of the celerifere was built by Baron Karl von Drais of Karlsruhe, Germany (Fig. 13-12). The rider of a Draisene kicked along with his feet, like someone riding a kiddie car (remember?), and turned the cumbersome two-wheeler by leaning in the desired direction. The Draisene became an almost instant success, costly, heavy, and clumsy though it was. The playboys of western Europe were soon kicking their way up and down the boulevards of major cities on what became known as the hobby horse. A hobby then, as today, inevitably develops into clubs, and hobby horse owners did just that—organized the sport into clubs, held races, and planned short tours (which had to be short, given the 100-pounds-plus weight of these bikes and the rough roads of the day).

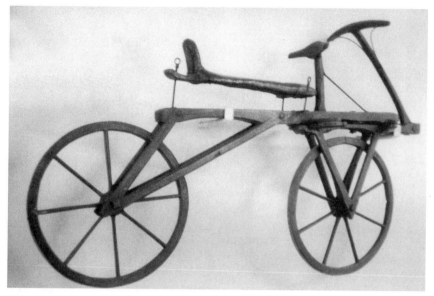

FIG. 13-11: Your author took this photo of a very early bicycle, circa 1791, on a visit to the Technical Museum in Milan, Italy.

FIG. 13-12: The original Draisene push bicycle, built by Baron Karl von Drais in 1817, on exhibit in the Breslau, Germany, museum.

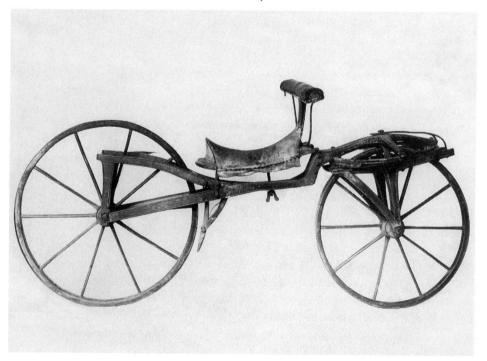

Bike technology advanced to the next logical stop, when crank arms and pedals were added to the Draisene, along with a steerer tube and handlebars so the new model could be steered by hand as well as by leaning, just as you can steer your bicycle today. The new version of the hobby horse was called a Boneshaker (Fig. 13-13), and I can believe it did just that. Steel-rimmed wooden wheels and a hard saddle mounted on a steel top tube certainly offered little by way of shock absorbance. By 1862, however, a more sophisticated, lighter, more comfortable version of the Boneshaker evolved that was also easier to steer (Fig. 13-14).

In 1872, bicycle development took a step backward, in my opinion, with the development of the high-wheeler. The next logical step in bike technology should have been the simple design of a steel diamond frame, along with the pedals and cranks already developed, and a chain to connect a chainwheel to the rear wheel. But the designers of the day simply created a Boneshaker with a bigger front wheel, again directly turned by pedals and cranks attached to it (Figs. 13-1, 13-7, and 13-8). The bigger the front wheel the faster the rider could go, the limitation being having legs long enough to

FIG. 13-13: The stiff wooden wheels and steel frame of this bicycle translated road shock to the rider of this aptly named Boneshaker. It was, however, the first bicycle to be equipped with pedals and cranks and so was very popular in the 1860s. Your author saw this model on a visit to the Technical Museum in Milan, Italy.

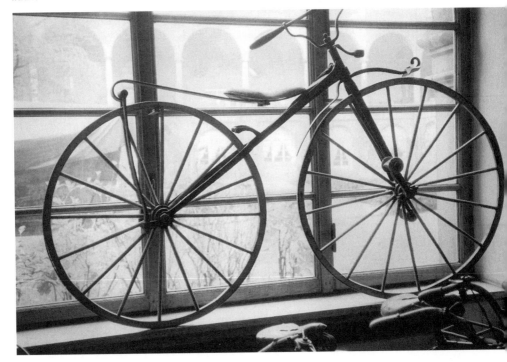

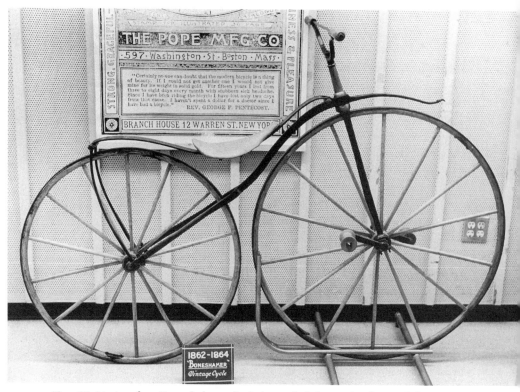

FIG. 13-14: Another Boneshaker, of a lighter, slightly more advanced design, was made in the United States and became a favorite with young men in the mid-1860s.

reach the pedals. This, by the way, is where today's archaic gear terminology comes from. We denote gears in inches, instead of in gear ratios. The more inches, the lower the gear ratio and the faster you can pedal today, if you have the muscle power (see Chapter 5 for more information on gearing). The high-wheeled machines were called Ordinaries, Penny Farthings, or velocipedes. Given the height of the rider above the saddle, the running start, and the hop needed to get up onto the saddle to get moving, the accident and injury potential of high-wheelers would, I am sure, be good as gold to plaintiff personal injury attorneys today.

A modicum of comfort came to the bicycle in 1888, when pneumatic rubber tires replaced steel and solid rubber tires. The air-filled bike tires were developed by veterinary surgeon J. B. Dunlop of Belfast, Ireland, when his son complained of the harsh ride of his new hard-tired trike. The good doctor made his first pneumatic tires out of rubber sheets and strips of linen. When his friend William Hume, president of the Belfast Cruiser's Cycling Club, persuaded Dr. Dunlop to make up a pair of pneumatic tires for his racing bicycle, and Mr. Hume then beat the crack racing cyclists of his day in a race on May 18, 1889, the age of pneumatic tires for bikes took off in earnest. The news of the new tires soon reached the bicycle world and by 1891 bicycles were routinely fitted with them. Dr. Dunlop was in business making his new tires for the general cycling public.

By 1895 the bicycle looked very much like the bikes of today, complete with chain drive and pneumatic tires (Fig. 13-15). Tandems were popular, but if you look closely at Fig. 13-16, you will see two rods connected to the rear handlebars so that the man in back could steer while the woman rode up front. I can just imagine the very justified outcry if today's tandems put the woman in such an inferior situation, one made worse by the fact that she rode in a more vulnerable location, up front. Certainly the man in back could not have had a clear view of oncoming road hazards, while the woman up front could do nothing about them though she could see them.

A shaft-drive transmission for bicycles was popular in 1896. Such bicycles were made by Victor Bicycle (Fig. 13-17) and by Pierce-Arrow, which later made very costly touring limousines for the wealthy.

Like history, technology sometimes repeats itself. For example, a cam-action brake introduced in 1935 (Fig. 13-18) operates on the same powerful cam principle as a similar brake designed by Charles Cunningham that found popularity on mountain bicycles in the 1980s. On the same note, a two-speed-capacity derailleur introduced in 1934 (Fig. 13-19) has its modern counter-

FIG. 13-15: A Cleveland women's bicycle of 1895 looks much like inexpensive bicycles of today. Harplike strings on the rear fender help keep flowing skirts from tangling in the spokes.

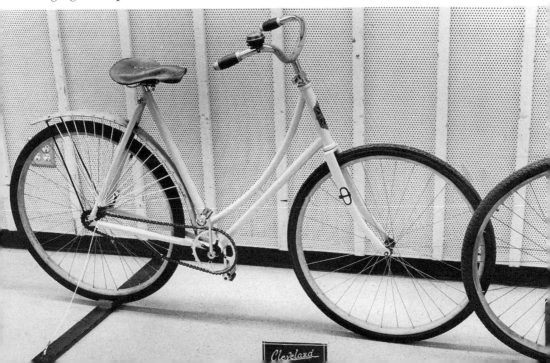

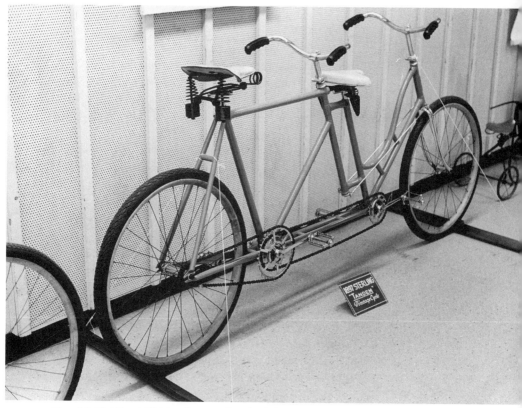

FIG. 13-16: This 1897 Sterling tandem had the woman up front, but the man in the rear controlled front-wheel steering by rods connecting the rear handlebars to the fork.

FIG. 13-17: Shaft-drive bicycles, such as this 1896 Victor model, eliminated the chain drive. Similar bicycles were also made by Pierce-Arrow, which later made luxury limousines.

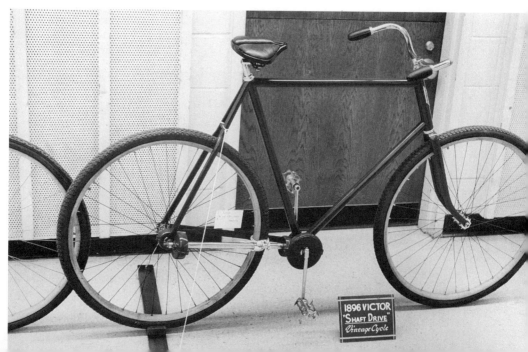

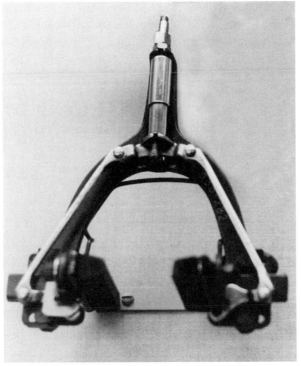

FIG. 13-18: Cam-action brakes like this one were popular in 1935. Similar designs are found today on mountain bicycles.

FIG. 13-19: An early derailleur, this one a two-speed model, helped cyclists make steep hills in 1934.

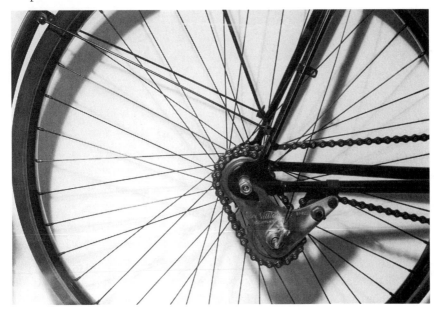

part in the eight-speed-capacity derailleur of today. The radial spoke pattern of some modern racing bicycle wheels had its predecessor in the spokes of a Boneshaker (Fig. 13-14). The epicyclic gear drive on an adult tricycle of 1890 (Fig. 13-20) was briefly popular on some bike models introduced in 1985.

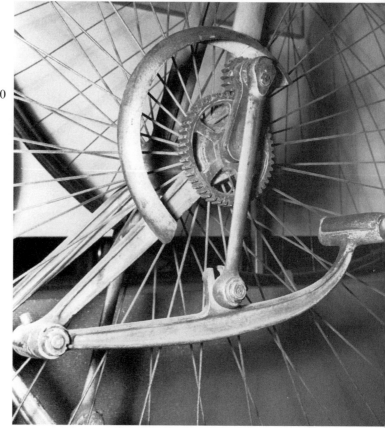

Fig. 13-20: An epicyclic gear drive on an 1890 tricycle.

Early Lights

Back before the automobile, bicyclists needed lights more to be able to avoid potholes, rocks, and the droppings of horses and cows than other cyclists, horses, and horse-drawn wagons. Early lights were candle-powered (Fig. 13-21), with lenses and prisms that amplified this feeble light source, something like the Fresnel lamp of a marine lighthouse. Acetylene lamps were popular by 1897 (Fig. 13-22). These lamps were indeed powerful. I put one on my road bike some years ago and was stopped by a policeman who was more curious than concerned about this strong beam coming from a bicycle. Battery-powered lights became popular around 1900 (Figs. 13-23 and 13-24).

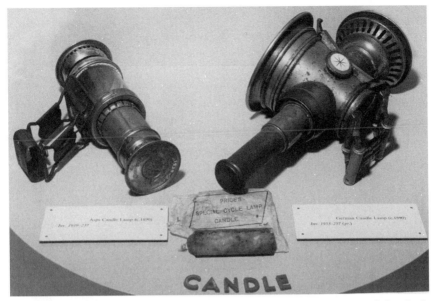

FIG. 13-21: Early bicycle lights were candle-powered, like these 1919 models, which had light-amplifying lenses like those on lighthouses.

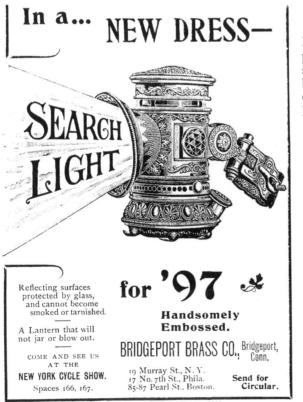

FIG. 13-22: More powerful bike lights, such as this one made by Bridgeport Brass Company, were acetylene-powered.

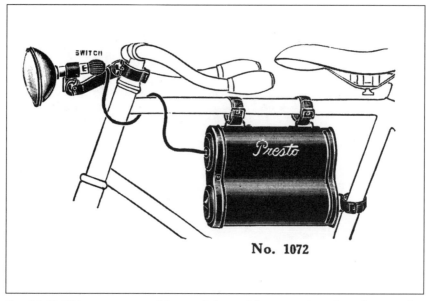

FIG. 13-23: This stem-mounted battery light, with batteries slung from the top tube, was popular in 1916, but its batteries were not rechargeable.

FIG. 13-24: This self-contained battery-powered light had side reflectors.

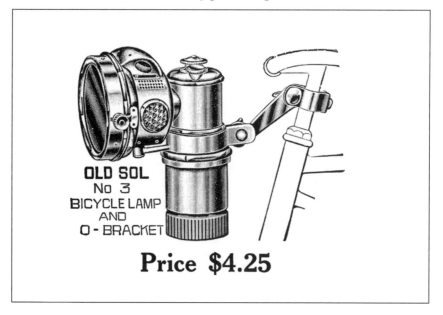

Materials

If you want to see a beautiful example of woodwork, take a look at the wooden rims on bicycles made up to around 1930. These rims are truly grand examples of the woodworker's art. They only had one problem. A good jolt over a pothole would fracture the wood, signifying a need for a new rim. Bike frames were mostly of mild steel tubing, though some, such as the Lum-in-num, made in St. Louis, were made of aluminum tubing. You can also see bamboo bike frames in museums such as the Smithsonian, in Washington, D.C.

Hostility, Then and Now

By the 1890s bicyclists were not exactly clogging the highways and byways of America, but they were out there. Unfortunately cyclists met lots of hostility from the noncyclist population. Possibly some of it was merited, when bikes spooked horses or mules (Fig. 13-7), as they still do today, when mountain bikes come silently down an off-road trail upon equestrians, do not sound a mild-sounding tinkle bell, and so cause horses to go off in a tizzy.

Farmers took personal delight in blocking the narrow roads of the day when bicyclists were spied, and went as slowly as possible to irritate the faster two-wheelers. Country bumpkins delighted in thrusting a stick into the spokes of a high-wheeler, resulting in disaster to the cyclist and guffaws from the pranksters. Horse-drawn vehicles were often deliberately sent careening into groups of cyclists, causing injury to the riders and damage to their bicycles. And in the early 1880s English restaurant and tea-shop owners often refused to serve cyclists, particularly females who wore what the owner of one establishment described as "outlandish and shocking costumes."

Such hostility was not as widespread in 1962 when I began bicycling to work from my home in Grosse Pointe, Michigan, 10 miles to my office in downtown Detroit, but it was there, believe me. Once a couple of adults leaned out the window of their taxi one early December day and wanted to know "What is your mommy gonna to buy you for next Christmas, sonny!" I've heard of yokels in Kentucky and in South Dakota who throw beer bottles at cyclists and try to run them off the road. Things don't change much in human nature.

Early Cycling Clubs

Bicycle clubs of the 1800s were formed for political as well as for social reasons, just as they are today. Cyclists back then wanted improved bicycle trails, as they do today. Cyclists wanted revisions of restrictive legislation then, just as mountain bikers want more freedom to ride mountain trails than is granted to them today. Bicycle clubs in the 1800s also wanted protection against wanton attacks by irate citizens, attacks that are not so widespread today, for which I and my millions of fellow cyclists are duly grateful.

In 1878 in England, regional cycling clubs joined forces and organized the British Touring Club. The BTC soon began publication of its own magazine, *The Bicycling Times.* In 1883 the BTC changed its name to the Cyclist's Touring Club (CTC) and its publication name to the *Gazette.* This magazine was an outspoken and fearless defender of cyclists and bicycling in England, although it was at times controversial; its editor was roundly denounced by some members, including those employed by bicycle manufacturers. During one meeting, at which the editor was being excoriated, George Bernard Shaw, an ardent cyclist and lifelong member of the club, arose to defend him. Mr. Shaw said, "Do you want it [the *Gazette*] to contain fact or fiction? You already have plenty of fiction in the advertising pages. . . . I want to raise a strong objection against what has been said as to raising the tone of the *Gazette.* What we want above all things is an abusive *Gazette.* If I wish to read a nice complimentary cycling paper—one that has a good word for everybody, for every dealer and seller, and every sort of kind of invention, I can easily buy it for a penny at any news shop. But we want something quite in the opposite direction in our *Gazette,* even if that publication does sometimes refer to a ladies' article as piffle. [Roars of laughter.] In my view," Shaw continued, "the gentlemen who object to ladies having to stand the same treatment as is meted out to men are the same people who object to ladies cycling together, and therefore I do not think they need be taken very seriously." George, born in 1856, died in 1950, living to the ripe old age of 94, so bicycling must have been good for him, as it is for all of us.

But the British Parliament reflected the electorate's attitude toward bicycling. The Highway and Railway Safety Act of 1878, issued by Parliament, gave the counties the power to regulate the use of bicycles. Local authorities promptly forbade cyclists from using public highways, or required them to pull over and stop whenever a horse-drawn vehicle appeared on the horizon.

However, the CTC's many politically influential members, as well as the many thousands of its rank and file members, had by 1893 enough clout to push the Local Government Act through Parliament, thereby abolishing the power of local counties to regulate bicycling. The CTC then, in rapid order, pushed through legislation providing for highway improvements, safe transport of bicycles on railroad baggage cars, and legal recourse against the antagonism of the noncycling public.

For example, a landmark case that drew national attention occurred when a member of the British nobility and an influential member of the CTC, Lady Harbeton, was refused service in the coffee room of the Hautboy Hotel in Surrey because of her dress. Hotel management offered to serve her in the ladies' parlor, an offer which Lady Harbeton rejected with much umbrage. The CTC leaped to her defense, took the case to court, and won an indictment against the hotel owners for "willfully and unlawfully neglecting to supply a traveler with victuals." A deciding exhibit in this case was a photo of Lady Harbeton in her riding garb, which, according to the CTC, showed an "elderly lady wearing a pair of exceedingly baggy knickerbockers reaching below the knees, and a jacket which came well over the hips and opened sufficiently to reveal the silk blouse underneath." Well, good for the CTC and good for Lady Harbeton. Harassment of women cyclists we did not need then, nor do we now.

The League of American Wheelmen

After a visit to the CTC's Liverpool headquarters, a group of American cyclists formed the League of American Wheelmen in Newport, Rhode Island, in 1880. Newport was then, and still is, where many of America's oldest and wealthiest families have their summer cottages (spell that "mansions"), which should give you an idea of the social status of cycling at that time. During its heyday the LAW was a force no politician could ignore. Famous men and women were members, including Orville and Wilbur Wright, who had owned a bicycle shop before building and flying the first airplane in the United States.

The league flexed its political muscle in 1884 when it made a test case out of the decision of Haddonfield, New Jersey, turnpike officials to bar bikes from that road. Turnpikes at the time were state roads used by horse-drawn vehicles (autos were 16 years away). Cyclists would have to use dung-strewn cowpaths or worse if they wanted to parallel that route. But with the backing of the league, its Philadelphia chapter sued the turnpike and won, forcing the turnpike authority to rescind its no-cycling stricture.

Take a lesson from the LAW and have your local cycling club put pressure on any government agency that threatens to force you off a safe road and onto one far less safe.

In another case, the LAW fought an 1879 restriction by the New York Board of Commissions that outlawed bicycles in New York City's Central Park, because, they said, bicycles were an eyesore and a menace to the citizenry. It took eight years of litigation before the governor of New York took matters into his own hands and overruled the board.

Long-Distance Touring in the 1880s

Think what it must have been like to cross the United States on a bicycle back in the 1880s. Primitive rutted roads, virtually nonexistent campgrounds, small towns without hotels or even restaurants. No roadside phone to call for help if your bike broke down. Little if any medical assistance if you needed it. High-wheelers of the day were hard to steer, heavy, and unresponsive, and had no gears to help you climb steep hills. The hard saddle and stiff frame did little to absorb road shock, which, given the rough roads of the day, must have been considerable. It took a hardy soul indeed to undertake such a venture.

Such a hardy soul was Thomas Stevens, who rode his high-wheeler from Oakland, California, all the way to Boston, Massachusetts, in 1884. Well, "rode" does not exactly describe his experience. As he tells it he sometimes pedaled, but often carried, pushed, dragged, and shoved his 75-pound steed through streams and fields, across mountains and deserts. His trip was not exactly a piece of cake. In one bar, rowdy cowpokes forced Stevens to ride his high-wheeler around a pool room, shooting at him as he rode. Once he was pursued by a pack of coyotes (I'd prefer the coyotes to the cowpokes, myself). To avoid being hit by a train while he was crossing a railroad trestle over a deep ravine he had to hang by one hand on the side of the trestle and hold his 75-pound high-wheeler with his other hand. That episode brought visions of Hollywood stuntmen to my mind, except that Stevens's case was for real. He forded flood-swollen rivers, barreled down the Rockies while his metal spoon brakes, in an effort to keep speed down, glowed red from friction. He was cursed by Erie Canal bargemen whose mules balked and reared (see Fig. 13-7) as he, that strange apparition, pedaled past. Stevens hit pay dirt from Chicago on, when he became a media celebrity, with frequent newspaper stories about his epochal ride as he progressed from the Windy City to Boston.

Other round-the-world bicycle treks, during the 1890s, drew national media attention because these journeys were so unusual and arduous, and bicycling at that time was almost a national obsession, so anything two-wheeled drew public interest. Some of these trips involved women. For example, a young American woman, Annie Londberry, set out one fine July morning in 1894 to tour the world. She left stony broke. She not only made it around the world but had $2,000 in her purse on her return, a sizeable amount in this days. Now *that's* a promoter!

Another woman, Fannie Bullock Workman, and her physician husband spent 10 years touring the world, starting in the late 1890s. Mrs. Workman was the daughter of a governor of Massachusetts and had inherited considerable wealth. Old photos show her mounted on her trusty Rover safety bicycle, clad always in a high-necked blouse, a voluminous skirt, and a pith helmet. The Workmans rode over the Atlas Mountains of northwest Africa, in southern Morocco, the highest peak of which is Tizi n'Taggarat, about 15,000 feet. I doubt they rode over that mountain, but there were other ranges that must have been a major challenge. Their trip also took them through the Sahara, a laudable feat by anybody's standards, even today.

Early Bicycle Racing

Start a hobby and men will turn it into a competitive event. Bicycling was no exception, even way back in 1817 when butt-busting Draisenes (Fig. 13-12) became popular. Young blades of that era took to racing them down the boulevards of Europe's major cities. The first official bicycle race involving comparatively modern two-wheelers was held in 1878 over a one-mile course. This race was won by Will R. Lipton in 3 minutes and 57 seconds, which translates to an average speed of about 16 mph. Not bad for 75-pound, solid-tired high-wheelers (Fig. 13-6).

A well-known professional bicycle racer, A. A. Zimmerman (who I mentioned earlier in this chapter), set a new world record for the half mile in 1 minute, 10¾ seconds, for an average speed of about 25 mph—on a 70-pound high-wheeler. Zimmerman was notorious for his training regimen, or rather, for his lack of one. He violated all the rules of training, carousing and drinking until the wee hours while his teammates slept. In one notable instance he climbed on his safety bicycle after having attended an all-night party and pedaled a paced mile in just 1 minute, 57⅖ seconds, for an average speed of about 31 mph, at the annual LAW meet in Asbury Park, New Jersey. Not a record, but hey, he was up all night. Zimmerman was truly a laid-back guy, never trying to beat a record or win a race by any more effort or speed than was necessary. Given his lifestyle, I can understand that.

Bicycle racing in the late 1890s was at least as big a business as it is today. Many pros became wealthy from their winnings and would undoubtedly have made even more money had they had product endorsement business managers as do world-famous racing cyclists today. By 1985 there were over 600 professional bicycle racers just in the United States, and even more than that in Europe.

Early track records are impressive even by today's standards. For example, in 1895, Constance Huret pedaled 529 miles, 585 yards in just 24 hours, which translates to an average speed of 20.5 mph over the 24 hours. In 1895 E. F. Lenert outran a fast race horse over a one-mile course, which he completed in just 95 seconds, at an average speed of a bit over 38 mph! And in 1899 Charles ("Mile-a-Minute") Murphy pedaled a record mile in 57.8 seconds behind a train. He pedaled on a boarded-over section of the Long Island Rail Road tracks at an average speed of 62.2 mph. It took six years for an automobile to break that record—a car driven by Barney Oldfield, a former racing cyclist, who pushed Henry Ford's "999" to a mile in 55.8 seconds, not much faster than Mile-a-Minute Murphy's pedaled mile record.

The Bicycle in War

Military logicians of the 1890s viewed the bicycle as an invaluable tool for scouting, outpost duties, messenger service, patrols, and convoys. *Harper's Weekly*, in a special bicycle issue of April 11, 1896, noted: "It is in rapidly moving considerable bodies of infantry that the bicycle will find its highest function in time of war. Fancy a force of infantry, independent of roads and railroads, moving in any direction, forty or fifty miles in one morning, and appearing on a field not weary and exhausted as after a two-days' march, but fresh and prepared to fight." Well, this writer sure would not be fresh and prepared to fight after a 50-mile A.M. ride. So I think maybe the bicycle could be the world's solution to the end of warfare. Let the fighters of the world hoist their derrieres onto their bikes, pedal away furiously for 50 miles or so between 9:00 A.M. and noon, and I bet there won't be much serious fighting, at least not right away. Better yet, have the soldiers bicycle another 100 miles till nightfall and maintain this morning and afternoon regimen until one side or the other is willing to call it quits.

The Italian army was the first to adopt the bicycle as a valued adjunct to military hardware. In 1870, each regiment was given four bicycles, each bike equipped with a brake, lantern, knapsack, rifle support, and a knapsack for carrying orders. The French army had elegant bikes that weighed only 23 pounds (see Fig. 13-4) with a hinged frame so they could be folded and carried slung over a soldier's back, if need be. In 1885, Austrian soldiers, carrying a full field kit (sounds heavy to me) were said to travel 100 miles a day on bicycles, thereby outdoing their cavalry, which was on horseback.

In America, the first military to use bicycles was the Connecticut National Guard. The U.S. Army used two side-by-side bicycles with a "mountain cannon" mounted between them. The army also used a tandem equipped to carry rifles, revolvers, and a field pack, as well as a tricycle fitted with a Colt rapid-fire machine gun.

Between 1890 and 1900 the U.S. Army taught soldiers how to ride, drill, and conduct field maneuvers on bicycles. The United States Military Wheelmen, a voluntary adjunct of the National Guard, did the same for its cyclists. One Lieutenant Whitney observed, in 1896, "The balance of power is so nicely adjusted, the chances in the coming conflict will be governed by efficiency in detailed preparation. The bicycle will weigh in the balance."

Brief History of All-Terrain (Mountain) Bicycling

All-terrain bicycling in the United States started in the early 1970s when a group of young people in Marin County, California—across the Bay from San Francisco—discovered the fun of bombing full tilt down the trails and fire roads of Mount Tamalpais. The bikes they rode were not conventional road-racing bikes. The preferred bike for riding down the 2,500-foot drop of Mount Tam was the same 60-pound balloon-tire bicycle that was so popular in the early 1930s. In fact, these bicycles became so popular that riders scoured bike shops in the area and picked them up for five dollars or so. The most sought-after ballooner was the old Schwinn Excelsior. This bike had one speed, a coaster brake, wide, flat handlebars, balloon tires that imitated those that were so popular on cars of that era, and an imitation gas tank complete with working horn, which also gave the bike overtones of a motorcycle. Kids loved this bike. As a bomber for tearing down the mountain the bike was amazingly quick and had good steering response, comfort, and stability.

Eventually the supply of these oldies but goodies ran dry, and those that were left began to break beyond the ability of frame repairers to patch. At about the same time, the mountain riders, who had to bum rides up to the top in pickup trucks, began trying to ride their heavy one-speed steeds to the peak of Mount Tam. But only the strongest could make it: Even though stripped of the imitation gas tank and the heavy steel rack, the bikes still weighed around 50 pounds. Finally, around 1975, Gary Fisher, a veteran road racer and today a manufacturer of mountain bicycles, added a multispeed derailleur transmission to the clunkers. Now these heavy old bikes could be ridden up to the top by everybody.

As these old frames wore out and fell by the wayside, premier frame builder and bicycle racer Joe Breeze built the first batch of some dozen true mountain bikes, using high-quality steel but borrowing frame geometry from the Schwinn Excelsior. The bikes were quickly snapped up and mountain bikers asked for more. This was in 1977, and the all-terrain bicycle, much as we know it today, was off and running. These early bikes weighed between 35 and 40 pounds.

Now that the frames were high-tech and strong, the problem was what to do about the wheels and tires. It took a while, but Joe Breeze and others, such as Tom Ritchey, who began to make mountain bikes in volume, persuaded Japanese manufacturers to make aluminum rims to fit the fat tires, cutting about four more pounds off the mountain bicycle. By 1979, the heavy, dead, unresponsive balloon tires of the Excelsior era were replaced by today's light, responsive, skinwall 26-inch tires that cut two more pounds off the mountain bike. Now these bikes were down to around 30 pounds, and racing versions were refined down to around 28 pounds. By 1979 Tom Ritchey was in large-volume production of high-quality mountain bicycles, and by 1980 just about every major bicycle manufacturer, in this country and abroad, either had begun making them domestically or was importing them under their own label from Japan and Taiwan. The rest is history.

During the nearly 200 years since the celerifere was introduced, the bicycle has progressed from a wealthy man's toy to everyman's vehicle of health, fun, and joy. There are faster ways to travel, but few more pleasant than by bicycle. Today there even is a modern version of the Pedersen bike originally patented in 1894. It's a Co-Ped (Fig. 13-25). This version costs from $1,475 to $2,000, depending on the model. For more data on the Co-Ped call 1-800-755-8671 or 1-312-876-1727.

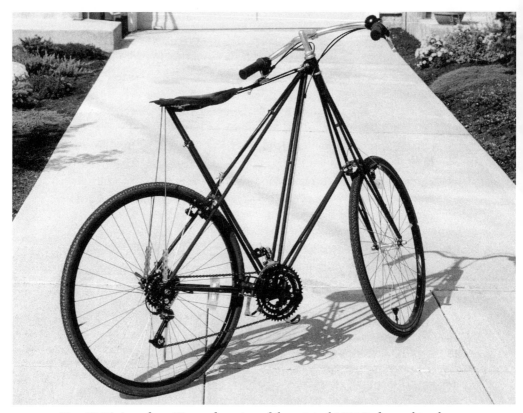

Fɪɢ. 13-25: A modern 10-speed version of the original 1894 Pedersen bicycle.

GLOSSARY

Alignment: Applies to the bicycle frame. Dropouts should be parallel; fork blades and stays parallel to the top tube; top tube centered between the stays; head tube parallel to the fork blades; fork blades parallel to each other; stays parallel to each other; seat tube parallel to the bottom bracket sides.

Ankling: Technique of pedaling in which the foot follows through nearly 360 degrees of pedal arc.

Bicycle computer: An electronic version of the mechanical bicycle odometer. The computer measures elapsed mileage for the day and total mileage for the trip, cadence, and miles per hour; some can measure pulse rate.

Binder bolt: Any bolt and nut that holds a part onto a bicycle, such as the binder bolt(s) for saddles, brakes, carriers, lights, generators, computers, derailleurs, cranks, and other bolted-on parts.

Bottom bracket assembly: Spindle, bearings, cones, cups, and locknut. The crank arms are attached to the spindle.

Bottom bracket hanger: The short round tube containing the bottom bracket assembly, to which the down tube, seat tube, and chain stays are attached.

Brake bridge: A tube mounted between the seat stays to which the rear brake is attached. May also hold fender mount and carrier mount.

Brake levers: Handlebar-mounted levers that control the brakes.

Cables: Flexible steel cables connecting brake levers to the brakes and shift levers to the front and rear derailleurs.

Cadence: Crank revolutions per minute, a measure of how fast the rider can spin the cranks. A good touring cadence would be 70 to 80 crank revolutions per minute for the casual touring cyclist, up to 100 or more for the trained racer.

Carrier: A metal rack fastened to the bicycle frame. A carrier can be fastened to seat stays or rear brake bridge, over the rear wheel, or to the fork crown and fork blades, over the front wheel. Carriers are also called racks. The term is also used for a carrier for the bicycle itself, mounted on the car roof or on the trunk door and rear bumper, or installed in the bed of a pickup truck.

Chain: The articulated drive unit connecting the chainwheel gears to the freewheel gears.

Chain stays: The frame tubing from the bottom bracket to the rear dropouts.

Chainwheels: The toothed gears attached to the bottom bracket spindle, which deliver pedal power to the freewheel gears. Chainwheels may be single, double, or triple.

Crank arm: The long shaft that is attached to the bottom bracket spindle and to which the pedals are attached.

Cyclometer: A mechanical device attached to a bike wheel to measure speed. An electronic device for measuring mileage, speed, and cadence.

Derailleur: From the French meaning "to derail" or shift. The rear derailleur shifts the chain from one freewheel cog to another, the front derailleur shifts the chain from one chainwheel to another.

Dishing: Describes truing the rear wheel so the rim is centered exactly between the hub axle locknuts—necessary because of the added width of the freewheel. In dishing, the rear-wheel rim is more toward the right hub flange, whereas the front-wheel rim, which is not dished, is centered between the hub flanges.

Down tube: The frame tube that is connected to the head tube and to the bottom bracket.

Dropouts: Slotted openings into which wheel hub axles fit. Hold front and rear wheels.

Fork: Consists of the fork blades, fork crown, front-wheel dropouts, and steering tube.

Head tube: The short tube to which are connected the top and down tubes and which holds the fork with its associated headset bearings, cups, cones, and locknut.

Hub: The front- and rear-wheel units that hold the wheel axle and to which are attached the spokes.

Panniers: A fancy word for bike packs and saddlebags.

Quick-release: A cam- and lever-actuated mechanism that permits quick and easy removal and installation of a bicycle wheel.

Saddle: The seat.

Seat post: A hollow tube sized to fit into the seat tube, designed to hold and support the saddle. Adjustable so saddle can be moved up or down.

Seat stays: Two hollow steel tubes attached at one end to the seat tube and at the other end to each of the rear-wheel dropouts. With the chain stays, they form the rear triangle of the bicycle frame.

BIBLIOGRAPHY

Books

Accident Facts, 124 pages. National Safety Council, 1993.

Alderson, Frederick. *Bicycling: A History,* 245 pages. Praeger Publishers, Inc., 1972.

Alexander, Don, and Ochowisc, Jim. *Tour de France '86: The American Invasion,* 192 pages. Alexander and Alexander, 1986.

Baker, Stannard J. *Bicycle Accident Investigation Manual,* 340 pages. The Traffic Institute, Northwestern University, 1980.

Behrman, Daniel. *The Man Who Loved Bicycles,* 130 pages. Harper's Magazine Press, 1973.

Bengtsson, Hans, and Atkinson, George, *Orienteering for Sport and Pleasure,* 224 pages. The Stephen Greene Press, 1977.

Bicycling: Its Rise and Development, 80 pages. Taplinger & Co., 1874.

Blomberg, Richard D., Hale, Allen, and Preusser, David F. *Conspicuity for Pedestrians and Bicyclists,* 180 pages. U.S. Department of Transportation, National Highway Traffic Safety Administration, 1984.

Boivin, Robert, and Pronovost, Jean-Francois. *The Bicycle: Global Perspectives,* 600 pages. Papers presented at the Conference Velo Mondiale, Montreal, Canada. Velo Quebec, 1992.

Borysewiczm, Edward. *Bicycle Road Racing,* 180 pages. Velo-News, 1985.

Brandt, Jobst. *The Bicycle Wheel,* 149 pages. Avocet, Inc., 1983.

Burke, Edward. *The Two-Wheeled Athlete,* 140 pages. Velo-News, 1986.

Burke, Edward, Perez, H. R., and Hodges, Patrick. *Inside the Cyclist,* 160 pages. Velo-News, 1979.

Burrell, Donald H. *The Stormwater Grate,* 36 pages. Report prepared by the Cincinnati Cycle Club for the City of Cincinnati Public Works and Traffic Safety Committee, 1983.

Code of Federal Regulations, Commercial Practices. Consumer Product Safety Commission, Part 1500 to 1512, January 1, 1988. U.S. Government Printing Office.

Counter, C. F. *The History and Development of Cycles,* 72 pages. British Science Museum Press, 1972.

Cyclist's Britain (contributions by about 25 authors), 306 pages. Hunter Publishing, 1985.

Darago, Vincent Stephen. *Regional Workshops on Bicycle Safety,* 68 pages. U.S. Department of Transportation, National Highway Traffic Safety Administration, 1978.

Demetriou, Angelos. *A Bikeway System for Highland Park, Illinois,* 130 pages. 1975.

Directory of Hostels in the U.S., 242 pages. American Youth Hostels, 1994.

Duncan, David N. *Pedaling the Ends of the Earth,* 272 pages. Fireside Books, Simon & Schuster, 1985.

Famous Cycling Videos. Five years of the Tour de France, many other exciting bike races in Europe, and mountain bike races in the United States. Famous Cycling Videos, 704 Hennepin Ave., Minneapolis, MN 55403, phone 1-800-359-3107.

Farny, Michael H. *New England over the Handlebars,* 174 pages. Little, Brown, 1975.

Ferguson, Gary. *Freewheeling: Bicycling the Open Road,* 194 pages. The Mountaineers, 1984.

Fleming, June. *Staying Found,* 159 pages. Vintage Books, 1982.

Forgery, William W., M.D. *Hypothermia, Death by Exposure,* 172 pages. ICS Books, 1985.

———. *Wilderness Medicine,* 124 pages. ICS Books, 1979.

Greenbank, Anthony. *The Book of Survival,* 250 pages. The New American Library, 1967.

Grossberg, Milton A. *Family Bike Rides,* 112 pages. Chronicle Books, 1982.

Guide for the Development of Bicycle Facilities, 44 pages. American Association of State Highway and Transportation Officials, 1991.

Hamill, James P. *Planning and Development of Bikeway Systems,* 26 pages. International City Management Association, 1973.

Hawkins, Gary, and Hawkins, Karen. *Bicycling in Europe,* 336 pages. Pantheon Books, 1980.

———. *Bicycling in the Western United States,* 360 pages. Pantheon Books, 1982.

Hayduk, Douglas. *Bicycle Metallurgy for the Cyclist,* 112 pages. Self-published, 1987.

Henderson, N. G., Armstrong, David, Burton, Beryl, Johnson, Gordon,

Porter, Hugh, Watson, John, and West, Les. *Cycling Year Books,* 128 pages. Pelham Books, 1971.

Higley, Donn C. *Pocketwise Tips on Use of the Compass, Man-Made and Natural,* 35 pages. Self-published, 1981.

Hinault, Bernard, and Genzling, Claude. *Road Racing: Technique and Training,* 208 pages. Velo-News, 1988.

Hurne, Ralph. *The Yellow Jersey,* 255 pages. Simon & Schuster, 1973.

International Hostelling. American Youth Hostels, 1993.

Jacobson, Michael. *Nutrition Scoreboard,* 102 pages. Center for Science in the Public Interest, 1973.

Jones, Phillip N. *Bicycling the Backroads of Northwest Oregon,* 192 pages. The Mountaineers, 1984.

Kals, W. S. *Land Navigation,* 230 pages. Sierra Club Books, 1983.

Kansas City Bikeways, 50 pages. Board of Parks and Recreation Commissioners, Kansas City, Kansas, 1980.

Kjellstrom, Bjorn. *Map & Compass,* 215 pages. Charles Scribner's Sons, 1976.

Kolin, Michael J., and de la Rosa, Denise. *The Custom Frame,* 274 pages. Rodale Press, 1979.

Leverte, Farley, Kara, Curry, and Curry, Sheila M. *Get Motivated!* Simon & Schuster, 1994.

Lobeck, Armin K. *Things Maps Don't Tell Us,* 160 pages. Macmillan, 1956.

Marr, Dick. *Bicycle Gearing: A Practical Guide.* The Mountaineers, 1989.

Matheny, Fred, *Solo Cycling: How to Train and Race Bicycle Time Trials,* 206 pages. Velo-News, 1986.

Matheny, Fred, and Grabe, Stephen. *Weight Training for Cyclists,* 80 pages. Velo-News, 1986.

Matson, Robert W. *North of San Francisco,* 276 pages. Celestial Arts, 1980.

McGonagle, Seamus. *The Bicycle in Life, Love, War, and Literature,* 142 pages. A. S. Barnes, 1968.

Merckx, Eddy. *The Fabulous World of Cycling,* 194 pages. Winning Publications.

Messina, John L. *Highway Design Liability,* 100 pages. The Association of Trial Lawyers of America, 1983.

Murphy, Tom A. *50 Northern California Bicycle Trips,* 126 pages. The Touchstone Press, 1972.

Paterek, Tim A. *The Paterek Manual for Bicycle Frame Builders,* 350 pages. The Framebuilders' Guild, 1985.

Platten, David. *The Outdoor Survival Handbook,* 160 pages. David and Charles, 1986.

Proudman, Robert D., and Rajala, Reuben. *Trail Building and Maintenance,* 2nd edition. Appalachian Mountain Club and the U.S. National Park Service (National Trails Program), 1981.

Roy, Karen E., and Rogers, Thurlow. *Fit & Fast: How to Be a Better Cyclist,* 166 pages. Vitesse Press, 1989.

Savage, Barbara. *Miles from Nowhere,* 324 pages. The Mountaineers, 1983.

Schubert, John. *The Tandem Scoop,* 112 pages. Burley Design Cooperative, 1993.

Selvi, Bettina. *Riding to Jerusalem,* 216 pages. Peter Bedrick Books, 1986.

Shimano Service Manual. Shimano American Corporation, 1993

Sjogarrd, Gisela, Nielsen, Bodil, Mikkelsen, Finn, Saltin, Benget, and Burke, Edmund R. *Physiology in Bicycling,* 110 pages. Movement Publications, 1982.

Sloane, Eugene A. *Sloane's Complete Book of All-Terrain Bicycles,* 285 pages. Simon & Schuster, 1985.

———. *Sloane's Handy Pocket Guide to Bicycle Repair,* 112 pages. Simon & Schuster, 1993.

———. *Sloane's New Bicycle Maintenance Manual,* 301 pages. Simon & Schuster, 1991.

Smith, Hempstone Oliver, and Berkeble, Donald H. *Wheels and Wheeling: The Smithsonian Institution Cycle Collection,* 104 pages. Smithsonian Institution Press, 1974.

Sterling E. M. *Trips and Trails Around the North Cascades,* 216 pages. The Mountaineers, 1978.

Sutherland, Howard, Allen, John S., Colaianni, Ed, and Hart, John Porter. *Sutherland's Handbook for Bike Mechanics,* 4th edition. Sutherland Publications, 1985.

Temple, R. Jarrell. *Bikeways,* 180 pages. National Recreation and Park Association, 1974.

Tobey, Eric, and Woklenburg, Richard. *Northeast Bicycle Tours,* 282 pages. Tobey Publishing Co., 1973.

Velox. *Velocipedes, Bicycles, and Tricycles: How to Make Them and How to Use Them,* 128 pages. S. R. Publishers, 1971 (originally published in 1869).

Walford, Roy, M.D. *Maximum Life Span,* 256 pages. Norton, 1983.

Watts, Alan. *Instant Weather Forecasting, 64 pages.* Dodd-Mead, 1968.

Whitnah, Dorothy L. *Point Reyes,* 114 pages. Wilderness Press, 1981.

Whitt, Frank Rowland, and Wilson, David Gordon. *Bicycling Science,* 364 pages. The M.I.T. Press, 1985.

Wilkerson, James A., M.D. *Medicine for Mountaineering,* 365 pages. The Mountaineers, 1975.

Willson, Janet. *Exploring by Bicycle: Southwest British Columbia, Northwest Washington,* 100 pages. Gundy's & Bernie's Guide Books, 1973.

Catalogs

Bikecology, President, Alan Goldsmith, 1515 Wilshire Blvd, Santa Monica, CA 90403-3900. Outside California, phone 1-800-282-BIKE. In California, phone 1-800-223-BIKE. Catalog of bicycles, frames, parts, components, clothing, exercisers, and more.

Bike Nashbar, 4111 Simon Rd., Youngstown, OH 44412-1343, phone 1-800-627-4227, FAX 1-800-458-1223. Excellent, well-thought-out catalog with a wide choice of just about every bicycle and bike component and accessory known to civilized man.

Campmor, Paramus, Box 999, Paramus, NJ 07653-0999. Outside New Jersey, phone 1-800-526-4784. In New Jersey, 1-201-445-5000. Free. Wide selection of high-quality camping gear.

L. L. Bean. Freeport, ME 04033, phone 1-800-221-4221. High-quality camp gear, clothing, bikes. The old standby.

Moss Tent Works, Inc., Mt. Mattie St., Camden, ME 04843, phone 1-207-236-8368. Super top-line tents by America's premier tentmaker. For the bike packer.

Palo Alto Bicycles, P.O. Box 1276, Palo Alto, CA 94302. Outside California, phone 1-800-227-8900. In California, phone 1-415-328-0128. Everything in bicycles.

Pedal Pushers, 1130 Rogero Rd., Jacksonville, FL 32211-5895. Outside Florida, phone 1-800-874-2453. In Florida, phone 1-800-342-7320. Good catalog, compiled by cyclists.

Performance Bicycle Shop. P.O. Box 2741, Chapel Hill, NC 27514, phone 1-800-334-5471. A beautifully put together catalog of bicycles, parts, components, accessories, clothing. Much help in parts selection.

Recreation Equipment, Inc., P.O. Box C-88125, Seattle, WA 98188, phone 1-800-426-4840. In Washington, phone 1-800-562-4894. For Canada, Hawaii, and Alaska, phone 1-206-575-3287. If you join their benefits program (fee five dollars) you receive a membership card, which, when used with orders, gives you a quite substantial discount. Catalog is free. Everything outdoors. Camping gear, bicycles, books, you name it, they have it.

Rhode Gear, 765 Allens Avenue, Providence, RI 02905, phone 1-800-HOT-GEAR. Excellent panniers and other equipment designed by this firm. Plus lots of parts, clothing, and other gear.

The Third Hand, P.O. Box 212, Mount Shasta, CA 96067, phone 1-916-926-2600 or 1-800-926-9904. The bike tool doesn't exist if it's not in their catalog. Plus small parts unavailable elsewhere.

Periodicals

Bicycle USA. 6707 Whitesone Road, Suite 209, Baltimore, MD 21207, $22 (nine issues). Official publication of the League of American Wheelmen, the oldest and best cycling organization in the United States.

Bicycle World. BG Publishing Co., P.O. Box 55729, Boulder, CO 80322-5729, phone 1-800-456-6501.

Bicycling. P.O. Box 7308, Red Oak, IA 51591-0308.

Mountain Bike Action. Hi-Torque Publications. P.O. Box 9502, Mission Hills, CA 91395-9985, phone 1-800-767-0345.

Recumbent Cyclist. Recumbent Cyclist Magazine, P.O. Box 58755, Renton, WA 98058-1755.

Sierra Club Bulletin. Editor, Francis Gendlin. 530 Buch Street, San Francisco, CA 94108, phone 1-415-981-8634, $29 (six issues). If you're a conservationist as well as a cyclist, subscribe to this magazine. Better yet, join the Sierra Club and get the magazine free. Annual dues are $29.

INDEX